COLOR ATLAS OF CONGENITAL MALFORMATION SYNDROMES

COLOR ATLAS OF
CONGENITAL
MALFORMATION
SYNDROMES

Michael Baraitser • Robin M Winter

MB CHB FRCP
Consultant Clinical Geneticist
Hospital for Sick Children
Great Ormond Street
London, UK

Professor of Clinical Genetics
and Dysmorphology
Institute of Child Health
University of London
London, UK

Mosby-Wolfe

London Baltimore Barcelona Bogotá Boston Buenos Aires Caracas Carlsbad, CA Chicago Madrid Mexico City Milan Naples, FL New York
Philadelphia St. Louis Seoul Singapore Sydney Taipei Tokyo Toronto Wiesbaden

Copyright © 1996 Times Mirror International Publishers Limited

Published in 1996 by Mosby-Wolfe, an imprint of Times Mirror International Publishers Limited

Printed by Grafos S.A. Arte sobre papel, Barcelona, Spain.

ISBN 0 7234 2073 4

For full details of all Times Mirror International Publishers Limited titles, please write to Times Mirror International Publishers Limited, Lynton House, 7–12 Tavistock Square, London WC1H 9LB, England.

A CIP catalogue record for this book is available from the British Library.

Library of Congress Cataloging-in-Publication Data applied for.

Project Manager:	Jeremy Theobald
Developmental Editor:	Jennifer Prast
Cover Design:	Lara Last
Production:	Jane Tozer
Index:	Nina Boyd
Publisher:	Richard Furn

CONTENTS

SYNDROMES WITH CRANIOSYNOSTOSIS

SYNDROMES DIAGNOSED THROUGH EYE ABNORMALITIES

SYNDROMES RECOGNISED THROUGH LIMB DEFECTS

SYNDROMES WITH SIGNIFICANT NEUROLOGICAL ABNORMALITIES

SYNDROMES WITH ENDOCRINE AND GROWTH ABNORMALITIES

SYNDROMES ASSOCIATED WITH PREDISPOSITION TO MALIGNANCY

SYNDROMES WITH METABOLIC DEFECTS

SYNDROMES WITH THE APPEARANCE OF PREMATURE AGEING

SYNDROMES WITH DERMATOLOGICAL ABNORMALITIES

SYNDROME ASSOCIATIONS

SYNDROMES CAUSED BY TERATOGENESIS

PREFACE

INTRODUCTION

Recent advances in molecular genetics have begun to make a significant contribution to the diagnosis of dysmorphic syndromes. In some instances, for example Prader–Willi and Angelman syndromes, the dysmorphologist can now hope to get help with the clinical diagnosis from the DNA laboratory. In other situations, for example Miller–Dieker (lissencephaly syndrome), the new technique of fluorescent in situ hybridisation (FISH) may confirm the diagnosis if a 17p deletion is found, or help to refine the correct recurrence risk if the test proves negative. Even in well known syndromes such as Williams syndrome, a microscopic deletion again using the FISH technique is proving to be an accurate way of diagnosing the more difficult cases. There have also been advances in other directions. The diagnosis of Smith–Lemli–Opitz syndromehas always caused problems but a biochemical test, i.e. a raised 7-dehydrocholesterol, has now been shown to be diagnostic and it remains likely that other dysmorphic syndromes will be found to have a biochemical basis.

Despite these promising advances in molecular biology and other areas, the diagnosis of the majority of the conditions mentioned in this book rests on clinical recognition and the method of diagnosis has not changed. Recognition is either immediate or if this fails the main features are identified and the literature is consulted. The purpose of this atlas is to help clinicians improve their immediate or 'gestalt' recognition and the conditions chosen are those that lend themselves to this process. They have distinct features and often have a recognisable facial appearance. The atlas can be consulted to match the features with those of the condition that the patient is thought to have. The description and references should be checked in all instances, as the other clinical features of the condition must also match before making a diagnosis.

THE CLINICAL APPROACH

As in all spheres of medicine, the initial stages in the diagnostic process involve taking a good history and carrying out a thorough clinical examination. This should include:-

a) **A detailed three generation pedigree**. Particular attention should be paid to other family members with malformations or retardation, even if they seem different from the proband's. These cases may give an indication of a balanced chromosome translocation segregating in the family, giving rise to different unbalanced translocation products. Details of any consanguinity should also be elicited.

b) **A detailed pregnancy history**. This should include information about drugs, alcohol and tobacco, and exposure to radiation or other potential teratogens. Any illness during pregnancy should be documented carefully, including information about hyperpyrexia or vomiting. Prenatal tests in the pregnancy, such as chorionic villus sampling (CVS) should be enquired of, as there has been a suggestion of limb and craniofacial defects where invasive procedures are carried out early in a pregnancy, particularly before 10 weeks.

c) **A detailed physical examination**. This must include a careful evaluation of any abnormal features observed in the patient, in comparison to other family members to assess, for example, whether they are simply family traits. Where appropriate, measurements should be made to document objectively features such as hypertelorism. Standard tables and graphs are available.

A working knowledge of a large number of syndromes often helps during the examination. For example, a child with synophrys and deafness may have Waardenburg syndrome. The inner canthal distance should be measured to assess the possibility of telecanthus, the eye should be carefully examined for evidence of heterochromia and depigmentation of hair and skin should be looked for.

Good clinical photographs are essential, especially to record abnormal facial features that cannot be described accurately in words. Photographs are also invaluable after the clinic when searching the literature or asking the opinion of experts. It is best to take a good camera down to the clinic, rather than rely on the medical photography department, as the clinician will often know the most appropriate features to photograph, and patients and their families are more likely to consent to an immediate photograph.

An attempt should be made to rank any abnormal features in order of importance. For example, fifth finger clinodactyly is unlikely to help in the diagnostic process as it is common in the general population, whereas an imperforate anus is not common, and is a key feature of several well documented syndromes.

d) **Investigations.** These should include, where appropriate, metabolic studies, radiographs, chromosome analysis and DNA studies. The more clinical detail that can be given to the laboratory, the more appropriate the tests will be. For example, there are numerous specialised techniques for examining chromosomes, including the increasing use of FISH using specific DNA probes. If the laboratory is to use these techniques, there has to be a suggested diagnosis so that the appropriate probes can be used. Care should be taken in accepting 'screening' tests as definitive. For example, the exact enzymes assayed in a 'white cell enzyme screen' should always be checked.

MAKING A DIAGNOSIS

Having gathered the clinical information, the general approach to a dysmorphic diagnosis is as follows:-

a) **Can you make a gestalt diagnosis?** Sometimes the facial features are instantly recognisable and the diagnosis can be made by pattern recognition. This approach is obviously perilous for the inexperienced and care must be taken to ensure that the other clinical features of the patient fit the diagnosis. For instance, if the facial features are suggestive of Cornelia de Lange syndrome the diagnosis becomes increasingly unlikely if the height and head circumference is normal and development is not significantly delayed. If the facial features are suggestive of Williams syndrome but the degree of retardation is severe then it may be necessary to reconsider the diagnosis.

b) **Choose a small number of the best handles.** If an immediate diagnosis cannot be arrived at, the clinical features of the patient should be evaluated to pick out the best diagnostic handles that may lead to a diagnosis. A good handle is defined as a clinical feature which does not overlap with common variation in the population. Choose handles which are not found in hundreds of syndromes, but which may be specific to a relatively few syndromes. Do, however, include those features without which a diagnosis would not be tenable, i.e. if your patient is mentally handicapped, then it wouldn't help to search for conditions without that feature.

Armed with three to five good handles, dysmorphology texts can be searched to find a match. Some of these have a 'gamut index' listing all syndromes with specific features (e.g. Jones; Gorlin *et al.*). This can be time consuming, and computer databases have been designed to facilitate searching for syndromes using combinations of key clinical features. The London Dysmorphology Database, developed by the current authors, is one such database (Winter and Baraitser). It is updated annually and is particularly useful when the dysmorphic features are distinct.

Many of the conditions seen by clinical dysmorphologists are simply not diagnosable. Most units diagnose about 40% of patients seen. It is always tempting to push a patient into a diagnostic category, but this must be resisted. Even the most experienced dysmorphologists in the world have to struggle to make a diagnosis in the majority of patients.

References

Gorlin RJ, Cohen MM, Levin LS (1990). *Syndromes of the head and neck*, 3rd edn. New York, Oxford: Oxford University Press.

Jones KL (1988). *Smith's Recognizable Patterns of Human Malformation*, 4th edn. Philadelphia, London, Toronto: W B Saunders.

Winter, R.M., Baraitser, M (1995). *The London Dysmorphology Database: A Computerised Database for the Diagnosis of Rare Dysmorphic Syndromes*. New York, Oxford: Oxford University Press.

ACKNOWLEDGEMENTS

The following people kindly provided photographs for the previous version of the book.

Dr Barbara Ansell
Dr Michael Bamford
Dr Nicholas Barnes
Professor Peter Beighton
Dr Caroline Berry
Dr Eric Blank
Professor John Burn
Dr Nicholas Cavanagh
Professor Michael Connor
Dr Martin Crawfurd
Dr M Daras
Dr Clare Davison
Dr Nicholas Dennis
Dr Michael Dillon
Professor Dian Donnai
Mr Oliver Fenton
Professor Malcolm Ferguson-Smith
Dr D W Fielding
Mr John Fixsen
Dr Christine Garrett
Professor Francesco Gianelli
Professor Robert Gorlin
Dr David Grant
Dr Christine Hall
Professor Anita Harding
Professor Peter Harper

Dr Roger Hitchings
Dr Peter Husband
Professor James Leonard
Dr Barry Lewis
Dr Michael Liberman
Dr Duncan Matthew
Dr Kay MacDermot
Dr Gerald McEnery
Professor Victor McKusick
Dr Peter Meinecke
Dr Milroy
Dr Patrick Mortimer
Professor Marcus Pembrey
Professor Michael Pope
Professor Michael Preece
Dr Michael Ridler
Dr Mary Rossiter
Dr Mary Seller
Dr S Stengel-Rutowski
Mr David Taylor
Dr James Taylor
Professor Richard Watts
Mr Peter Webb
Dr John Wilson
Dr Mark Winter

The authors would like to thank the following people for the provision of the figures listed in the current text.

20C–E Courtesy of Dr M Porteous
24B Courtesy of Dr VM Der Kaloustian
25A and B Couresty of Dr RJ Gorlin
26A and B Courtesy of Dr IK Temple
27A and E Courtesy of Dr N Niikawa
27C and D Courtesy of Dr N Philip
31C Courtesy of Dr AOM Wilkie
38A and B Courtesy of Dr EA Haan
53A and B Courtesy of Dr DW Fielding
62A–C Courtesy of Dr JL Tolmie
64A and B Courtesy of Dr VM Der Kaloustian
65A and B Courtesy of Dr KD MacDermot
65C–E Courtesy of Dr RE Stevenson
68A Courtesy of Dr TR Gollop
76A and B Courtesy of Prof D Donnai
82B Courtesy of Dr CJR Curry
83A–D Courtesy of Dr R Salonen
92A and D Courtesy of Drs RJ Gorlin and S Jurenka
94B and C Courtesy of Dr RCM Hennekam
95B Courtesy of Drs O Callaghan and ID Young
96B Courtesy of Mr D Taylor
98C–E Courtesy of Dr UG Froster
99A and B Courtesy of Dr RF Mueller
102A and B Courtesy of Dr I Buntinx
104A–C Courtesy of Dr G Camera
106A and B Courtesy of Dr D Kumar
110A and B Courtesy of Dr M Daras
112A–D Courtesy of Dr Prof Young
118B Courtesy of Dr ME Gillin
122C Courtesy of Dr A Verloes
151A Courtesy of Prof P Beighton
160A–C Courtesy of Dr GS Pai
163C and D Courtesy of Dr PA Tilsley
165A–D Courtesy of Dr AE Donnenfeld

167A–D Courtesy of Prof P Beighton
179 Courtesy of Mr D Taylor
180 Courtesy of Dr LA Alsing
186C Courtesy of Dr WB Dobyns
187A–C Courtesy of Dr R Salonen
201A and B Courtesy of Dr S Stengel-Rutkowski
210 Courtesy of Mr D Taylor
212A and B Courtesy of Dr G Neri
214A Courtesy of Dr RJ Gorlin
215A and B Courtesy of Mr D Taylor
216A–D Courtesy of Dr RJ Gorlin
228A Courtesy of Prof RWE Watts
230A Courtesy of Dr VM Der Kaloustian
231 Courtesy of Prof HR Wiedemann
236 Courtesy of Dr RJ Gorlin
238B Courtesy of Dr Norton
239D Courtesy of Dr Insley
240B and C Courtesy of Dr P Meinecke
245A and B Courtesy of Dr AE Fryer
247B Courtesy of Drs LI Al-Gazali and D Donnai
247C Courtesy of Dr JJ Hoo
249A and C Courtesy of Dr RJ Gorlin
253A and B Courtesy of Dr RJ Gorlin
253C Courtesy of Prof GB Winter
256 Courtesy of Dr I Winship
261 Courtesy of Dr K Suzomori
269A–C Courtesy of Dr R Phillips
270A Courtesy of Dr S Alexander
271A and B Courtesy of Dr A Verloes
273A Courtesy of Dr DL Viljoen
275 Courtesy of Dr D Atherton
276A–C Courtesy of Dr DL Rimoin
280 Courtesy of Dr RJ Gorlin

Without the generous help from the photographic department at the Hospital for Sick Children, Great Ormond Street, this atlas could not have been produced.

Permission has been obtained from the copyright holders listed below for the use of the following figures:

REPRINTED WITH THE PERMISSION OF OXFORD UNIVERSITY PRESS

216A–D Gorlin RJ. *Syndromes of the Head and Neck.* **373**:12-16.
270A Gorlin RJ. *Syndromes of the Head and Neck.* **491**:13-110.

REPRINTED WITH THE PERMISSION OF JOHN WILEY & SONS LTD.

30A,B Clark RD, Baraitser M. *Am J Med Genet* 1987, **26**:13–16.
43A Patton MA, Baraitser M, Nickolaides K. *Prenatal Diagn* 1986, **6**:109–116.
68A Gollop TR. *Am J Med Genet* 1981, **10**:409–412.
82A,B Curry CJR, Carey JC, Holland JS *et al. Am J Med Genet* 1987, **26**:45–57.
160A–C Pai GS, Macpherson RI. *Am J Med Genet* 1988, **29**:929–936.
165A–D Donnenfeld AE, Conrad KA, Roberts NS *et al. Am J Med Genet* 1987, **27**:159–173.
212A,B Neri G, Martini–Neri ME, Katz BE *et al. Am J Med Genetics* 1984, **19**:195–207
247C Hoo JJ, Kapp–Simon K, Rollnick B, Chao M. *Am J Med Genet* 1991, **40**:290–293.
261 Suzumori K, Kanzaki T. *Prenatal Diagn* 1991, **11**:451-457.
271A,B Verloes A, Mulliez N, Gonzales M *et al. Am J Med Genet* 1992, **43**:539–547.

REPRINTED WITH THE PERMISSION OF THE BMJ PUBLISHING GROUP

1A Wilkie AOM, Gibbons RJ, Higgs DR, Pembrey ME. *J Med Genet* 1991, **28**:738–741.
20C,D Porteous MEM, Goudie DR. *J Med Genet* 1991, **28**:44–47.
32A,B Thompson EM, Baraitser M. *J Med Genet* 1987, **24**:129–143.
34A–E Oley C, Baraitser M. *J Med Genet* 1988, **25**:47–51.
36A Winter RM. *J Med Genet* 1986, **23**:11–13.
37A,B,D Thompson E, Pembrey ME. *J Med Genet* 1985, **22**:192–201.
40A,B Baraitser M, Brett EM, Piesowicz AT. *J Med Genet* 1983, **20**:210–212.
45A,C Hurst J, Baraitser M. *J Med Genet* 1988, **25**:133–138.
47B,D Hurst JA, Baraitser M. *J Med Genet* 1989, **26**:45–48.
62A–C Galea P, Tolmie JL. *J Med Genet* 1990, **27**:784–787.
88B, 88C, 88E, 89 Baraitser M. *J Med Genet* 1986, **23**:116–119.
90B,D,E Baraitser M, Burn J, Fixsen J. *J Med Genet* 1983, **20**:65–67.
80A,B Levy P, Baraitser M. *J Med Genet* 1991, **28**:338–341.
87A–D Holder SE, Winter RM. *J Med Genet* 1993, **30**:310–313.
90A Burn J, Dezateux C, Hall CM *et al. J Med Genet* 1984, **21**:189–192.
95A,B O'Callaghan M, Young ID. *J Med Genet* 1990, **27**:457–461.
97A–D Burn J, Winter RM, Baraitser M *et al. J Med Genet* 1984, **21**:331–340.
98C–E Froster–Iskenius UG. *J Med Genet* 1990, **27**:320–326.
99A, 99C Al–Gazali LI, Farndon P, Burn J *et al. J Med Genet* 1990, **27**:42–47.
104A–C Camera G, Ferraiolo G, Leo D *et al. J Med Genet* 1993, **30**:65–69.
107A,B Winter RM, Donnai D. *J Med Genet* 1989, **26**:417–420.
117A–E Thompson EM, Donnai D, Baraitser M *et al. J Med Genet* 1987, **24**:733–749.
133A,B Temple IK, Thompson EM, Hall CM *et al. J Med Genet* 1989, **26**:457–460.
161A,B Winter RM. *J Med Genet* 1989, **26**:772–775.
164B–E Hennekam RCM. *J Med Genet* 1991, **28**:262–266.
181A Baraitser M, Carter CO, Brett EM. *J Med Genet* 1983, **20**:64–75.
198A,C,F Winter RM, Patton MA, Challener J *et al. J Med Genet* 1989, **26**:320–325.
199C,D Donnai D, Thompson E *et al. J Med Genet* 1989, **26**:447–451.
200C Winter RM, Baraitser M, Grant DB *et al. J Med Genet* 1984, **21**:124–128.
204A–C Thompson EM, Hill S, Leonard JV, Pembrey ME. *J Med Genet* 1987, **24**:232–234.

234E Patton MA, Giannelli F, Francis AJ *et al. J Med Genet* 1989, **26**:154–159.
237A,B Baraitser M, Insley J, Winter RM. *J Med Genet* 1988, **25**:53–56.
247B Al–Gazali LI, Donnai D, Berry SA *et al. J Med Genet* 1988, **25**:773–778.
265C–F Tse K, Temple IK, Baraitser M. *J Med Genet* 1990, **27**:752–755.
281A–C,E Oley CA, Baraitser M, Grant DB. *J Med Genet* 1988, **25**:147–157.

REPRINTED WITH THE PERMISSION OF MUNKSGAARD INTERNATIONAL PUBLISHERS

32C,D Thompson EM, Baraitser M, Lindenbaum RH. *Clin Genet* 1985, **27**:582–594
63A–D Baraitser M, Winter RM, Brett EM. *Clin Genet* 1983, **24**:257–265.
106A,B Kumar D, Curtis D, Blank CE. *Clin Genet* 1984, **25**:68–72.
167A–D Goldblatt J, Wallis C, Viljoen DL *et al. Clin Genet* 1987, **31**:19–24.
182D Baraitser M, Patton M, Lam STS *et al. Clin Genet* 1987, **31**:323–330.
256 Winship I, Young K, Martell R *et al. Clin Genet* 1991, **39**:330–337.

REPRINTED WITH THE PERMISSION OF CHAPMAN & HALL LTD.

26A–C Temple IK. *Clin Dysmorphol* 1992, **1**:17–21.
27C,D Philip N, Meinecke P, David A *et al. Clin Dysmorphol* 1992, **1**:63–77.
68B Reardon W, Winter RM, Taylor D, Baraitser M. *Clin Dysmorphol* 1994, **3**:70–74.
72A,B Gibbs ML, Wilkie AOM, Winter RM *et al. Clin Dysmorphol* 1994, **3**:132–138.
245A,B Fryer AE. *Clin Dysmorphol* 1992, **1**:99–102.

REPRINTED WITH THE PERMISSION OF BLACKWELL SCIENCE, INC.

238B Norton KI, Glicklich M, Kupchik G *et al. Dysmorph Clin Genet* 1990, **4**:57–62.

REPRINTED WITH THE PERMISSION OF ELSEVIER SCIENCE, INC.

110A,B Harden CL, Tuchman AJ, Daras M. *Pediatr Neurol* 1991, **7**:302–304.

REPRINTED WITH THE PERMISSION OF SPRINGER-VERLAG GMBH AND CO. KG

94B,C Hennekam RCM. *Eur J Pediatr* 1987, **146**:94–95.

REPRINTED WITH THE PERMISSION OF THE AMERICAN MEDICAL ASSOCIATION

25A Gorlin RJ, Anderson RC, Blaw M. *Am J Dis Child* 1969, **117**:652–662.
64A Der Kaloustian VM, Sinno AA, Nassar SI. *Am J Dis Child* 1972, **124**:716–718.

REPRINTED WITH THE PERMISSION OF THE AMERICAN SOCIETY OF NEURORADIOLOGY

186B Dobyns WB, McCluggage CW. *Am J Neuroradiol* 1985, **6**:545–550.

REPRINTED WITH THE PERMISSION OF BLACKWELL SCIENCE LTD.

96B Taylor D, Ed. *Pediatric Ophthalmology*, Blackwell Scientific Press, Oxford, 1991:635.
163C,D Tilsley DA, Burden PW. *Br J Dermatol* 1981, **105**:331–336.

REPRINTED WITH THE PERMISSION OF THE OPTHALMIC PUBLISHING COMPANY

247A Ladenheim J, Metrick S. *Am* J Ophthalmol 1956, **41**:1059–1062.

CHROMOSOMAL DISORDERS

The diagnosis is often suggested by 'immediate recognition' or 'gestalt' in a hypotonic neonate, rather than an analysis of individual characteristics. There is a short nose, with a flat nasal bridge, upslanting palpebral fissures and prominent epicanthic folds. The mouth is small and the tongue appears large. The occiput is flat and there may be three fontanelles. The neck is short. A heart lesion is present in about 40% of cases and A-V canal defects predominate. Duodenal atresia is common. Dermatoglyphic analysis reveals single palmar creases, fifth finger clinodactyly with a single flexion crease, an excess of ulnar loops on the fingertips, a displaced palmar axial triradius and an open field pattern in the hallucal area.

Genetic aspects: 95% of cases have regular trisomy 21, about 3% of cases have mosaicism and 2% have translocations. A 14;21 Robertsonian translocation is the most common. A small percentage of translo-cation cases have an isochromosome for the long arm of chromosome 21–t(21q;21q). Parents of translocation cases should have their chromosomes checked to rule out a balanced translocation (in about a half of these cases the parental chromosomes will be normal).

Maternal non-disjunction is responsible for 95% of trisomic cases. The risk of a liveborn infant with Down syndrome increases with the age of the mother (see Table 1).

In women under 40 years the recurrence risk after one child with regular trisomy 21 is about 1% for a baby with some form of trisomy (trisomy 21 would be the most common). If the mother carries a 14;21 translocation recurrence risks are 10% and if the father carries such a translocation the risks are 2%. In the rare t(21q;21q) translocation cases where one parent carries the translocation chromosome recurrence risks are 100%.

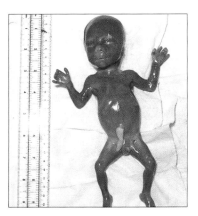

1A There is difficulty in making the diagnosis in a fetus.

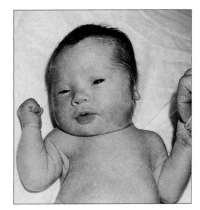

1B–1G Note the up-slanting palpebral fissures, epicanthic folds, prominent tongue, small nose with flat nasal bridge and small ears. The mother in C has mosaic Down syndrome.

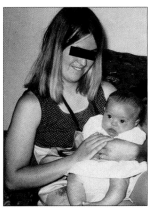

1C

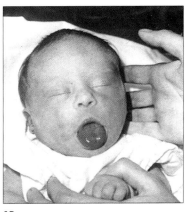

1D

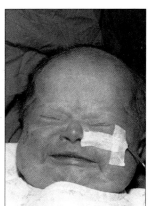

1E

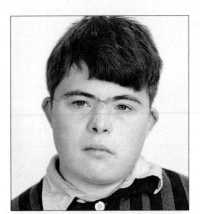

1F

1G

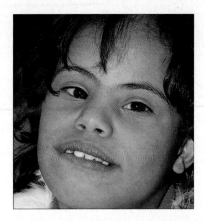

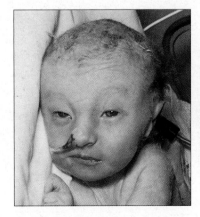

1H There is a longitudinal crease in the hallucal area indicating a wide sandle gap.

Table 1

Maternal Age	Liveborn Risk of Down Syndrome
25 years	1 in 1300
35 years	1 in 380
38 years	1 in 180
40 years	1 in 100
45 years	1 in 45

TRISOMY 18 (EDWARDS SYNDROME)   2A–2E

This condition occurs with a frequency of 1 in 5 000 live births. A maternal age effect is demonstrable and the sex ratio is F:M, 4:1. There is low birthweight. There is a prominent occiput, narrow palpebral fissures and a small chin. In the hands the nails are small and the second and fifth fingers overlap the middle two. In the feet the profile of the sole is convex and the heel prominent (a 'rocker-bottom foot'). This appearance is caused by a vertical talus. 10–20% of cases have other malformations such as a cleft lip, exomphalos or radial aplasia. Congenital heart defects and other internal malformations such as a horseshoe kidney are common. 30% of cases die within 2 months and 90% die before 1 year. Long-term survivors might have mosaicism.

Genetic aspects: Most cases have regular trisomy 18. The risk of recurrence after one affected child with a standard trisomy is about 1% for a baby with some form of trisomy (trisomy 21 would be the most common).

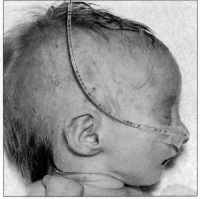

2A and 2B Note small chin, low-set ears, prominent occiput, short palpebral fissures.

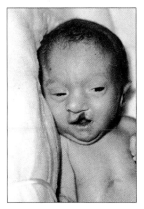
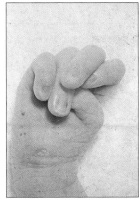
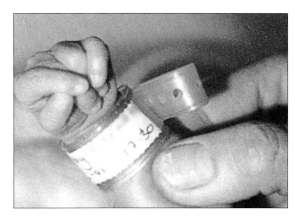

2C Note cleft lip and short sternum.

2D and 2E Note overlapping fingers with small nails.

TRISOMY 13 (PATAU SYNDROME)   3A–3F

The clinical picture at birth includes cleft lip and palate (sometimes an agenesis of the premaxilla with holoprosencephaly), microcephaly, scalp defects, microphthalmia with the eyes closely placed together, post-axial polydactyly, rocker-bottom feet and genital abnormalities. Other useful diagnostic features include forehead haemangiomas. Cardiac, renal and central nervous system malformations are common. 45% of cases die within the first month, 70% die within 6 months, and 86% within 12 months. Few survive beyond 5 years.

Genetic aspects: 75–80% of cases are simple trisomies. 20% of cases have translocations. A few cases are mosaic. The risk of recurrence after one affected child with a standard trisomy is about 1% for a baby with some form of trisomy (trisomy 21 would be the most common).

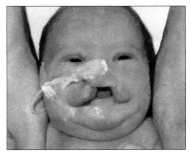

3A–3E Note microcephaly, low hairline, scalp defects, sloping forehead, microphthalmos, bilateral cleft lip and palate, broad nasal bridge, and abnormal low-set ears.

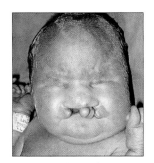
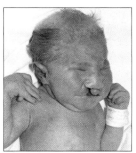

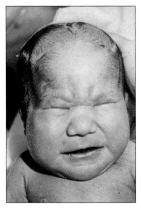
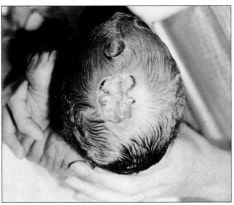
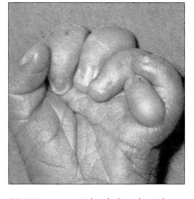

3F Note post-axial polydactyly with overlapping fingers.

3D   **3E**

PARTIAL TRISOMY 22   4A–4D

This is not usually a full trisomy, although this has been reported. Trisomy 22 (non-mosaic) has a live birth incidence of between 1 in 30 000 and 1 in 50 000. The main clinical features of non-mosaic trisomy 22 are growth and mental retardation, microcephaly, hypertelorism, epicanthic folds, antimongoloid eye-slant – all very non-specific features.

More frequently seen is trisomy 22 as a consequence of a 3;1 meiotic segregation from a parent with a (11q23;22q11) balanced translocation. In tetrasomy 22q11 (Cat-Eye syndrome) there are four copies of the 22q11 region because of a small supernumerary marker chromosome. The clinical features are a coloboma of the iris, pre-auricular pits and tags, anal abnormalities (a covered anus, anal atresia or an anteriorly placed anus), congenital heart defects, kidney anomalies and variable mental retardation, although intelligence can be normal.

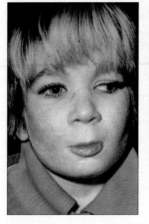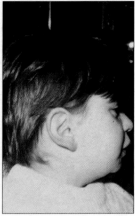

4A and 4B Note the long philtrum, pre-auricular pits, large ear and micrognathia.

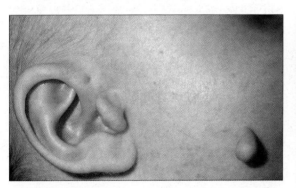

4C Note pre-auricular ear tag.

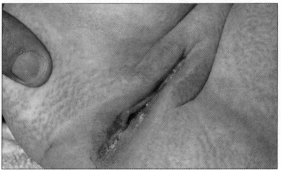

4D Note anteriorly placed anus.

TRISOMY 8 MOSAICISM   5A–5C

In this condition the clinician may have to recognise the phenotype and suggest a skin biopsy in order to make the diagnosis.

The main clinical clues to the diagnosis are:
- Deep skin crease in palms and soles
- Expressionless face with hypertelorism and deep-set eyes
- Multiple skeletal abnormalities including a small or absent patellae
- A long narrow trunk
- Mild to moderate mental retardation.

Genetic aspects: Most cases are thought to result from a post zygotic non-disjunction and recurrence risks are likely to be very small. About two-thirds of cases have a low frequency mosaicism and the diagnosis can easily be missed.

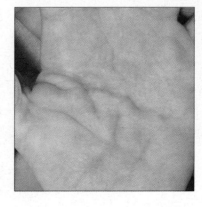

5A–5C Note the deep palmar and plantar creases.

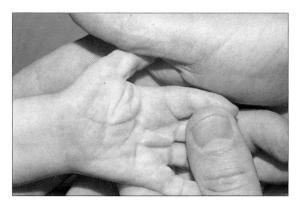

5B

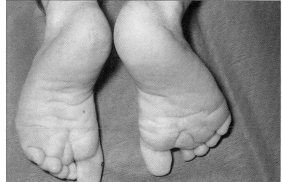

5C

9p TRISOMY

6A–6C

Full trisomy 9 is not usually viable although the mosaic situation might be. Individuals with 9p trisomy have three copies of the short arm of chromosome 9. The commonest features are intrauterine growth retardation, mental retardation, microcephaly and congenital heart defects, especially a VSD. Facially, the eyes are small and deep-set, and there is a thin protruding upper lip with a bulbous nose. But the main clue to the diagnosis is the hand, in which there is severe shortening and clinodactyly of the fifth finger with often only one flexion crease.

Genetic aspects: Parental chromosomes should be examined for balanced translocations.

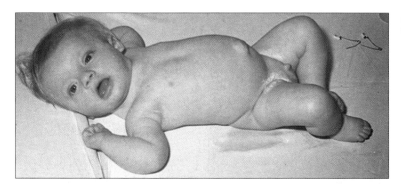

6A and 6B Note deep-set eyes and thin upper lip.

6B

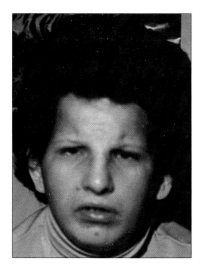

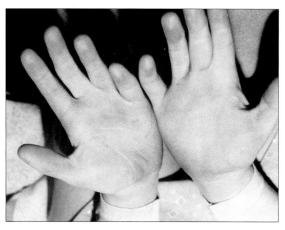

6C Note severe clinodactyly and brachymesophalangy of the fifth fingers.

5p– (CAT CRY SYNDROME)

This condition has a frequency of about 1 in 50 000 live births. It is characterised clinically by a cat-like cry from birth (although this might disappear later in life), microcephaly and a 'moon face' (full cheeks, hypertelorism, epicanthic folds and a flat nasal bridge). The phenotype changes with age and the face becomes more elongated. Mental retardation is usually severe.

Genetic aspects: Deletions are *de novo* in about 85% of cases, and although the size of the deletion is variable, the phenotype is probably related to a deletion of band 5p15. Parental chromosomes should always be examined and if they are normal recurrence risks are about 1%.

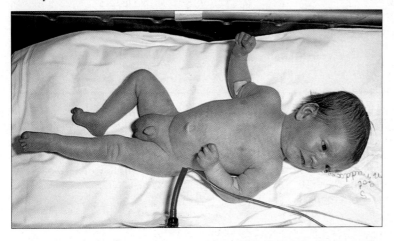

7A–7D Note the round face in the newborn, wide-spaced eyes, epicanthic folds. Note also elongation of the face that occurs in later childhood and adulthood.

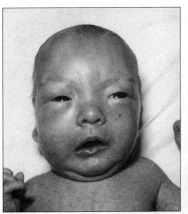

7B

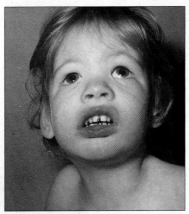

7C

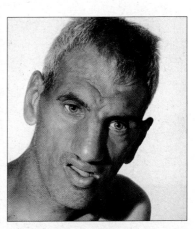

7D

4p– (WOLF–HIRSCHHORN SYNDROME)

The face is characteristic and is said to resemble a Greek helmet (the combination of frontal bossing with a high hairline, a prominent glabella and parallel borders to the nose). The other important clinical feature is a short and well formed philtrum and there may be a non-midline cleft. The philtral pillars are often prominent. Low birth-weight, pre-auricular pits, simple ears, iris colobomas and scalp defects are common. At least a one-third of patients die within the first year of life, mostly with conditions secondary to complications associated with severe hypotonia and developmental delay. Survivors are usually profoundly retarded.

Genetic aspects: The majority of cases are sporadic. Parental chromosomes should always be checked for a balanced translocation.

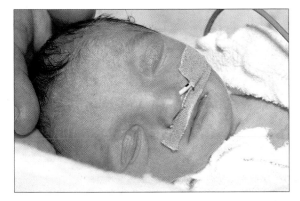

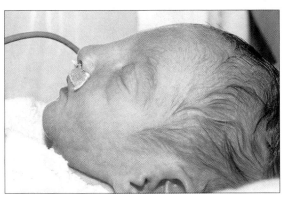

8A–8C Note the hypertelorism and prominent glabella giving a 'Greek Warrior Helmet' appearance. In addition the ears are simple, the philtrum short and clefting is present in **8C**.

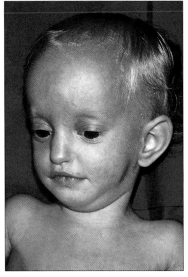

8B

8C

18q– SYNDROME

9A–9B

This is one of the more common deletion syndromes and well over 100 patients have been reported. The profile is characteristic in that there is mid-facial hypoplasia, with deep-set eyes. Pre-auricular pits are common. The mouth is carp-shaped, meaning that the upper lip has a tented appearance and the lower jaw seems to jut forwards. The philtrum is short and smooth and the ears have a narrow or atretic exter-nal auditory canal. At least one-quarter of patients have a congenital heart defect and the external genitalia are often abnormal (hypospadias is common). Mental retardation is variable.

Genetic aspects: About three-quarters of patients have a *de novo* deletion, but parental chromosomes should always be examined.

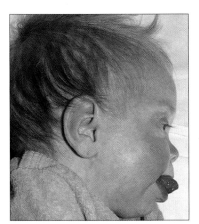

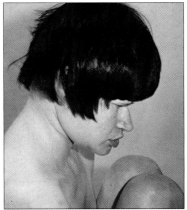

9A–9B Note the mid-facial hypoplasia, prominent chin and everted lower lip.

13q– SYNDROME

The clinical phenotype depends on the breakpoints. The retinoblastoma gene is at 13q14 and deletions distal to this are not at risk. The diagnosis is not possible on phenotypic examination alone. The only clue to the diagnosis in a dysmorphic child with developmental delay and a facial appearance which is non specific, but suggestive of a chromosomal abnormality, is the hypoplasia of the thumbs. The facial features include trigonocephaly, microcephaly, a broad nasal root, hypertelorism and epicanthic folds. A congenital heart defect is present in about one-half of all cases and occasionally an imperforate anus has been described. Retardation is usually severe.

Genetic aspects: Mostly sporadic. Parental chromosomes should always be examined.

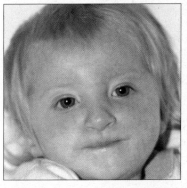 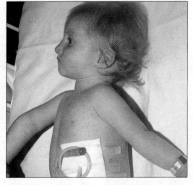 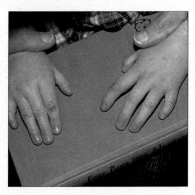

10A–10C The face is not diagnostic but the thumb hypoplasia in **10C** is characteristic of this deletion syndrome.

TURNER SYNDROME

Presentation in infancy is with short stature, extra folds of skin in the neck (the webbing develops later), wide-spaced nipples, pedal oedema and a congenital heart defect (mostly a coarctation). There are minor dysmorphic facial features such as a narrow maxilla, a small chin, a curved upper lip and a straight lower lip and prominent ears. An increased carrying angle at the elbows might be seen in older girls as will the shield shaped chest and wide-spaced nipples. The other important consideration is the gonadal dysgenesis, causing absent or delayed and scanty menstruation and infertility.

Genetics aspects: Most cases have an XO karyotype in every cell. It is likely that those who menstruate are mosaic and skin biopsy may be necessary to detect this. The commonest mosaic patterns are 45,X /46,XX and 45,X/47,XXX. In both of these situations the phenotype can be mild. Cases with a 45,X/46,XY karyotype usually have female genitalia, although ambiguity is occasionally seen. In these individuals the presence of a cell line with a Y chromosome causes a 30% risk of a dysgerminoma or a gonadoblastoma in a streak gonad. These individuals should therefore be considered for removal of their gonads.

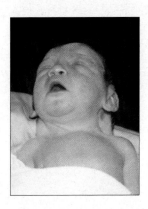

11A–11F Note the severe neck webbing (or in the fetus, nuchal oedema with hydrops), the short neck and low hairline.

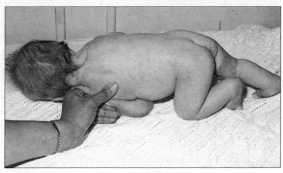

11B

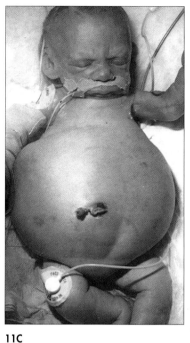

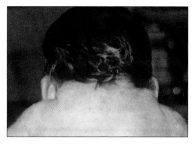

11D

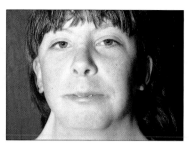

11E

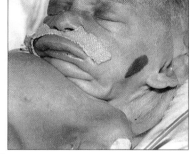

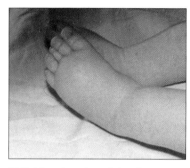

11C

11F

11G Note there is pedal oedema.

KILLIAN–PALLISTER MOSAIC SYNDROME

12A–12G

It is necessary to recognise this condition clinically, as it can be diagnosed only by looking at skin chromosomes, and this is not routinely done when the blood karyotype is normal. Patients have mosaic tetrasomy for the short arm of chromosome 12. The facial features are coarse, with a broad forehead, normal OFC, apparent hypertelorism, sagging cheeks and a droopy mouth. The upper lip is prominent. The hair is sparse, especially over the temporal areas. Supernumerary nipples are commonly found. Birth-weight is often normal. Hypopigmented macules, and even a swirly hyperpigmentation, as seen in Ito syndrome, can be found. Mental retardation can be severe.

Genetics aspects: As all cases are chromosomal mosaics, recurrence risks are small.

References

Daniel A, Kelly TE, Gollin SM *et al.* (1987). Isochromosome 12p mosaicism (Pallister-Killian syndrome): report of 11 cases. *Am J Med Genet* **27**:257–274.

Quarrell OWJ, Hamill MA, Hughes HE (1988). Pallister-Killian mosaic syndrome with emphasis on the adult phenotype. *Am J Med Genet* **31**:841–844.

Reynolds JF, Daniel A, Kelly TE *et al.* (1987). Isochromosome 12p mosaicism (Pallister mosaic aneuploidy or Pallister-Killian syndrome): report of 11 cases. *Am J Med Genet* **27**:257–274.

Schinzel A (1991). Syndrome of the month. Tetrasomy 12p (Pallister-Killian syndrome). *J Med Genet* **28**:122–125.

Warburton D, Anyane-Yeboa K, Francke U (1987). Mosaic tetrasomy 12p: four new cases, and confirmation of the chromosomal origin of the supernumerary chromosome in one of the original Pallister-mosaic syndrome cases. *Am J Med Genet* **27**:275–284.

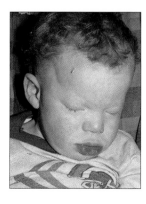

12A–12G Note the heavy facial features with sagging cheeks and full lips. The hair is sparse over the temporal regions.

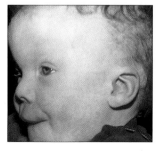

12B

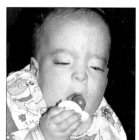

12C

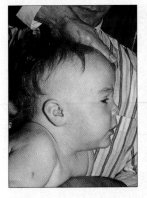 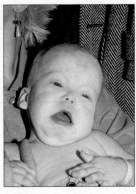 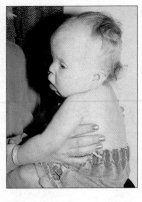 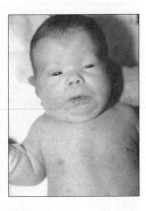

12D **12E** **12F** **12G**

SMITH–MAGENIS SYNDROME 13

The behaviour pattern might suggest the diagnosis. Self-destructive behaviour such as onychotillomania (pulling out of nails) and polyembolokoiamania (the insertion of foreign bodies into orifices), wrist biting and head banging are common. Many patients have a disturbed sleep pattern, having difficulty either falling asleep or staying asleep. There may be phenotypic overlap with Prader–Willi syndrome with short stature and obesity.

Genetic aspects: This is a microdeletion syndrome involving 17p11.2. The chromosomal region involved includes that duplicated in Charcot–Marie–Tooth disease type IA. FISH may be necessary to detect the deletion in those patients whose phenotype suggests the diagnosis.

References

Greenberg F, Guzzetta V, de Oca-Luna RM *et al.* (1991). Molecular analysis of the Smith–Magenis syndrome: a possible contiguous-gene syndrome associated with del(17)(p11.2). *Am J Hum Genet* **49**:1207–1218.

Kondo I, Matsuura S, Kuwajima K *et al.* (1991). Diagnostic hand anomalies in Smith-Magenis syndrome: four new patients with del(17)(p11.2p11.2). *Am J Med Genet* **41**:225–229..

Smith ACM, McGavran L, Robinson J *et al.* (1986). Interstitial deletion of (17)(p11.2p11.2) in nine patients. *Am J Med Genet* **24**:393–414.

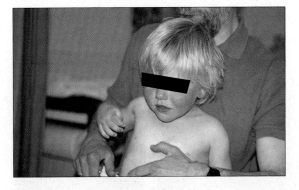

13 The face is round, the hair fair and the fingers short.

TRIPLOIDY 14A–14C

This is a common chromosomal abnormality in first trimester miscarriages and occurs with a frequency of 1–3% of human conceptuses. The rare cases who proceed to term usually die in the early post-natal period. Longer term survival usually indicates mosaicism. The clinical features include hypertelorism, a prominent forehead, a broad nose, and 3–4 syndactyly of the fingers and 2–3 syndactyly of the toes. The fingers and toes may have bulbous tips and there may be clinodactyly. Mosaic individuals can show body asymmetry and linear and whorled skin pigmentation or depigmentation.

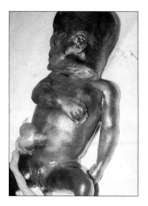 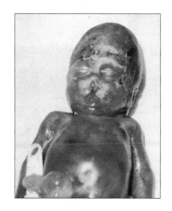 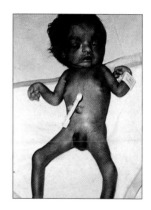

14A–14C Note short sternum, low-set ears, micrognathia, syndactyly of third and fourth fingers and genital anomalies. Note also hypotelorism, midline cleft lip and rudimentary nose (pre-maxillary agenesis).

XXX SYNDROME 15

There are few significant phenotypic characteristics of triple X females, and although some patients have late puberty, amenorrhoea, and infertility, the majority do not have these problems and are fertile. As a group there is a reduction in IQ. Prospective studies have shown a mean verbal IQ of 85.3, a mean performance IQ of 88.3 and a full scale IQ range of 64–110.
Genetic aspects: Nearly always a sporadic non-disjunction. No XXX daughter of an XXX mother has been reported, but it might still be pertinent to offer pre-natal diagnosis.

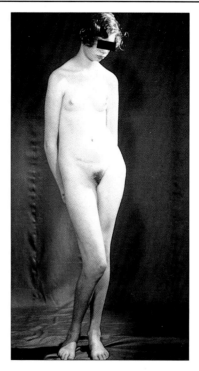

15 Note slender body habitus.

XXY (KLINEFELTER) 16

Although this condition has a frequency of about 1 in 1000 in a newborn males, presentation is usually much later. The main clinical features are a reduction of IQ by about 10–15 points, small testes (penile growth is normal in 77% at puberty and at the lower end of normal in the remaining boys), gynecomastia in about half the patients and occasional breast cancer. Patients are of average or above average height and adult males have a female distribution of body fat. Facial hair growth is sparse and body hair is scanty. The males are usually sterile.

Mean verbal IQ is 93.5, mean performance IQ 96.7 and full scale IQ range 67–131.

Genetic aspects: Most (90%) have the XXY karyotype in every cell, and about 10% are mosaics. XXXY and XXYY males are similar to those with Klinefelter syndrome, but have a greater degree of retardation. In one study of XXYY males the mean IQ was 60 and the range 55 to 75. XXXY and XXXXY males may be more severely retarded and radioulnar synostosis may be a feature.

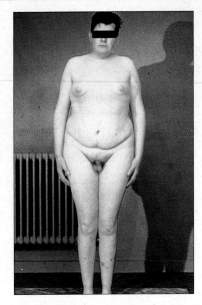

16 Note the female fat distribution, gynaecomastia, and female secondary sexual hair distribution in this XXY male.

XYY SYNDROME 17

Most males with this karyotype are phenotypically normal. Prospective studies have shown a mean verbal IQ of 100.2, and a mean performance IQ of 104.3. In one prospective study remedial help at school was required for 54% of the boys compared to 18% of controls.

Behaviour problems in childhood resulting in medical referral occurred in 50% of cases compared to 25% for XXX and XXY. As to the longer term outcome in terms of behaviour, this is not yet known and whereas there might still be an excess of criminality amongst XYY males the type of crime committed (theft and arson have been mentioned) is no different from that committed by XY males.

Genetic aspects: Sporadic. Decreased spermatogenesis and subfertility have been noted, but many males have had normal offspring.

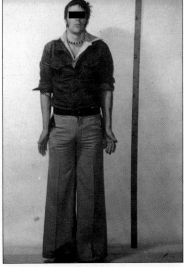

17 Note the tall stature and muscular build.

XXXX SYNDROME 18A–18B

The dysmorphic features are mild and are said by some to look a little like those of Down syndrome. Retardation is a little more severe than in those with XXX and less severe than those with XXXXX and the mean IQ is in the vicinity of 60. The facial features are not diagnostic.

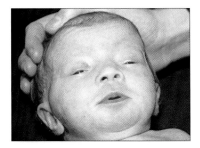

18A Note the face is not diagnostic although some authors suggest that there is a resemblance to Down syndrome.

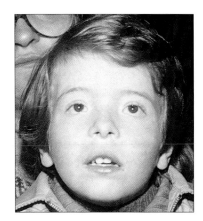

18B Note wide-set eyes, low-set nasal bridge, epicanthus, mandibular prognathism, low-set ears and short neck in this XXXXY male.

XXXXX (THE PENTA X SYNDROME)

Patients with this chromosomal constitution are said to look a little like Down syndrome children but the overall appearance is different despite the upslanting palpebral fissures. The other useful feature from a diagnostic point of view is the presence of a radio-ulnar synostosis. Other dysmorphic features include a broad flat nose, hypertelorism, epicanthic folds, a prominent jaw, hypogenitalism and mental retardation.

FRAGILE X-LINKED MENTAL RETARDATION   19A–19D

This occurs in 1 in 2000–3000 liveborn males and is characterised clinically by relative macrocephaly or normocephaly, a long face, big ears and a prominent jaw. The latter features may become more obvious with age. The dysmorphic features are seldom severe and many males in the past were referred to as having "pure" mental retardation. The retardation is variable, and a specific language disorder, hyperactivity and seizures are common features. Testicular size may be increased in the postpubertal period.

Genetic aspects: All mothers of isolated males must be assumed to be carriers and about one-third of carrier females are retarded, although more mildly than affected males. Only 30–50% of carrier females show fragile sites. The well documented phenomenon of phenotypically normal transmitting males whose daughters can have affected sons is explained by the finding of an unstable p(CCG)n trinucleotide repeat sequence in the responsible gene (FMR-1). Affected individuals have greater than 200 copies of this repeat, normal individuals have ~6–60 copies and normal transmitting males ~6–200 copies. Very rarely patients may have a deletion of the FMR-1 gene.

Dennis *et al.* reported two families with mild developmental delay, absence of the Martin-Bell phenotype, expression of a fragile site at Xq27.3, but no detectable insert in the FMR-1 gene. Flynn *et al.* have shown that the fragile site in these families (FRAXE) is distal to the site associated with FMR-1 (FRAXA).

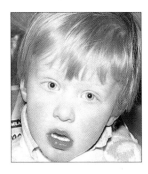
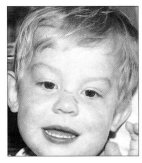
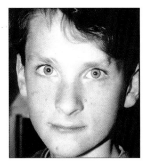
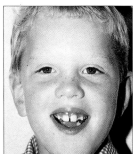

19A–19D Males with Fragile X syndrome. Note normal appearance of facies although the ears are relatively prominent and the face is long.

References

Bundey S, Webb TP, Thake A, Todd J (1985). A community study of severe mental retardation in the west Midlands and the importance of the fragile X chromosome in its aetiology. *J Med Genet* **22**:258–266.

Dennis NR, Curtis G, Macpherson JN, Jacobs PA (1992). Two families with Xq27.3 fragility, no detectable insert in the FMR-1 gene, mild mental impairment, and absence of the Martin-Bell phenotype. *Am J Med Genet* **43**:232–236.

Flynn GA, Hirst MC, Knight SJL et al. (1993). Identification of the FRAXE fragile site in two families ascertained for X-linked mental retardation. *J Med Genet* **30**:97–100.

Gedeon AK, Baker E, Robinson H et al. (1992). Fragile X syndrome without CCG amplification has an FMR-1 deletion. *Nature Genetics* **1**:341–344.

Goldson E, Hagerman RJ (1992). The fragile X syndrome. *Dev Med Child Neurol* **34**:826–832.

Hagerman RJ, Jackson C, Amiri K et al. (1992). Girls with fragile X syndrome: physical and neurocognitive status and outcome. *Pediatrics* **89**:395–400.

Oostra BA, Jacky PB, Brown WT, Rousseau F (1993). Guidelines for the diagnosis of fragile X syndrome. *J Med Genet* **30**:410–413.

SYNDROMES RECOGNISED THROUGH FACIAL FEATURES

AARSKOG SYNDROME 20A–20E

The main features are short stature, hypertelorism, short hands and feet, a shawl scrotum and a characteristic facial appearance. There is hypertelorism and ptosis with a broad forehead, down-slanting palpebral fissures, a short snub nose and a long philtrum. The shawl scrotum is characterised by a scrotal fold encircling the base of the penis and the fold is like a gothic arch, rather than the usual rounded arch seen commonly in normal boys. Mental retardation is present in only a minority of cases and is seldom severe. Other useful signs are joint laxity, mild skin syndactyly, splayed toes with bulbous tips, delayed bone age and occasionally hypoplastic terminal phalanges.

Genetic aspects: X-linked dominant. Most cases have been males and transmission can occur through mildly affected females. However, male to male transmission has been reported in some families (Grier *et al.*). Porteous *et al.* (1992) mapped the gene by linkage analysis to Xp11.2-Xq13 and the gene has now been isolated (Pasteris *et al.*).

References

Aarskog D (1970). A familial syndrome of short stature associated with facial dysplasia and genital anomalies. *J Pediatr* **77**:856–861.

Bawle E, Tyrkus M, Lipman S, Bozimowski D (1984). Aarskog syndrome: full male and female expression associated with an X-autosome translocation. *Am J Med Genet* **17**:595–602.

Friedman JM. Umbilical dysmorphology (1985). The importance of contemplating the belly button. *Clin Genet* **28**:343–347.

Grier RE, Farrington FH, Kendig R et al. (1983). Autosomal dominant inheritance of the Aarskog syndrome. *Am J Med Genet* **15**:39–46.

Pasteris NG, Cadle A, Logie LJ et al. (1994). Isolation and characterization of the faciogenital dysplasia (Aarskog-Scott syndrome) gene: a putative Rho-Rac guanine nucleotide exchange factor. *Cell* **79**:669–678.

Porteous MEM, Goudie DR (1991). Syndrome of the month. Aarskog syndrome. *J Med Genet* **28**:44–47.

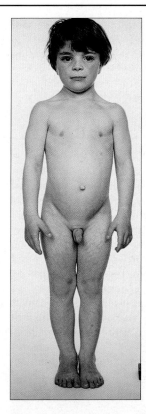 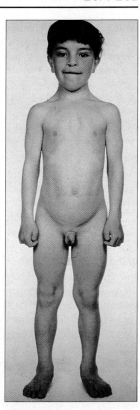

20A Note round face, ptosis and shawl scrotum.

20B Brother of patient in **20A**. Note cleft lip.

Porteous MEM, Curtis A, Lindsay S et al. (1992). The gene for Aarskog syndrome is located between DXS255 and DXS566 (Xp11.2-Xq13). *Genomics* **14**:298–301.

Van De Vooren MJ, Niermeijer MF et al. (1983). The Aarskog syndrome in a large family, suggestive for autosomal dominant inheritance. *Clin Genet* **24**:439–445.

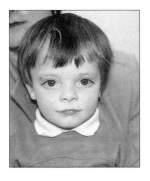

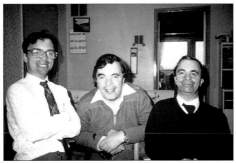

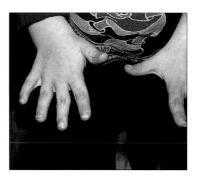

20C Note round face and mild hypertelorism.

20D Three brothers with Aarskog syndrome.

20E Note hyperextension at interphalangeal joints and mild skin syndactyly of fingers.

ROBINOW (FETAL FACE) SYNDROME   21A–21D

Mesomelic limb shortening is usually (but not always) apparent. The facial features are said to resemble those of a fetus, with a prominent forehead, hypertelorism, a wide mouth and a small nose with anteverted nostrils. There may be significant gum hypertrophy. Other features include a micropenis in males, hydronephrosis or urinary tract infections, cleft lip and palate, and hemivertebrae.

Genetic aspects: Autosomal dominant and recessive families have been reported.

References

Bain MD, Winter RM, Burn J (1986). Robinow syndrome without mesomelic 'brachymelia': a report of five cases. *J Med Genet* **23**:350–354.

Butler MG, Wadlington WB (1987). Robinow syndrome: report of two patients and review of the literature. *Clin Genet* **31**:77–85.

Schonau E, Pfeiffer RA, Schweikert HU *et al.* (1990). Robinow or 'fetal face' syndrome in a male infant with ambiguous genitalia and androgen receptor deficiency. *Eur J Pediatr* **149**:615–617.

Schorderet DF, Dahoun S, Defrance I *et al.* (1992). Robinow syndrome in two siblings from consanguineous parents. *Eur J Pediatr* **151**:586–589.

Teebi AS (1990). Autosomal recessive Robinow syndrome. *Am J Med Genet* **35**:64–68.

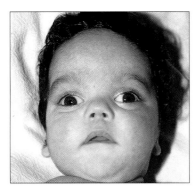

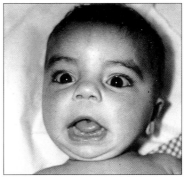

21A and 21B Note the high broad forehead, short upturned nose, long philtrum and large mouth.

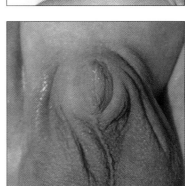

21C Note the gum hypertrophy.

21D Note micropenis.

NOONAN SYNDROME

The main features are short stature, a short neck with webbing or redundancy of the skin, cardiac anomalies (particularly PS, ASD, VSD, PDA and hypertrophic cardiomyopathy). Left ventricular thickening can be progressive and may not be present at birth. Other features include a characteristic chest deformity with a pectus carinatum superiorly and a pectus excavatum inferiorly, wide-spaced nipples and a characteristic facial appearance which changes significantly with age. In the newborn period the main features are hypertelorism, a downward eye-slant, low-set posteriorly rotated ears, a deeply grooved philtrum and a broad nasal tip. In later infancy the eye-slant may become horizontal and the facies can become coarser. In adults the facies may be more subtle. Mild retardation is seen in 35% of cases.

A bleeding diathesis can be part of the condition. Sharland *et al.* (1992) studied 72 affected individuals and found 29 with a prolonged activated partial thromboplastin time with partial factor XI:C, XII:C or VIII:C deficiencies in 36 patients.

The incidence has been estimated to be between 1 in 1000 and 1 in 2500 live births.

Genetic aspects: Autosomal dominant with variable expression. The gene maps to 12q.

References

Allanson JE (1987). Syndrome of the month: Noonan syndrome. *J Med Genet* **24**:9–13.

Allanson JF, Hall JG, Hughes HF *et al.* (1985). Noonan syndrome: the changing phenotype. *Am J Med Genet* **21**:507–514.

De Haan M, van De Kamp JJP *et al.* (1988). Noonan syndrome: partial factor XI deficiency. *Am J Med Genet* **29**:277–282.

Fryer AE, Holt PJ, Hughes HE (1991). The cardio-facio-cutaneous (CFC) syndrome and Noonan syndrome: are they the same? *Am J Med Genet* **38**:548–551.

Ranke MB, Heidermann P, Knupfer C *et al.* (1988). Noonan syndrome: growth and clinical manifestations in 144 cases. *Eur J Pediatr* **148**:220–227.

Sharland M, Burch M, McKenna WM *et al.* (1992). A clinical study of Noonan syndrome. *Arch Dis Child* **67**:178–183.

Sharland M, Morgan M, Smith G *et al.* (1993). Genetic counselling in Noonan syndrome. *Am J Med Genet* **45**:437–440.

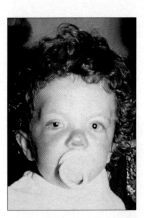

22A–22H Note the wide-spaced eyes, ptosis, down-slanting palpebral fissures, posteriorly rotated ears, low posterior hairline, short stature and short curly hair. The girls in **22C** and **22D** are sisters. The case in **22E** and **22F** shows overlap with Costello syndrome.

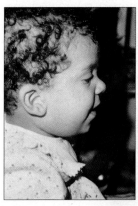

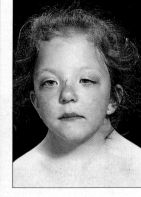

22B

22C

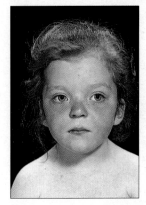

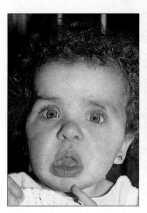

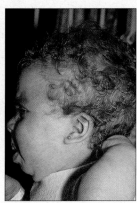

22D

22E

22F

22G

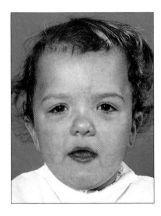

22H

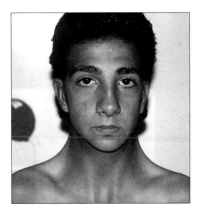

CARDIO-FACIO-CUTANEOUS (CFC) SYNDROME

23A–23C

The facial features are similar to Noonan syndrome, but may be coarser, and the hair is especially sparse, friable and curly. The head is relatively large when compared with overall body size and there is a noticeable bi-temporal constriction. The cardiac features are variable, but a pulmonary stenosis is the most common, next being an ASD. The skin is dry, and hyperkeratotic lesions develop, especially over the extensor surfaces. An enlarged liver and spleen have been found and many patients have been investigated for a possible storage disorder. It remains uncertain whether this is a separate entity.

Genetic aspects: Most cases have been isolated. Fryns *et al.* reported a possible dominant family, but the affected individuals did not have as severe manifestations as some other cases in the literature and this family may suggest further evidence of a 'Noonan–CFC spectrum'.

References
Baraitser M, Patton MA (1986). A Noonan-like short stature syndrome with sparse hair. *J Med Genet* **23**:161–164.
Bottani A, Hammerer I, Schinzel A (1991). The cardio-facio-cutaneous syndrome: report of a patient and review of the literature. *Eur J Pediatr* **150**:486–488.
Fryer AE, Holt PJ, Hughes HE (1991). The cardio-facio-cutaneous (CFC) syndrome and Noonan syndrome: are they the same? *Am J Med Genet* **38**:548–551.
Fryns JP, Volcke P, Van den Berghe H (1992). The cardio-facio-cutaneous (CFC) syndrome: autosomal dominant inheritance in a large family. *Genetic Counseling* **3**:19–24.
Reynolds JF, Neri G, Herrmann JP *et al.* (1986). New multiple congenital anomalies/mental retardation syndrome with cardio-facio-cutaneous involvement - the CFC syndrome. *Am J Med Genet* **25**:413–427.
Somer M, Peippo M, Aalto-Korte K *et al.* (1992). Cardio-facio-cutaneous syndrome: three additional cases and review of the literature. *Am J Med Genet* **44**:691–695.

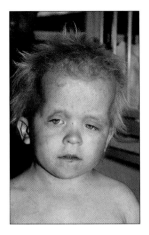
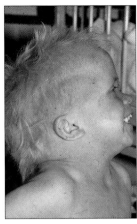
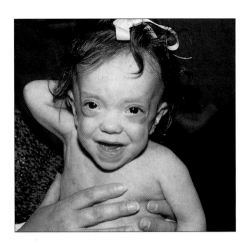

23A and 23B Note short stature, ptosis, webbed neck, sparse hair and pectus carinatum.

23C Note broad forehead, hypertelorism, and sparse hair.

COSTELLO SYNDROME

There is overlap between this condition and Noonan and CFC syndromes. The hallmarks of Costello syndrome are the presence of nasal papillomata which develop towards the end of the first decade and the presence of loose skin, especially over the hands and feet, which can be present from birth. Indeed, some children have been diagnosed as having cutis laxa congenita. Perioral and perianal papillomata and hyperkeratosis of the palms and soles may also been seen. The facial appearance becomes coarser with age and significant mental retardation can be a feature. A high birth-weight, a vertical talus, dislocated hips and acanthosis nigricans appear to be part of the condition.

Genetic aspects: Most cases are sporadic but parents should be examined for Noonan-like features.

References

Borochowitz Z, Pavone L, Mazor G et al. (1992). New multiple congenital anomalies: mental retardation syndrome (MCA/MR) with facio-cutaneous-skeletal involvement. *Am J Med Genet* **43**:678–685.

Costello JM (1977). A new syndrome: mentally subnormality and nasal papillomata. *Aust Paediatr J* **13**:114–118.

Der Kaloustian VM, Moroz B, McIntosh N et al. (1991). Costello syndrome. *Am J Med Genet* **41**:69–73.

Martin RA, Jones KL (1991). Delineation of the Costello syndrome. *Am J Med Genet* **41**:346–349.

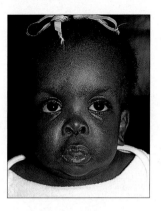
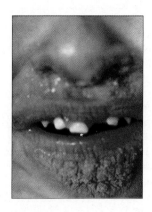
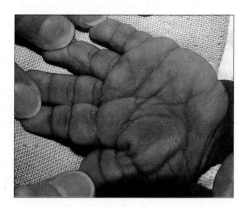

24A Note the sagging skin over the face, wide-spaced, down-slanting palpebral fissures and prominent lips.

24B The characteristic papillomata develop later in childhood.

24C There is excess skin over the palms.

LEOPARD SYNDROME

The acronym LEOPARD stands for Lentigines (multiple), Ocular hypertelorism, Pulmonary stenosis, Abnormalities of genitalia, Retardation of growth and Deafness (sensorineural) (Gorlin *et al.*). The lentigines are small (less than 5mm) dark brown spots, concentrated on the face and upper trunk. They develop at an earlier age than freckles, and unlike the latter do not increase in number on exposure to the sun. Cardiac abnormalities include mild pulmonary stenosis, subaortic stenosis, or other abnormalities. There is widening of the QRS complex with bundle branch block, abnormal P-waves and prolongation of the P-R interval. Genital abnormalities include hypogenitalism and hypospadias. Height is usually below the 25th centile, but is not severely affected. Sensorineural deafness is variable, ranging from normal to severe. There is also an association with granular cell schwannomas.

Genetic aspects: Autosomal dominant.

References

Gorlin RJ, Anderson RC, Moller JH (1971). The leopard (multiple lentigines) syndrome revisited. *Laryngoscope* **81**:1674–1681.

Nordlund JJ, Lerner AB, Braverman IM, McGuire JS (1973). The multiple lentigines syndrome. *Arch Dermatol* **107**:259–261.

Peter JR, Kemp JS (1990). LEOPARD syndrome: death because of chronic respiratory insufficiency. *Am J Med Genet* **37**:340–341.

Pickering D, Laski B, MacMillan DC, Rose V (1971). 'Little leopard' syndrome. Description of three cases and review of 24. *Arch Dis Child* **46**:85–90.

Ruiz-Maldonado R, Trevizo L, Tamayo L et al. (1983). Progressive cardiomyopathic lentiginosis: report of six cases and one autopsy. *Pediatr Dermatol* **1**:146–153.

Seuanez H, Mane-Garzon F, Kolski R (1976). Cardio-cutaneous syndrome (the "LEOPARD" syndrome). Review of the literature and a new family. *Clin Genet* **9**:266–276.

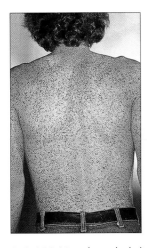
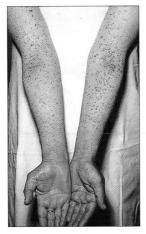
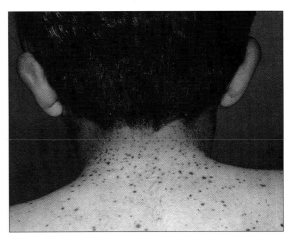

25A–25C Note the multiple lentigenes.

CHAR SYNDROME

26A–26C

The upper lip has a pronounced convex curve, with the central part almost touching the nose, and both upper and lower lips are prominent and slightly everted. The nose itself has a broad tip and the ears are prominent and low set. Ptosis and wide-spaced eyes are characteristic. The teeth are wide-spaced and the palate high-arched. Speech is impaired because of an inability to close the lips, development can be mildly delayed. Patent ductus arteriosus and an absent phalanx of the fifth finger, together with lack of flexion of distal interphalangeal joints, are further features of the condition.

Genetic aspects: Autosomal dominant.

References

Char F (1978). Peculiar facies with short philtrum, duck-bill lips and low-set ears – a new syndrome? *BDOAS* **14**:303–305.
Temple IK (1992). Char syndrome (unusual mouth, patent ductus arteriosus, phalangeal anomalies). *Clin Dysmorphol* **1**:17–21.

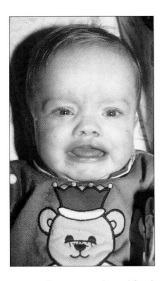
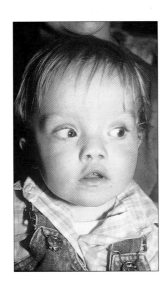
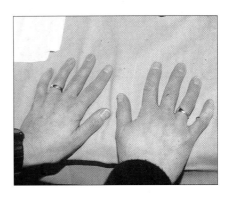

26C Clinodactyly is part of the clinical picture.

26A and 26B Note broad forehead, flared eyebrows, hypertelorism, short philtrum and triangular mouth.

KABUKI MAKE-UP SYNDROME

This is a mental retardation syndrome with short stature and a characteristic face, which is reminiscent of the make-up worn by actors in Kabuki theatre. The lateral third of the lower lid is everted and the palpebral fissures are long. The eyebrows are long and may have a central gap. The nasal tip is broad, the ears and ear lobes prominent and the palate cleft or high-arched. The fifth finger is short and there is persistence of the fetal finger pads. There are mild radiological changes in the vertebrae. Joint hypermobility, ptosis and hypotonia appear to be more frequent in European patients. Craniosynostosis may be an occasional feature. The mental retardation is usually moderate to mild.

Genetic aspects: Unknown, but to date most cases have been sporadic.

References

Kuroki Y, Katsumata N, Eguchi T *et al.* (1987). Precocious puberty in Kabuki makeup syndrome. *J Pediatr* **110**:750–752.

Niikawa N, Kuroki Y, Kajii T *et al.* (1988). Kabuki make-up (Niikawa-Kuroki) syndrome: a study of 62 patients. *Am J Med Genet* **31**:565–590.

Philip N, Meinecke P, David A *et al.* (1992). Kabuki make-up (Niikawa-Kuroki) syndrome: a study of 16 non-Japanese cases. *Clin Dysmorphol* **1**:63–77.

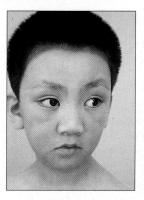 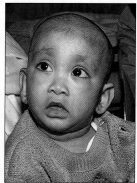 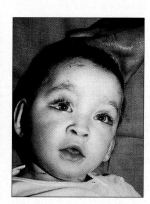

27A–27C Note the typical long palpebral fissures and everted lower lids. The eyebrows are arched with sparse lateral halves. The ears are often prominent.

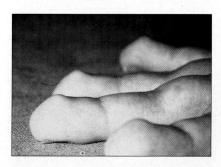 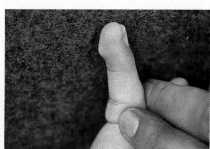

27D and 27E Note the prominent fingertip pads (fetal pads).

WILLIAMS SYNDROME

The facial features consist of periorbital fullness, medial eyebrow flare, a stellate iris pattern, a flat nasal bridge, a flat malar region with full cheeks and lips, and a wide mouth with a long smooth philtrum. The facies may become coarser with age. The characteristic heart defect is a supravalvular aortic stenosis or a peripheral pulmonary artery stenosis. Renal artery stenosis can occur. Hypercalcaemia may be difficult to document by the time the child has developed the full clinical features, but occasionally it is severe and persists. Enamel hypoplasia, strabismus and inguinal hernias are common.

Genetic aspects: Most cases are sporadic but autosomal dominant transmission has been reported. Ewart *et al.* identified hemizygosity of the elastin gene at 7q11 in four familial and five sporadic cases of Williams syndrome.

References

Burn J (1986). Syndrome of the month: Williams syndrome. *J Med Gen* **23**:389–395.

Ewart AK, Morris CA, Atkinson D *et al.* (1993). Hemizygosity at the elastin locus in a developmental disorder, Williams syndrome. *Nature Genetics* **5**:11–16.

Halladie-Smith KA, Karas S (1988). Cardiac anomalies in Williams–Beuren syndrome. *Arch Dis Child* **63**:809–813.

Jones KL (1990). Williams syndrome: an historical perspective of its evolution, natural history, and etiology. *Am J Med Genet* **Suppl.6**:89–96.

Lopez-Rangel E, Maurice M, McGillivray B, Friedman JM (1990). Williams syndrome in adults. *Am J Med Genet* **44**:720–729.

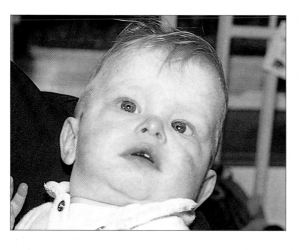

28A–28E A series of pictures showing Williams syndrome at different ages.

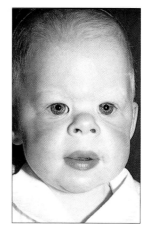

28B

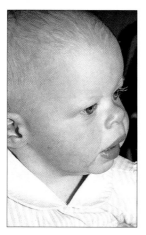

28C

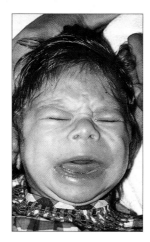

28D

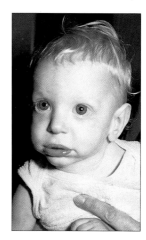

28E

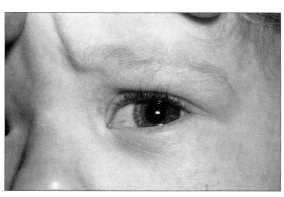

28F and 28G Note the stellate iris pattern.

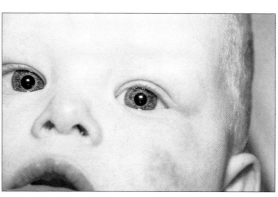

28G

COFFIN–LOWRY SYNDROME

This X-linked syndrome is recognisable in males, who are usually severely retarded and have a characteristic facial appearance. There is hypertelorism with down-slanting palpebral fissures, the nose is usually broad, and the mouth is large and bow-shaped with prominent everted lips. The head circumference may be small and there is often fullness of the upper lids, especially at their lateral margins. The ears appear to be large and many case reports refer to a long philtrum. Pectus carinatum or excavatum has been commented on and a severe kyphoscoliosis develops in older patients. Radiologically there might be degenerative changes in the spine, tufting of the distal phalanges, and poor modelling of the middle phalanges, as well as pseudo-epiphyses of the metacarpals. An almost pathognomonic sign is the pudgy, tapering digits.

Genetic aspects: X-linked. Female carriers often have minor facial features (coarseness), characteristic (tapering) fingers and, in some cases, can have mild mental retardation. The locus maps to Xp22.

References

Gilgenkrantz S, Mujica P, Gruet P *et al.* (1988). Coffin-Lowry syndrome: a multicenter study. *Clin Genet* **34**:230–245.

Hanauer A, Alembik Y *et al.* (1988). Probable localisation of the Coffin-Lowry locus in Xp22.2-p22.1 by multipoint linkage analysis. *Am J Med Genet* **30**:523–530.

Hunter AGW, Partington MW, Evans JA (1982). The Coffin-Lowry syndrome. Experience from four centers. *Clin Genet* **21**:321–335.

Wilson WG, Kelly TE (1981). Early recognition of the Coffin-Lowry syndrome. *Am J Med Genet* **8**:215–220.

Young ID (1988). Syndrome of the month. The Coffin-Lowry syndrome. *J Med Gen* **25**:344–348.

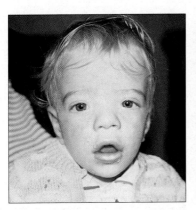
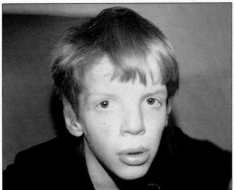
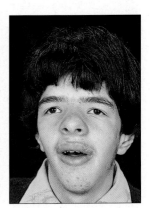

29A–29C Note the thick lips, bulbous nose with thick nasal alae, ptosis and down-slanting palpebral fissures.

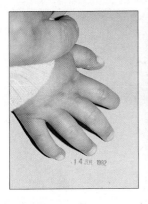
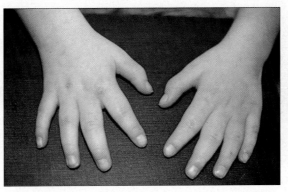
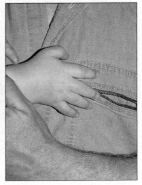

29D–29F Note the sausage-shaped tapering fingers.

ATKIN-FLAITZ SYNDROME 30A–30B

This is a rare form of X-linked mental retardation. Affected males are macrocephalic and have large square foreheads, prominent supra-orbital ridges, wide-spaced, down-slanting palpebral fissures, broad nasal tips and thick lower lips. There is a prominent gap between the upper incisors and a prominent mid-line groove of the tongue. The diagnosis can be difficult – some of the original cases resembled Coffin–Lowry syndrome whereas other affected family members did not.

Genetic aspects: Apparently X-linked with some manifestations in females.

References
Atkin JF, Flaitz K, Patil S, Smith W (1985). A new X-linked mental retardation syndrome. *Am J Med Genet* **21**:697–705.
Clark RD, Baraitser M (1987). A new X-linked mental retardation syndrome (Letter). *Am J Med Genet* **26**:13–16.

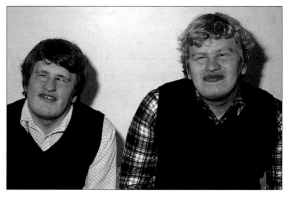

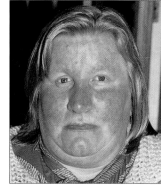

30B Carrier mother showing similar but milder features.

30A Note two large males with macrocephaly and obesity.

ALPHA THALASSAEMIA–MENTAL RETARDATION (NON-DELETION) 31A–31C

This interesting entity causes mental retardation with haematological evidence of haemoglobin H disease. Clinically there is short stature, microcephaly, hypertelorism, a flat face with a depressed nasal bridge, epicanthic folds, macrostomia, small teeth, and a V-shaped upper lip or short philtrum with an everted lower lip. Seizures are a feature. Cryptorchidism or hypogonadism is common and some of the males have ambiguous genitalia and have been brought up as female. All cases have been male, apart from a phenotypic female in the original report who had a 46,XY karyotype. One case had hemivertebrae.

The diagnosis is confirmed by demonstrating haematological features of alpha thalassaemia. HbH bodies, present in 1–40% of red cells, must be demonstrated by staining with 1% brilliant cresyl blue (see Logie *et al.* for technical details).

Genetic aspects: The condition is X-linked recessive. Female carriers can often be shown to have HbH inclusions in red cells. The gene maps to Xq12-Xq21 (Gibbons *et al.*).

References
Cole TRP, May A, Hughes HE (1991). Alpha thalassaemia/mental retardation syndrome (non-deletional type): report of a family supporting X linked inheritance. *J Med Gen* **28**:734–737.
Gibbons RJ, Wilkie AOM, Weatherall DJ, Higgs DR (1991). A newly defined X linked mental retardation syndrome associated with alpha thalassaemia (Review). *J Med Gen* **28**:729–733.
Gibbons RJ, Suthers GK, Wilkie AOM et al. (1992). X-linked alpha-thalassemia/mental retardation (ATR-X) syndrome: localization to Xq12-q21.31 by X inactivation and linkage analysis. *Am J Hum Genet* **51**:1136–1149.
Logie LJ, Gibbons RJ, Higgs DR et al. (1994). Alpha thalassaemia mental retardation (ATR-X): an atypical family. *Arch Dis Child* **70**:439–440.
Wilkie AOM, Zeitlin HC, Lindenbaum RH et al. (1990). Clinical features and molecular analysis of the alpha thalassemia/mental retardation syndromes. II. Cases without detectable abnormality of the alpha globin complex. *Am J Hum Genet* **46**:1127–1140.

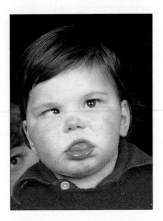 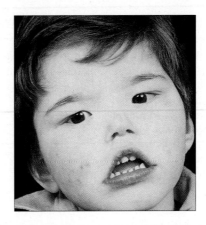 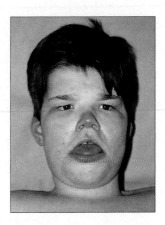

31A–31C Note the prominent everted lower lip, V-shaped upper lip and the short upturned nose.

FG SYNDROME

This is a form of X-linked mental retardation with rather 'soft' dysmorphic features. Affected males will be floppy at birth, have relative macrocephaly, develop severe constipation which might lead to a suspicion of Hirschsprung's disease, and eventually be found to be moderately to severely mentally handicapped. Most males have a broad forehead with an upsweep of the frontal hairline (cowlicks) or posterior hairline. The face is droopy due to severe hypotonia. An anal stenosis or an anteriorly placed anus may be present. Failure to thrive and death in infancy are other features. It is worth looking for prominent fetal finger pads. It is diagnostically helpful to find an agenesis of the corpus callosum. This syndrome can be difficult to diagnose as the individual features are 'soft' and by no means specific to the condition.

Genetic aspects: X-linked. Some female carriers have a broad forehead and a frontal cowlick and can be slow.

References
Opitz JM, Kaveggia EG, Adkins WN (1982). Studies of malformation syndromes of humans XXXIIIC. The FG syndrome - further studies on three affected individuals from the FG family. *Am J Med Genet* **12**:147–154.
Opitz JM, Richieri-Costa A et al. (1988). FG syndrome update 1988: note of five new patients and bibliography. *Am J Med Genet* **30**:309–328.
Thompson E, Baraitser M (1987). Syndrome of the month: FG syndrome. *J Med Gen* **24**:139–143.
Thompson EM, Baraitser M, Lindenbaum RH (1985). The FG syndrome: seven new cases. *Clin Genet* **27**:582–594.

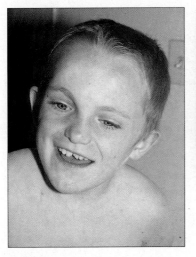 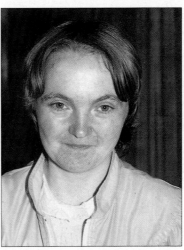

32A and 32B Note 'cowlicks' in child and his mother. Head circumference is normal to large.

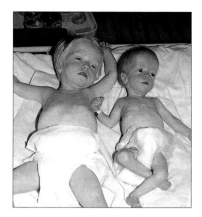

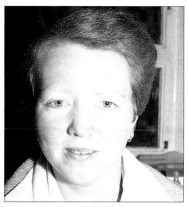

32C and 32D The mother of these two boys has a broad forehead and a frontal cowlick.

BORJESON–FORSSMAN–LEHMANN SYNDROME 33

The clinical features are mental retardation, hypotonia, obesity, microcephaly, a coarse facial appearance with 'fatty' cheeks, ptosis, occasional cataracts, prominent supraorbital ridges with deep-set eyes, and large ears. Both the penis and the testes are small and secondary sexual characteristics are delayed. Affected males are of small stature and usually have a delayed bone age. Radiologically, the proximal femoral and humeral heads might be small and scoliosis occurs in some.

Genetic aspects: X-linked recessive. The gene has been localized to Xq26-27.

References

Ardinger HH, Hanson JW, Zellweger HU (1984). Borjeson-Forssman-Lehmann syndrome: further delineation in five cases. *Am J Med Genet* **19**:653–664.

Dereymaeker AM, Fryns JP et al. (1986). The Borjeson-Forssman-Lehmann syndrome. A family study. *Clin Genet* **29**:317–320.

Mathews KD, Ardinger HH et al. (1989). Linkage localization of Borjeson-Forssman-Lehmann syndrome. *Am J Med Genet* **34**:470–474.

Robinson LK, Jones KL, Culler F et al. (1983). The Borjeson-Forssman-Lehmann syndrome. *Am J Med Genet* **15**:457–468.

Turner G, Gedeon A, Mulley J et al. (1989). Borjeson-Forssman-Lehmann syndrome: clinical manifestations and gene localization to Xq26-27. *Am J Med Genet* **34**:463–469.

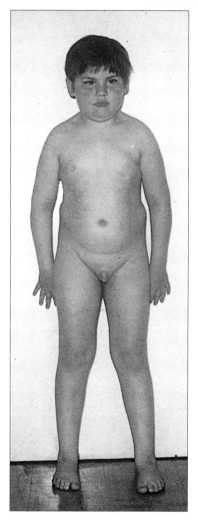

33 Note obesity, gynaecomastia, hypogenitalism, and round face with narrow palpebral fissures.

BLEPHAROPHIMOSIS–PTOSIS–EPICANTHUS INVERSUS SYNDROME

In this condition there is a reduced horizontal diameter of the palpebral fissures, droopy eyelids and a fold of skin which runs from the lower lids medially and upwards. Telecanthus is found in the majority of patients and the eyelid skin is smooth. The nasal bridge is flat and the ears might be simple, protruding or cup-shaped. Intelligence is mostly normal although mild mental retardation has been reported. However, it should be noted that early motor milestones might erroneously be thought to be delayed because of hypotonia and backwards head tilt. There is an increased frequency of menstrual irregularity and infertility in females and some authors designate this as type I in families where there is transmission by males only. In type II, transmission is through both sexes.

Genetic aspects: Autosomal dominant. Several cases with chromosomal rearrangements have suggested localization of the gene to 3q23.

References

Fujita H, Meng J, Kawamura M *et al.* (1992). Boy with a chromosome del (3)(q12q23) and blepharophimosis syndrome. *Am J Med Genet* **44**:434–436.

Fukushima Y, Wakui K, Nishida T, Ucoka Y (1991). Blepharophimosis sequence and de novo balanced autosomal translocation [46,XY,t(3;4)(q23;p15.2)]: possible assignment of the trait to 3q23. *Am J Med Gen* **40**:485–487.

Oley C, Baraitser M (1988). Blepharophimosis, ptosis, epicanthus inversus syndrome (BPES syndrome). *J Med Gen* **25**:47–51.

Zlotogora J, Sagi M, Cohen T *et al.* (1983). The blepharophimosis, ptosis and epicanthus inversus syndrome: delineation of two types. *Am J Hum Genet* **35**:1020–1027.

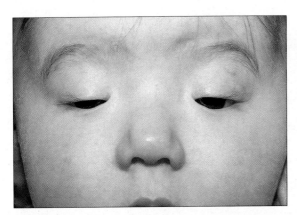
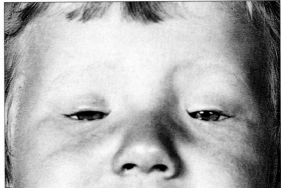

34A–34E Note blepharophimosis, ptosis and epicanthus inversus. These features are less prominent in adulthood.

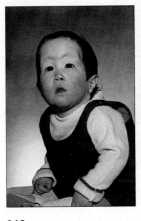
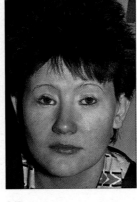
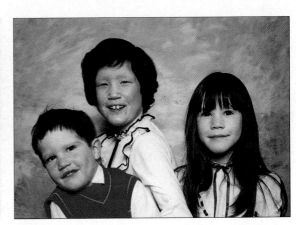

34C **34D** **34E**

DE LANGE SYNDROME

This mental retardation syndrome is characterised by low birth-weight in the majority, short stature, microcephaly, and generalised hirsutism resulting in synophrys, a hairy forehead, hairy ears and marked hair whorls on the posterior trunk and arms. The nose is short, the nostrils anteverted and flared, and there is a long philtrum and a thin upper lip with a midline beak. Feeding difficulties, irritability, a deep hoarse cry, and increased tone in the limbs are common early problems. Upper limb defects are common and vary from proximally placed thumbs to absence deformities and ectrodactyly.

The existence of a milder form of the condition, sometimes with autosomal dominant inheritance, is still controversial.

Genetic aspects: Concordance in monozygotic twins and affected siblings with the classic form has occasionally been reported, but most cases are sporadic.

Ireland *et al.* reported a convincing case with a 3q26:17q23 *de novo* translocation.

References

Baraitser M, Papavasiliou AS (1993). Mild de Lange syndrome – does it exist? *Clin Dysmorphol* **2**:147–150.

Filippi G (1989). The de Lange syndrome. Report of 15 cases. *Clin Genet* **35**:343–363.

Greenberg F, Robinson LK (1989). Mild Brachmann-de Lange syndrome: changes of phenotype with age. *Am J Med Gen* **32**:90–92.

Hawley PP, Jackson LG, Kurnit DM (1985). 64 patients with Brachmann-de Lange syndrome: a survey. *Am J Med Gen* **20**:453–459.

Ireland M, English C, Cross I *et al.* (1991). A de novo translocation t(3;17)(q26.3;q23.1) in a child with Cornelia de Lange syndrome. *J Med Gen* **28**:639–640.

Ireland M, Burn J (1993). Cornelia de Lange syndrome - photo essay. *Clin Dysmorphol* **2**:151–160.

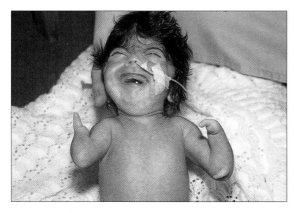
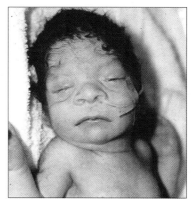

35A–35E Note generalised hirsutism, synophrys, anteverted nostrils, long philtrum, thin upper lip, small jaw, downturned angle of the mouth and limb defects including ectrodactyly.

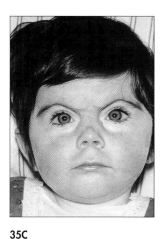
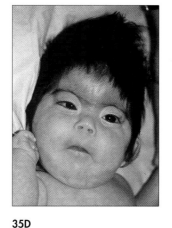
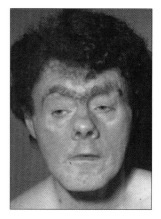

35C   35D   35E

DUBOWITZ SYNDROME

These children are short, microcephalic, and have sparse hair, telecanthus, ptosis, blepharophimosis and prominent epicanthic folds. The nasal tip is broad, the jaw is small and three-quarters of the patients have either prominent or mildly dysplastic ears. A palatal abnormality is a frequent finding but it varies between a high-arched palate and a cleft. With time the face elongates, and the nasal bridge becomes more prominent and almost continuous with the forehead. The supraorbital ridges are hypoplastic with sparse arched eyebrows. Intrauterine growth retardation is one of the cardinal features and the average birth-weight is 2.3kg. Severe and unusual eczema is another cardinal feature. Early feeding difficulties are not uncommon and mild to moderate retardation, rather than severe retardation, occurs. This is a gestalt diagnosis – firm diagnostic criteria should be adhered to.

Genetic aspects: Autosomal recessive.

References

Dubowitz V (1965). Familial low birth-weight dwarfism with an unusual facies and a skin eruption. *J Med Genet* **2**:12–17.

Orrison WW, Schnitzler ER, Chun RWM (1980). The Dubowitz syndrome: further observations. *Am J Med Genet* **7**:155–170.

Parrish JM, Wilroy RS (1980). The Dubowitz syndrome: the psychological status of ten cases at follow-up. *Am J Med Genet* **6**:3–8.

Winter RM (1986). Syndrome of the month: Dubowitz syndrome. *J Med Genet* **83**:11–13.

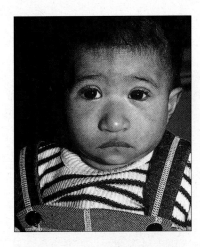

36A–36E Note the ptosis, blepharophimosis and prominent epicanthic folds. The head and jaw are small and the nasal tip is broad.

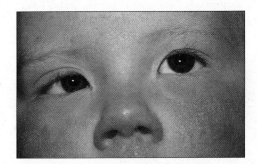

36B

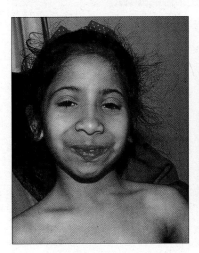

36C

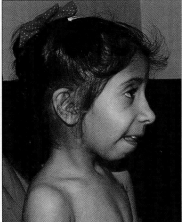

36D

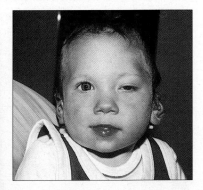

36E

SECKEL SYNDROME (BIRD-HEADED DWARFISM)   37A–37D

The main diagnostic criteria are severe intrauterine growth retardation (average birth-weight 1543 grams at term), severe microcephaly (average -8.7 SD), short stature (average -7.1 SD), retarded bone age and moderate to severe mental retardation. The face is characteristic with a receding forehead, protruding eyes, a large beaked nose, a receding chin and down-slanting eyes. Dislocation of the radial head is common, as are fifth finger clinodactyly, absent ear lobes, and teeth abnormalities. The stance can be abnormal with fixed flexion at the hips and knees.

Genetic aspects: Autosomal recessive.

References

Harper RG, Orti E, Baker RK (1967). Bird-headed dwarfs (Seckel's syndrome). A familial pattern of developmental, dental, skeletal, genital and central nervous system anomalies. *J Pediatr* **70**:799–804.

Majewski F, Goecke T (1982). Studies of microcephalic primordial dwarfism I: approach to a delineation of the Seckel syndrome. *Am J Med Genet* **12**:7–21.

Szalay GC (1974). Seckel syndrome. *J Med Genet* **11**:216.

Thompson E, Pembrey ME (1985). Seckel syndrome: an overdiagnosed syndrome. *J Med Genet* **22**:192–201.

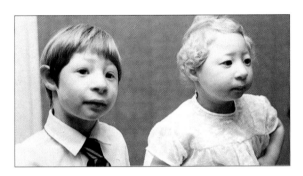

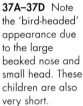

37A–37D Note the 'bird-headed' appearance due to the large beaked nose and small head. These children are also very short.

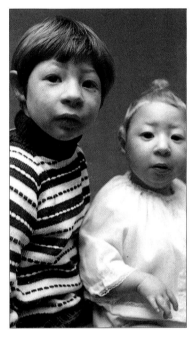

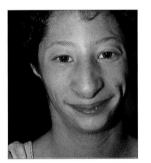

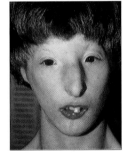

37C   **37D**   **37B**

OSTEODYSPLASTIC PRIMORDIAL DWARFISM TYPE I   38A–38B

The main features are low birth-weight dwarfism, extreme microcephaly, a prominent nose and eyes, sparse scalp hair, a short neck, short limbs with dislocation of the elbows and hips, relatively broad hands and feet, and dry hyperkeratotic skin. Radiographs reveal shortening and bowing of the humeri and femora in type I and elongated clavicles, cleft cervical arches, lumbar platyspondyly, hypoplastic iliac wings and a horizontal acetabulum.

This syndrome was first described by Majewski *et al.* who subdivided similar cases into types I, II and III. Winter *et al.* argued that types I and III may reflect the appearance of the same condition at different ages.

Genetic aspects: The inheritance pattern is likely to be autosomal recessive.

References

Majewski F, Stoeckenius M, Kemperdick H (1982). Studies of microcephalic primordial dwarfism III: an intrauterine dwarf with platyspondyly and anomalies of pelvis and clavicles - osteodysplastic primordial dwarfism type III. *Am J Med Genet* **12**:37–42.

Meinecke P, Passarge E (1991). Microcephalic osteodysplastic primordial dwarfism type I/III in siblings. *J Med Genet* **28**:795–800.

Winter RM, Wigglesworth J, Harding BN (1985). Osteodysplastic primordial dwarfism: report of a further patient with manifestations similar to those seen in patients with types I and III. *Am J Med Genet* **21**:569–574.

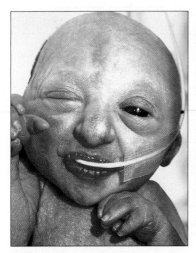
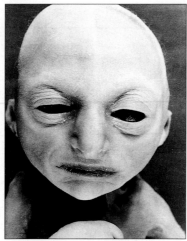

38A and 38B Note microcephaly, alopecia, with sloping forehead, prominent eyes, large nose and small pointed chin.

MICROCEPHALY (AUTOSOMAL RECESSIVE)

39A–39E

There appears to be a form of 'true' autosomal recessive microcephaly. Affected individuals have a very small vault to the skull but the face is of normal size. The ears appear large and the forehead is sloping. Motor milestones are generally good and seizures or other neurological abnormalities are not a major part of the condition. The diagnosis is made from the characteristic clinical features in the absence of any environmental causes for microcephaly. Further supporting evidence would be a CAT scan that did not show major structural abnormalities of the brain.

Genetic aspects: Autosomal recessive. In single cases with consistent clinical features the recurrence to siblings risk is about 10%.

References
Chervenak FA, Rosenberg J *et al.* (1987). A prospective study of the accuracy of ultrasound in predicting fetal microcephaly. *Obstet Gynecol* **69**:908–910.
Jaffe M, Tirosh E, Oren S (1987). The dilemma in prenatal diagnosis of idiopathic microcephaly. *Dev Med Child Neurol* **29**:187–189.
Opitz JM, Holt MC (1990). Microcephaly: general considerations and aids to nosology. *J Cranio Gen Dev Bio* **10**:175–204.
Pescia G, Nguyen-The H, Deonna T (1983). Prenatal diagnosis of genetic microcephaly. *Prenatal Diagn* **3**:363–365.

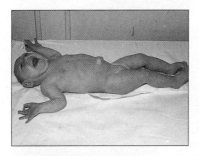
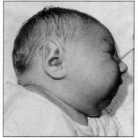
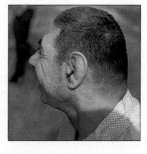

39A–39C Note the small head with receding forehead and the disproportion between the normal sized face and the small cranium.

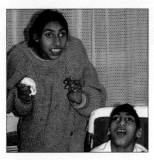
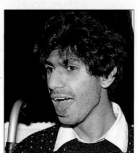

39D–39E Note two sibling pairs with microcephaly and more severe neurological problems.

MICROCEPHALY–INTRACRANIAL CALCIFICATION   40A–40C

There are several sibships reported with individuals manifesting microcephaly, intracranial calcification and mental retardation. Syndromes to consider in the differential diagnosis are Aicardi–Goutieres, fetal CMV, Cockayne and Fahr. There is danger in making the diagnosis of intrauterine infection after the birth of the first child, in the absence of direct evidence.

Genetic aspects: Autosomal recessive. The reports are rather heterogeneous. Baraitser *et al.* described two brothers with spasticity, seizures and calcification of the white matter and thalami. Burn *et al.* described two siblings, the offspring of Turkish Cypriot second cousins, with lissencephaly, polymicrogyria, massive calcification throughout the brain and corneal clouding.

References

Baraitser M, Brett EM, Piesowicz AT (1983). Microcephaly and intracranial calcification in two brothers. *J Med Genet* **20**:210–212.

Burn J, Wickramasinghe HT, Harding B *et al.* (1986). A syndrome with intracranial calcification and microcephaly in two siblings, resembling intrauterine infection. *Clin Genet* **30**:112–116.

Ishitsu T, Chikazawa S, Matsuda I (1985). Two siblings with microcephaly associated with calcification of cerebral white matter. *Jpn J Hum Genet* **30**:213–217.

Jervis GA (1954). Microcephaly with extensive calcium deposits and demyelination. *J Neuropath Exp Neur* **13**:318–329.

Melchior JC, Bendon CE, Yakovlev PI (1960). Familial idiopathic cerebral calcifications in childhood. *Arch Dis Child* **99**:787–803.

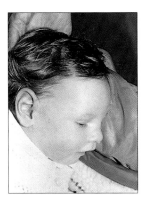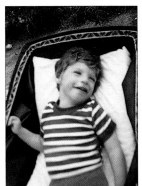

40A–40B Siblings with microcephaly.

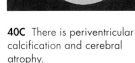

40C There is periventricular calcification and cerebral atrophy.

MICROCEPHALY–LYMPHOEDEMA   41A–41B

Crowe and Dickerman described a male and his maternal uncle who both had microcephaly and peripheral oedema. The mother of the child and her mother and maternal aunt had lymphoedema. Inheritance was assumed to be X-linked or autosomal dominant. There is an association between lymphoedema and microcephaly in the autosomal dominant syndrome described by Jarmas *et al.*, however, falciform retinal folds are also present in that syndrome.

Feingold and Bartoshesky reported two isolated boys aged 9 years and 2 years with microcephaly, lymphoedema and unusual retinal pigmentation. The elder boy was described as having areas of reticulated chorioretinal atrophy with mottled pigmentation. Atrophic yellow spots in the fundi and mild optic atrophy were also seen. The younger patient had somewhat similar findings.

Genetic aspects: Uncertain but likely to be autosomal dominant.

References

Crowe CA, Dickerman LH (1986). A genetic association between microcephaly and lymphedema. *Am J Med Genet* **24**:131–135.

Feingold M, Bartoshesky L (1992). Microcephaly, lymphedema, and chorioretinal dysplasia: a distinct syndrome? *Am J Med Genet* **43**:1030–1031.

Jarmas, AL, Weaver, DD, Ellis, FD Davis A (1981). Microcephaly, microphthalmia, falciform retinal folds, and blindness. *Am J Dis Child* **135**:930–933.

Leung AKC (1985). Dominantly inherited syndrome of microcephaly and congenital lymphedema. *Clin Genet* **27**:611–612.

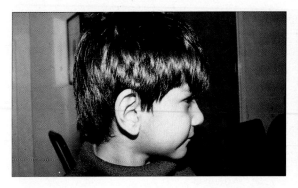
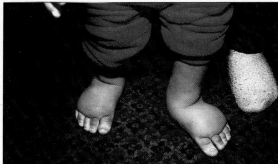

41A and 41B Note microcephaly and lymphoedema of the feet.

CUTIS VERTICIS GYRATA-MENTAL RETARDATION 42

Cutis verticis gyrata is characterised by the presence of scalp-folds and furrows, giving the scalp a corrugated appearance. It has been reported in individuals with both normal and decreased intelligence. The exact age of onset is uncertain but it is likely not to be present at birth. When mental retardation occurs it is usually severe, and may be associated with microcephaly and seizures.

Genetic aspects: Of 47 Swedish cases, 46 were males (Akesson, 1964) and consanguinity was not uncommon. However, all cases were single.

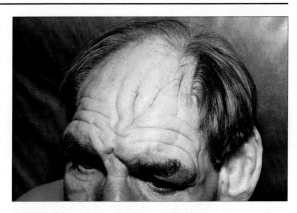

42 Note microcephaly and furrowing and folding of the scalp.

References

Akesson HO (1964). Cutis verticis gyrata and mental deficiency in Sweden. I. Epidemiological and clinical aspects. *Acta Medica Scand* **175**:115–127.

Akesson HO (1965). Cutis verticis gyrata and mental deficiency in Sweden. II. Genetic aspects. *Acta Medica Scand* **177**:459–464.

Diven DG, Tanus T, Raimer SS (1991). Cutis verticis gyrata. *Int J Dermatol* **30**:710–712.

Felding I, Feingold M (1988). Cutis verticis gyrata. *Am J Dis Child* **142**:305–306.

Rasmussen SA, Frias JL (1989). Cutis verticis gyrata: a proposed classification. *Dysmorph Clin Genet* **3**:97–102.

Schepis C, Palazzo R, Ragusa RM et al. (1989). Association of cutis verticis gyrata with fragile X syndrome and fragility of chromosome 12 (Letter). *Lancet* **2**:279.

G (OPITZ-FRIAS) SYNDROME 43A–43B

The main features are hypertelorism, hypospadias, and swallowing difficulties. The nasal bridge is flat. Other characteristic features include a laryngeal cleft, an imperforate or ectopic anus, a cleft lip and/or palate and fetal hydrops. About half the cases have delayed development, but seldom severely so, and males might be more severely affected than females. Guion-Almeida and Richieri-Costa reported a series of 12 male cases with midline CNS abnormalities, including Dandy–Walker malformation, an enlarged cisterna magna, an enlarged fourth ventricle and agenesis of the corpus callosum.

Genetic aspects: Autosomal dominant, but males are more severely affected than females.

References

Bershof JF, Guyuron B, Olsen MM (1992). G syndrome: a review of the literature and a case report. *J Craniomaxillo Surg* **20**:24–27.

Guion-Almeida ML, Richieri-Costa A (1992). CNS midline anomalies in the Opitz G/BBB syndrome: report on 12 Brazilian patients. *Am J Med Genet* **43**:918-928.

Opitz JM (1987). G syndrome (hypertelorism with oesophageal abnormality and hypospadias, or hypospadias-dysphagia, or "Opitz-Frias" or "Opitz-G" syndrome) - perspective in 1987 and bibliography. *Am J Med Genet* **28**:275–286.

Tolmie JL, Coutts N, Drainer IK (1987). Congenital anal anomalies in two families with the Opitz G syndrome. *J Med Genet* **24**:688–691.

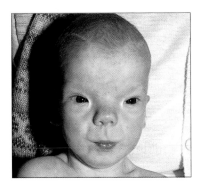 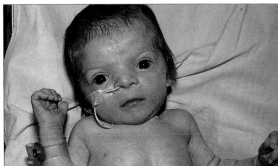

43A and 43B
Note the hypertelorism, widow's peak and broad nasal root.

FRONTONASAL DYSPLASIA

44A–44D

The main features are marked hypertelorism in conjunction with a broad nasal tip which is frequently cleft. Notching of the alae nasi might be a feature. The occurrence of a widow's peak and an occasional anterior encephalocele emphasises the midline nature of this syndrome. Other involvement of the CNS is unusual, although mental retardation and an agenesis of the corpus callosum have been described. Lipoma of the corpus callosum and a frontal encephalocele have also been reported. An anterior cranium bifidum may be detected on skull X-ray. The condition is also known as the median cleft face syndrome.

Genetic aspects: Most cases are sporadic, but there have been rare apparently dominant pedigrees (Fryburg *et al.*)

References
Bakken AF, Aabyholm G (1976). Frontonasal dysplasia. Possible hereditary connection with other congenital defects. *Clin Genet* **10**:214–217.
Fryburg JS, Persing JA, Lin KY (1993). Frontonasal dysplasia in two successive generations. *Am J Med Genet* **46**:712–714.
Grubben C, Fryns JP, de Zegher F, Van den Berghe H (1990). Anterior basal encephalocele in the median cleft face syndrome. Comments on nosology and treatment. *Genetic Counseling* **38**:103–109.
Moreno Fuenmayor H (1980). The spectrum of frontonasal dysplasia in an inbred pedigree. *Clin Genet* **17**:137–142.
Pascual-Castroviejo I *et al.* (1985). Fronto-nasal dysplasia and lipoma of the corpus callosum. *Eur J Pediatr* **144**:66–71.

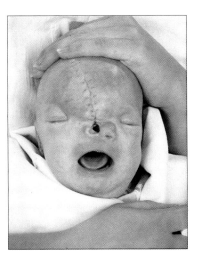

44A–44D Note hypertelorism, bifid, and broad nasal tip, with a gap where an anterior encephalocele was present in **44A**.

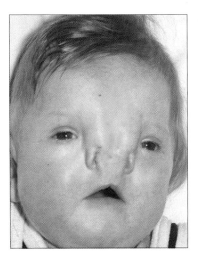

44B

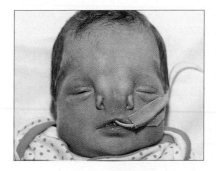

44C

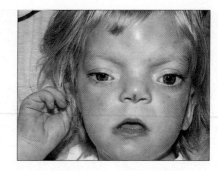

44D

CRANIOFRONTONASAL DYSPLASIA   45A–45D

This condition combines the features of frontonasal dysplasia with craniosynostosis. The clinical features are marked hypertelorism, a broad bifid nose, frontal bossing (which might be asymmetrical), a low posterior hairline with an anterior widow's peak, and occasionally a cleft lip and palate. If the palate is intact it is often high. The teeth are widely spaced and there is mal-eruption. Neck webbing, rounded shoulders, abnormal clavicles and raised scapulae are all features. In the limbs there is often longitudinal splitting of the nails, occasionally skin syndactyly, and the fingers and toes might be deviated distally. Most children have normal intelligence, although mild delay has been reported. Radiographs of the skull show premature coronal synostosis.

Genetic aspects: This is uncertain. Parent to child transmission has been shown but there is a predominance of affected females. Autosomal dominant inheritance with some sex limitation seems likely.

References

Grutzner E, Gorlin RJ (1988). Craniofrontonasal dysplasia: phenotypic expression in females and males and genetic considerations. *Oral Surg* **65**:436–444.

Kapusta L, Brunner HG, Hamel BCJ (1992). Craniofrontonasal dysplasia. *Eur J Pediatr* **151**:837–841.

Kumar D, Clark JW, Blank CE, Patton MA (1986). A family with craniofrontonasal dysplasia, and fragile site 12q13 segregating independently. *Clin Genet* **29**:530–537.

Morris CA, Palumbos JC, Carey JC (1987). Delineation of the male phenotype in craniofrontonasal syndrome. *Am J Med Genet* **27**:623–631.

Natarajan U, Baraitser M, Nicolaides K, Gosden C (1993). Craniofrontonasal dysplasia in two male siblings. *Clin Dysmorphol* **2**:360–364.

Sax CM, Flannery DB (1986). Craniofrontonasal dysplasia: clinical and genetic analysis. *Clin Genet* **29**:508–515.

Young ID (1987). Syndrome of the month: craniofrontonasal dysplasia. *J Med Genet* **24**:193–196.

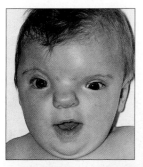

45A–45D Note the combination of frontonasal dysplasia (hypertelorism, bifid nasal tip) with craniosynostosis.

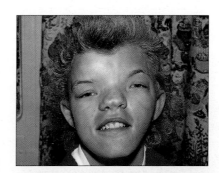

45B

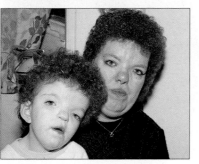

45C

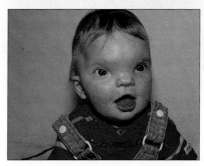

45D

HYPERTELORISM–MICROTIA–CLEFTING 46A–46B

In this condition there is hypertelorism, cleft lip and palate and malformed ears. The degree of hypertelorism is more severe than would otherwise be expected in isolated cleft lip and palate. The nasal root is broad. Both sisters reported by Bixler *et al.* (1969) had microcephaly and were mentally handicapped. They also had congenital cardiac defects, one an endocardial cushion defect, and the other an ASD. There was also a degree of hypoplasia of the thenar eminences and both had renal defects.

Genetic aspects: Possibly autosomal recessive.

References
Baraitser M (1982). The hypertelorism microtia clefting syndrome. *J Med Genet* **19**:387–388.

Bixler D, Christian JC, Gorlin RJ (1969). Hypertelorism, microtia and facial clefting: a newly descibed syndrome. *Am J Dis Child* **118**:495–500.

Bixler D, Christian JC, Gorlin RJ (1969). Hypertelorism, microtia and facial clefting: a new inherited syndrome. *BDOAS* **5**:77–81

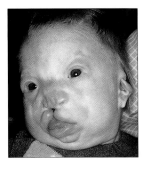
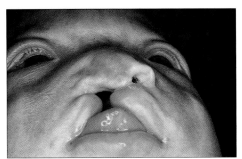

46A and 46B Note the hypertelorism, cleft lip and palate, and small malformed ears.

JOHANSON–BLIZZARD SYNDROME 47A–47F

Facially, this condition is characterised by very hypoplastic alae nasi, and there are areas of aplasia cutis congenita on the scalp. The hair grows in an unusual fashion and is often spiky and difficult to comb. The initial clinical problem may be failure to thrive due to exocrine insufficiency of the pancreas. Mental retardation is usually a feature, albeit often mild, but there have been cases with normal intelligence. Hypothyroidism, which commonly occurs, does not seem to be correlated positively with mental retardation. All children should be followed up from an audiological point of view because sensorineural hearing loss is common. Despite adequate treatment, growth is usually slow.

Genetic aspects: Autosomal recessive.

References
Gershoni-Baruch R, Lerner A, Braun J et al. (1990). Johanson-Blizzard syndrome: clinical spectrum and further delineation of the syndrome. *Am J Med Genet* **35**:546–551.

Gould NS, Paton JB, Bennett AR (1989). Johanson-Blizzard syndrome: clinical and pathological findings in two siblings. *Am J Med Genet* **33**:194–199.

Hurst JA, Baraitser M (1989). Johanson-Blizzard syndrome. *J Med Genet* **26**:45–48.

Johanson AJ, Blizzard RM (1971). A syndrome of congenital aplasia of the alae nasi, deafness, hypothyroidism, dwarfism, absent permanent teeth, and malabsorption. *J Pediatr* **79**:982–987.

Moeschler JB, Polak MJ, Jenkins JJ et al. (1987). The Johanson-Blizzard syndrome: a second report of full autopsy findings. *Am J Med Genet* **26**:133–138.

Zerres K, Holtgrave E-A (1986). The Johanson-Blizzard syndrome: report of a new case with special reference to the dentition and review of the literature. *Clin Genet* **30**:177–183.

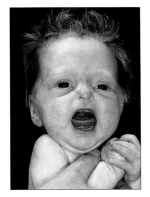

47A–47F Note the considerable hypoplastic alae nasi, and small nose. The hair is unruly with areas of aplasia cutis on the scalp.

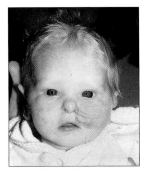
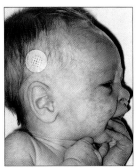

47B **47C**

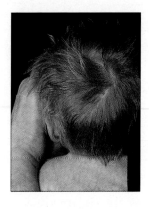

47D

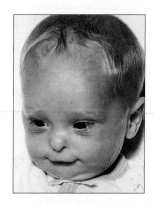

47E

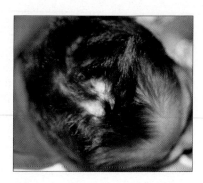

47F

VAN DER WOUDE – CLEFT LIP/PALATE; LIP PITS　　　　　　　48

About 50% of gene carriers have cleft lip or palates (one-third cleft palate alone; two-thirds cleft lip with or without cleft palate). 80% have symmetrical pits or eminences of the lower lip. These are usually situated at the vermilion border on either side of the midline. Microforms consist of verrucous eminences of the lower lip. Hypodontia is present in 10–20% of gene carriers.

The incidence of gene carriers is about 1 in 33 600. About 2% of cases of cleft lip/palate are thought to caused by Van der Woude syndrome.

Genetic aspects: Autosomal dominant. The gene maps to 1q32-41.

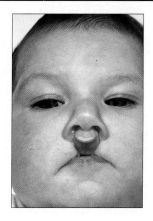

48 Note the bilateral cleft lip with lip pits on the lower lip.

References

Bocian M, Walker AP (1987). Lip pits and deletion 1q32-41. *Am J Med Genet* **26**:437–444.

Murray JC, Nishimura DY, Buetow KH *et al.* (1990). Linkage of an autosomal dominant clefting syndrome (Van der Woude) to loci on chromosome 1q. *Am J Hum Genet* **46**:486–491.

Schinzel A, Klausler M (1986). Syndrome of the month: the van der Woude syndrome (dominantly inherited lip pits and clefts). *J Med Genet* **23**:291–294.

ARTERIO–HEPATIC DYSPLASIA (ALAGILLE SYNDROME)　　　　　49

The main features of this sydrome are intrahepatic cholestasis, congenital heart disease, and skeletal and ocular anomalies. In most cases there is a paucity of intrahepatic bile ducts (occasionally extrahepatic as well) resulting in prolonged neonatal jaundice (91%), although a quarter develop jaundice later in infancy (Mueller *et al.*). The cardiac lesions (85%) are predominantly peripheral pulmonary stenosis but might include pulmonary valve stenosis, partial anomalous venous drainage or atrial and ventricular septal defects. Various degrees of anterior chamber defect (particularly posterior embryotoxon) might occur as well as a pigmentary retinopathy (88%). The skeletal changes consist of hemi or butterfly vertebrae (87%) and there may be shortening of the distal phalanges, radius or ulna. Short stature is common (50%) and there is occasional mental retardation (16%). The forehead is prominent, the eyes deep set and the nose long with a flattened tip. It has been suggested that the facial features are secondary to the prolonged effects of bile duct obstruction.

In general the liver abnormalities resolve with age although occasional cases can have more severe hepatic problems leading to early death.

Genetic aspects: Autosomal dominant families have been reported. Some cases have been shown to have a deletion of the short arm of chromosome 20.

References

Alagille D, Estrada A, Hadchouel M *et al.* (1987). Syndromic paucity of interlobular bile ducts (Alagille syndrome or arterio-hepatic dysplasia): review of 80 cases. *J Pediatr* **110**:195–200.

Dahms BB, Petrelli M, Wyllie R *et al.* (1982). Arteriohepatic dysplasia in infancy and childhood: a longitudinal study of six patients. *Hepatology* **2/3**:350–358.

Desmaze C, Deleuze JF, Dutrillaux AM *et al.* (1992). Screening of microdeletions of chromosome 20 in patients with Alagille syndrome. *J Med Genet* **29**:233–235.

Johnson BL (1990). Ocular pathologic features of arteriohepatic dysplasia (Alagille's syndrome). *Am J Ophthalmol* **110**:504–512.

Mueller RF (1987). The Alagille syndrome (arteriohepatic dysplasia). *J Med Genet* **24**:621–626.

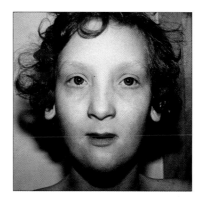

49 Note prominent forehead, deep-set eyes with up-slanting palpebral fissures, and straight nose with prominent nasal bridge.

VELO-CARDIO-FACIAL SYNDROME   50A–50B

This syndrome combines cardiac anomalies with an unusual facial appearance, cleft palate (often sub-mucous), short stature, mental retardation and long, thin, hyperextensible fingers. The face is characterised by a prominent nose with a squared-off nasal tip and notched alae nasi, micrognathia, microcephaly (sometimes), and occasionally ocular abnormalities (up-slanting palpebral fissures, microphthalmia, strabismus, cataracts, small optic discs and tortuous retinal vessels). The cardiac anomalies can include ventriculo-septal defects, pulmonary stenosis and double outlet right ventricle. Shprintzen *et al.*, (1992) reported that over 10% of their original cases had developed personality disturbance in adolescence or later evidence of chronic schizophrenia with paranoid delusions.

Genetic aspects: There is a considerable overlap with DiGeorge syndrome and the majority of patients can be shown to have 22q11 deletions at the molecular level (Driscoll *et al.*, Scambler *et al.*). Autosomal dominant pedigrees have been reported.

References

Driscoll DA, Spinner NB, Budarf ML *et al.* (1992). Deletions and microdeletions of 22q11.2 in velo-cardio-facial syndrome. *Am J Med Genet* **44**:261–268.

Goldberg R, Motzkin B, Marion R *et al.* (1993). Velo-cardio-facial syndrome: a review of 120 patients. *Am J Med Genet* **45**:313–319.

Scambler PJ, Kelly D, Lindsay E *et al.* (1992). Velo-cardio-facial syndrome associated with chromosome 22 deletions encompassing the DiGeorge locus. *Lancet* **1**:1138–1139.

Shprintzen RJ, Goldberg R, Golding-Kushner KJ, Marion RW (1992). Late-onset psychosis in the velo-cardio-facial syndrome (Letter). *Am J Med Genet* **42**:141–142.

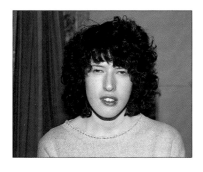 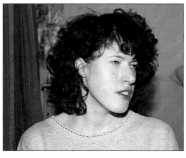

50A and 50B Note prominent nose, pinched nasal tip, short philtrum and up-slanting palpebral fissures.

FREEMAN–SHELDON SYNDROME (WHISTLING FACE SYNDROME)   51A–51C

The descriptive title for the syndromes comes from the appearance of the mouth, which is puckered with a groove below the lower lip. The nose is characterised by colobomata of the nares. The philtrum is long and the eyes are deep set. There may be a bony ridge on the forehead above the eyebrows. The other cardinal features are camptodactyly with ulnar deviation of the fingers, talipes equinovarus and severe scoliosis. Intelligence is usually normal. In general the muscles are thin and there is evidence of an underlying myopathy.

Genetic aspects: Autosomal dominant in most cases. However, there is probably a rare autosomal recessive form, which is difficult to distinguish, but which may be more severe (Dallapiccola *et al.*).

References

Dallapiccola B, Giannotti A *et al.* (1989). Autosomal recessive form of whistling face syndrome in siblings. *Am J Med Genet* **33**:542–544.

Fitzsimmons JS, Zaldua V, Chrispin AR (1984). Genetic heterogeneity in the Freeman-Sheldon syndrome: two adults with probable autosomal recessive inheritance. *J Med Genet* **21**:364–368.

Sanchez JM, Kaminker CP (1986). New evidence for genetic heterogeneity of the Freeman-Sheldon syndrome. *Am J Med Genet* **25**:507–511.

Vanek J, Janda J, Amblerova V, Losan F (1986). Freeman-Sheldon syndrome: a disorder of congenital myopathic origin? *J Med Genet* **23**:231–236.

Wettstein A, Buchinger G, Braun A (1980). A family with whistling-face-syndrome. *Hum Genet* **55**:177–189.

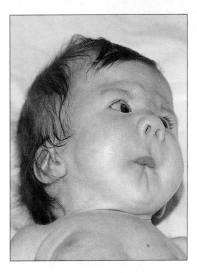

51A Note blepharophimosis, hypoplastic alae nasi, long philtrum, small mouth with puckered lips, and H-shaped depression below lower lip.

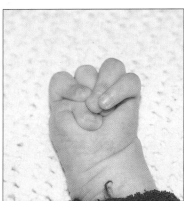

51B Note contractures with ulnar deviation of the fingers.

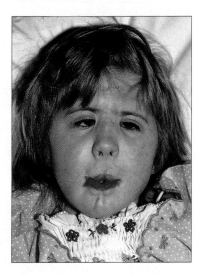

51C Same patient at a later age.

CEREBRO-COSTO-MANDIBULAR SYNDROME

The clinical appearance is of a child with severe Pierre Robin association (a very small jaw, a U-shaped cleft palate and glossoptosis). The mandible may appear almost absent. Microcephaly occurs in only 20% of cases. Radiographs reveal posterior rib gaps and missing ribs. Mental retardation occurs in about half of those who survive. Early death occurs in 40% of cases, due mainly to respiratory difficulties. Survivors are short, have epicanthic folds, and the rib gaps might heal partially and give rise to pseudoarthroses.

Genetic aspects: Affected siblings with apparently normal parents have been reported (Hennekam *et al.*, Drossou-Agakidou *et al.*). However, there is also a dominantly inherited form of cerebro-costo-mandibular syndrome which has speech delay, but a normal head circumference and a normal IQ (Leroy *et al.*, Merlob *et al.*). In general the two types cannot be distinguished clinically. In isolated cases the parents must be X-rayed.

References

Clarke EA, Nguyen VD (1985). Cerebro-costo-mandibular syndrome with consanguinity. *Pediatr Radiol* **15**:264–266.

Drossou-Agakidou V, Andreou A, Soubassi-Griva V, Pandouraki M (1991). Cerebrocostomandibular syndrome in four siblings, two pairs of twins. *J Med Genet* **28**:704–707.

Hennekam RCM, Beemer FA, Huijbers W *et al.* (1985). The cerebro-costo-mandibular syndrome: third report of familial occurrence. *Clin Genet* **28**:118–121.

Leroy JG, Devos EA, Bulcke VIJ *et al.* (1981). Cerebro-costo-mandibular syndrome with autosomal dominant inheritance. *J Pediatr* **99**:441–443.

Merlob P, Schonfeld A, Grunebaum M *et al.* (1987). Autosomal dominant cerebro-costo-mandibular syndrome: ultrasonographic and clinical findings. *Am J Med Genet* **26**:195–202.

Tachibana K, Yamamoto Y, Osaki E (1980). Cerebro-costo-mandibular syndrome - a case report and review of the literature. *Hum Genet* **54**:283–286.

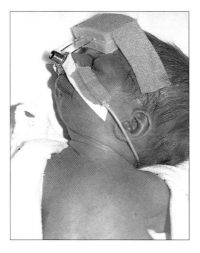
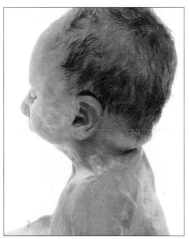
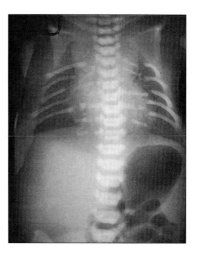

52A and 52B Note severe micrognathia.   **52B**

52C Note the rib gaps.

BRANCHIO-OCULO-FACIAL SYNDROME (HAEMANGIOMATOUS BRANCHIAL CLEFTS)   53A–53B

This unusual disorder is characterised by a pseudo-cleft of the upper lip that may look like a repaired cleft. The philtrum may be short and true clefts also occur. The nose is broad and asymmetric, there is lacrimal duct obstruction and a branchial sinus or reddened skin lesion behind the ear might be seen. The latter has been shown to represent ectopic thymic tissue. Colobomata of the iris and/or retina are common, and auricular and lip pits are also frequent. Some of those affected are short and mildly mentally retarded. Premature greying of the hair is a further unusual feature. Some cases have unilateral renal agenesis.

Genetic aspects: Autosomal dominant.

References
Fielding DW, Fryer AE (1992). Recurrence of orbital cysts in the branchio-oculo-facial syndrome. *J Med Genet* **29**:430–431.
Fujimoto A, Lipson M, Lacro RV *et al.* (1987). New autosomal dominant branchio-oculo-facial syndrome. *Am J Med Genet* **27**:943–951.
Hall BD, deLorimier A, Foster LH (1983). A new syndrome of hemangiomatous branchial clefts, lip pseudoclefts, and unusual facial appearance. *Am J Med Genet* **14**:135–138.
Lin AE, Losken HW, Jaffe R, Biglan AW (1991). The branchio-oculo-facial syndrome. *Cleft Palate-Craniofac J* **28**:96–102.

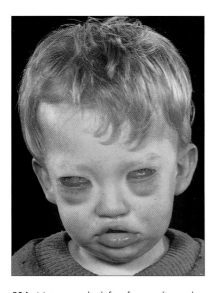
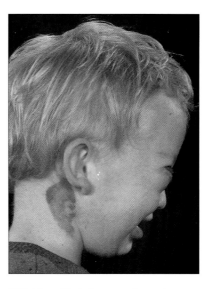

53A Note pseudoclefts of upper lip and orbital cysts.

53B Note skin lesion posterior to the ear.

BRANCHIO-OTO-RENAL (BOR) SYNDROME   54A–54D

This syndrome is characterised by hearing loss with a significant sensorineural component, structural changes to the external middle and internal ear consisting mainly of atresia of the canals, cup-shaped anteverted pinnae and occasionally severe hypoplasia of the external ear, and bilateral absence of the ossicles. Bilateral or unilateral pre-auricular pits or skin tags are found. The pre-auricular pits are characteristically found on the helix. In the neck there is a branchial cleft sinus or fistula and there might be facial asymmetry or a facial palsy. The lacrimal duct is frequently blocked. The renal abnormalities are variable. Duplication of the collecting system, megaureter due to obstruction at the uretero-pelvic junction, reflux and unilateral or bilateral renal aplasia or hypoplasia have all been described.

Genetic aspects: Autosomal dominant. Smith *et al.* and Kumar *et al.* localized the gene to proximal 8q.

References

Carli R, Binshtock M, Abeliovich D *et al.* (1983). The branchio-oto-renal syndrome: report of bilateral renal agenesis in three siblings. *Am J Med Genet* **14**:625–627.

Chitayat D, Hodgkinson KA, Chen M-F *et al.* (1992). Branchio-oto-renal syndrome: further delineation of an underdiagnosed syndrome. *Am J Med Genet* **43**:970–975.

Heimler A, Lieber E (1986). Branchio-oto-renal syndrome: reduced penetrance and variable expressivity in four generations of a large kindred. *Am J Med Genet* **5**:15–27.

Kumar S, Kimberling VVJ, Kenyon JB *et al.* (1992). Autosomal dominant branchio-oto-renal syndrome - localization of a disease gene to chromosome 8q by linkage in a Dutch family. *Hum Molec Genet* **1**:491–496.

Smith RJH, Coppage KB, Ankerstjerne JKB *et al.* (1992). Localization of the gene for branchio-oto-renal syndrome to chromosome 8q. *Genomics* **14**:841–844.

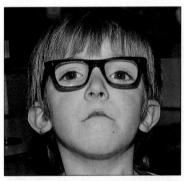
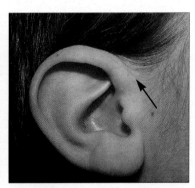

54A and 54B Note prominent, cup-shaped ears with a pit on the anterior part of the helix (arrow).

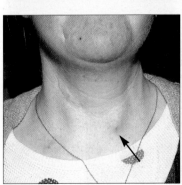
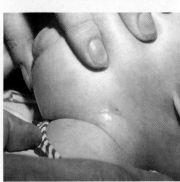

54C and 54D Note branchial cyst in mother (arrow) and branchial sinus in child.

GOLDENHAR (FACIO-AURICULO-VERTEBRAL) SYNDROME   55A–55F

This condition affects the face asymmetrically. The ears are small and malformed, often with pre-auricular ear tags in a line between the front of the ear and the side of the mouth, and there is macrostomia and failure of formation of the mandibular ramus and condyle. Cervical vertebral and cardiac anomalies are common. An epibulbar dermoid is usually insisted on as a diagnostic feature. Where this is absent, the term first and second branchial arch syndrome is perhaps preferable. Where the face is affected on only one side without an epibulbar dermoid then the term hemifacial microsomia has been used. Severe central nervous system involvement is rare but hydrocephalus, microcephalus, encephalocele and mental retardation have been described.

Genetic aspects: Most cases are sporadic. However, inheritance is uncertain – irregular dominant families have been described (Robinow *et al.*, Rollnick *et al.*).

References

Bassila MK, Goldberg R (1989). The association of facial palsy and/or sensorineural hearing loss in patients with hemifacial microsomia. *Cleft Palate J* **26**:287–291.

Cohen MM Jr, Rollnick BR, Kaye CI (1989). Oculoauriculovertebral spectrum: an updated critique. *Cleft Palate J* **26**:276–286.

Morrison PJ, Mulholland HC, Craig BG, Nevin NC (1992). Cardiovascular abnormalities in the oculo-auriculo-vertebral spectrum (Goldenhar syndrome). *Am J Med Genet* **44**:425–428.

Robinow M, Reynolds JF, Fitzgerald J et al. (1986). Hemifacial microsomia, ipsilateral facial palsy, and malformed auricle in two families: an autosomal dominant malformation. *Am J Med Genet* **Suppl.2**:129–133.

Rollnick BR, Kaye CI (1983). Hemifacial microsomia and variants: pedigree data. *Am J Med Genet* **15**:233–253.

Rollnick BR, Kaye CI, Nagatoshi K et al. (1987). Oculoauriculovertebral dysplasia and variants: phenotypic characteristics of 294 patients. *Am J Med Genet* **26**:361–376.

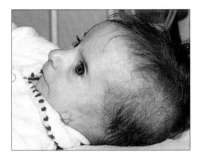

55A Note the malformed ear.

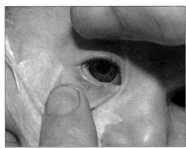

55B Subconjunctival dermoid in the same patient.

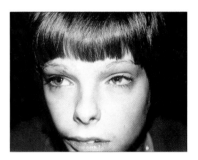

55C There is facial asymmetry and an epibulbar dermoid.

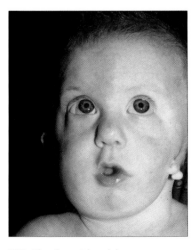

55D The dermoid and the major ear malformation can be on opposite sides.

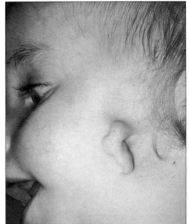

55E Note the small jaw and malformed ear.

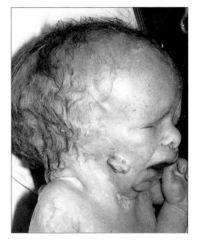

55F Hydrocephalus is an occasional feature.

TREACHER COLLINS SYNDROME (MANDIBULOFACIAL DYSOSTOSIS)   56A–56D

The main features are symmetrical facial abnormalities consisting of malformed ears, malar hypoplasia, a coloboma of the lateral part of the lower lid, mandibular hypoplasia, a cleft palate and sensorineural deafness. There can be extreme variability of expression, even within the same family.

Genetic aspects: Autosomal dominant and the gene has been mapped to 5q31-33 (Dixon *et al.*, 1991).

References

Dixon MJ, Read AP, Donnai D *et al.* (1991). The gene for Treacher Collins syndrome maps to the long arm of chromosome 5. *Am J Hum Genet* **49**:17–22.

Dixon MJ, Marres HAM, Edwards SJ *et al.* (1994). Treacher Collins syndrome: correlation between clinical and genetic linkage studies. *Clin Dysmorphol* **3**:96–103.

Kreiborg S, Dahl E (1993). Cranial base and face in mandibulofacial dysostosis. *Am J Med Genet* **47**:753–760.

Nicolaides KH, Johansson D, Donnai D *et al.* (1984). Prenatal diagnosis of mandibulofacial dysostosis. *Prenatal Diagn* **4**:201–205.

Rogers BO (1964). Berry-Treacher Collins syndrome a review of 200 cases. *Br J Plast Surg* **17**:109.

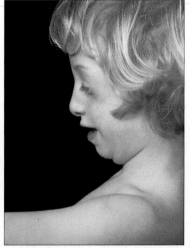

56B

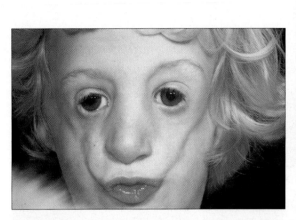

56A–56D Note the down-slanting palpebral fissures, coloboma of the lower eyelids, malar and mandibular hypoplasia and symmetrical malformation of the ear.

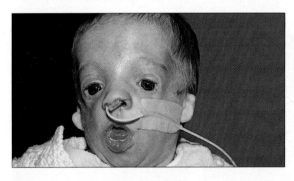

56C

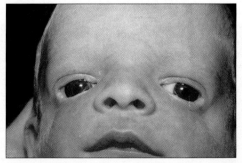

56D

SYNDROMES WITH CRANIOSYNOSTOSIS

CROUZON SYNDROME (CRANIOFACIAL DYSOSTOSIS)   57A–57D

This is one of the most common forms of the craniosynostosis syndromes. It is characterised by premature closure of the coronal sutures, and facially by mid-facial hypoplasia, proptosis secondary to shallow orbits, mild hypotelorism, a beak-shaped nose and a small jaw. Severe cases might show a clover-leaf skull.

Intelligence is usually normal. The shape of the skull is usually brachycephalic, but can be scaphocephalic depending on the order of premature closure of the sutures. Complications include optic atrophy and deafness. The other sutures, which include the sagittal and lambdoid, might also be prematurely fused.

Genetic aspects: Autosomal dominant. Preston *et al.* mapped the locus to 10q25-26 and Reardon *et al.* demonstrated mutations in the fibroblast growth factor receptor 2 (FGFR2) gene.

References

Cohen MM Jr (1986). Craniosynostosis: Diagnosis, Evaluation, and Management. New York: Raven Press.

Cohen MM Jr, Kreiborg S (1992). Birth prevalence studies of the Crouzon syndrome: comparison of direct and indirect methods. *Clin Genet* **41**:12–15.

Menashe Y, Baruch GB *et al.* (1989). Exophthalmus - prenatal ultrasonic features for diagnosis of Crouzon syndrome. *Prenatal Diagn* **9**:805–808.

Navarrete C, Pena R, Penaloza R, Salamanca F (1991). Germinal mosaicism in Crouzon syndrome. A family with three affected siblings of normal parents. *Clin Genet* **40**:29–34.

Preston RA, Post JC, Keats BJB *et al* (1994). A gene for Crouzon craniofacial dysostosis maps to the long arm of chromosome 10. *Nature Genetics* **7**:149–153.

Reardon W, Winter RM, Rutland P *et al.* (1994). Mutations in the fibroblast growth factor receptor 2 gene cause Crouzon syndrome. *Nature Genetics* **8**:98–103.

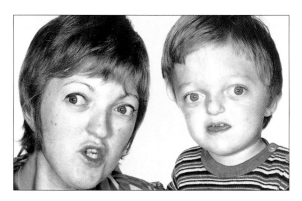

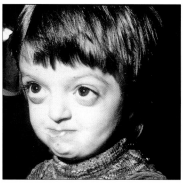

57A–57D Note the prominent forehead, proptosis, hypertelorism, hooked nose and small jaw. The young boy in school uniform is the grandfather of **57C**.

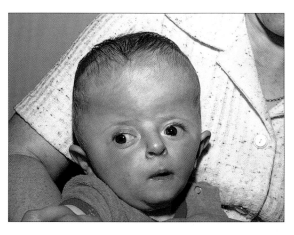

57C

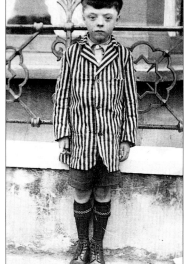

57D

APERT SYNDROME – ACROCEPHALOSYNDACTYLY TYPE I

58A–58E

Cohen *et al.* (1992) estimated that Apert syndrome has a birth prevalence of about 1 in 65 000 and accounts for 4.5% of all cases of craniosynostosis. At birth all the cranial sutures are abnormal, apart from the lambdoidal, and the head is tower-shaped, flat from front to back with a prominent forehead.

The eyes are prominent, the nose beaked and the palate high, narrow and sometimes cleft. The hands are characteristic with fusion of digits two to five and sometimes including the thumb – the so-called mitten hand. The nails on the fingers might be fused. The toes are similarly affected and pre-axial polydactyly of the feet is occasionally seen. Fusion of cervical vertebrae, usually C5–6, is present in about 70% of cases. A study by Patton *et al.* showed that about 50% of affected individuals are mentally retarded, although earlier studies had suggested a higher figure. Neuropathological studies can show polymicrogyria, hypoplastic white matter and heterotopic grey matter.

Genetic aspects: Autosomal dominant, although most cases are fresh mutations. Mutations have been demonstrated in the FGFR2 gene (Wilkie *et al.*, 1995).

References

Cohen MM Jr (1986). *Craniosynostosis: Diagnosis, Evaluation, and Management.* New York: Raven Press.

Cohen MM Jr, Kreiborg S (1990). The central nervous system in the Apert syndrome. *Am J Med Genet* **35**:36–45.

Cohen MM Jr, Kreiborg S (1991). Genetic and family study of the Apert syndrome. *J Cranio Gen Dev Bio* **11**:7–17.

Cohen MM Jr, Kreiborg S, Lammer EJ et al. (1992). Birth prevalence study of the Apert syndrome. *Am J Med Genet* **42**:655–659.

Kreiborg S, Barr M Jr, Cohen MM Jr (1992). Cervical spine in the Apert syndrome. *Am J Med Genet* **43**:704–708.

Patton MA, Goodship J et al. (1988). Intellectual development in Apert's syndrome: a long term follow-up of 29 patients. *J Med Genet* **25**:164–168.

Wilkie AOM, Slaney SF, Oldridge M et al. (1995). Apert syndrome results from localized mutations of FGFR2 and is allelic with Crouzon syndrome. *Nature Genetics* **9**:165–172.

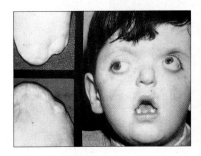
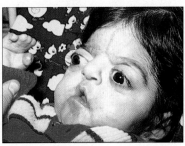
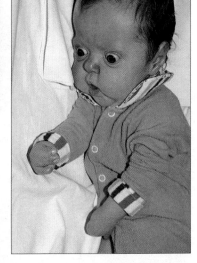

58A–58C Note the unusual head shape characterised by brachycephaly, acrocephaly, proptosis, mid-facial hypoplasia and a beaked nose.

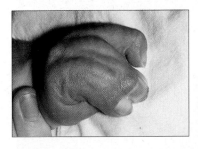
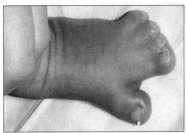

58C

58D–58E Syndactyly of fingers and toes is also characteristic.

PFEIFFER SYNDROME – ACROCEPHALOSYNDACTYLY TYPE V   59A–59H

The main features are craniostenosis, broad thumbs and great toes, and variable soft tissue syndactyly. In the feet the halluces are characteristically in the varus position. Craniostenosis usually affects the coronal sutures, but a clover-leaf skull can also be seen. The facies resemble Crouzon syndrome. Radiographs of the hands and feet reveal brachymesophalangy, broad distal phalanges, deformed proximal phalanges of the thumbs and great toes, symphalangism and a broad or duplicated first metatarsal. Cohen recognises three

subtypes. Type 1 is the classic form as reported by Pfeiffer. Type 2 has a clover-leaf skull together with ankylosis of the elbows. Type 3 is similar to type 2, but without a clover-leaf skull and with severe proptosis. Types 2 and 3 have a poor prognosis.

Genetic aspects: Autosomal dominant. Mutations in the FGFR1 gene have been demonstrated in some type 1 families (Muenke *et al.*) and in the FGFR2 gene in cases with features of the type 2 phenotype (Rutland *et al.*).

References

Cohen MM Jr. Pfeiffer syndrome update, clinical subtypes, and guidelines for differential diagnosis. *Am J Med Genet* 1993;**45**:300–307.

Martsolf JT, Cracco JB, Carpenter GG *et al*. Pfeiffer syndrome. An unusual type of acrocephalosyndactyly with broad thumbs and great toes. *Am J Dis Child* 1971;**121**:257–262.

Muenke M, Schell U, Hehr A *et al*. A common mutation in the fibroblast growth factor receptor 1 gene in Pfeiffer syndrome. *Nature Genetics* 1994;**8**:269–274.

Rutland P, Pulleyn LJ, Reardon W *et al*. Identical mutations in the FGFR2 gene cause both Pfeiffer and Crouzon syndrome phenotypes. *Nature Genetics* 1995;**9**:173–176.

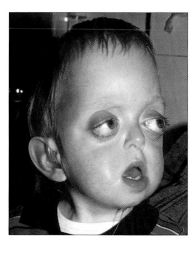
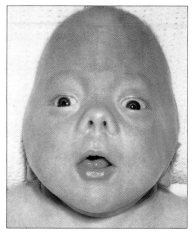
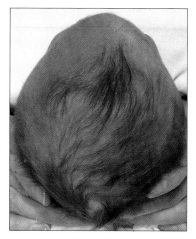

59A–59C Note the acrocephalic skull shape and prominent eyes.

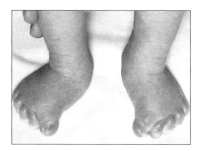

59D Note the broad, deviated great toes.

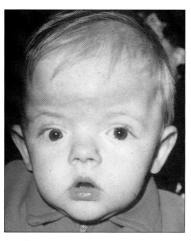

59E A child with Pfeiffer syndrome.

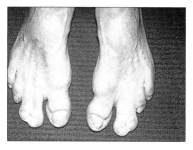

59F Feet of the affected grandfather to **59E**

59G and 59H A clover-leaf skull is not infrequently seen as part of Pfeiffer syndrome.

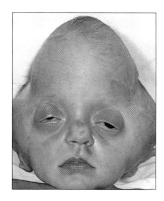
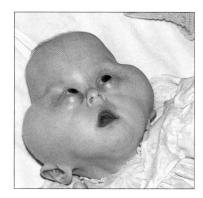

SAETHRE–CHOTZEN – ACROCEPHALOSYNDACTYLY TYPE III 60A–60I

The facies are asymmetric with brachycephaly, a broad forehead, ptosis, a beaked nose, loss of the frontonasal angle, and low-set ears with folded pinnae and prominent cruri. Parietal foramina may be present. Minor abnormalities of the hands and feet are frequent consisting of soft tissue syndactyly, mild brachydactyly, clinodactyly and hallux valgus. Craniostenosis, usually of the coronal sutures, can be demonstrated in about 90% of patients. Expression is variable.

Genetic aspects: Autosomal dominant. The gene maps to 7p21.

References
Brueton LA, van Herwerden L, Chotai KA, Winter RM (1992). The mapping of a gene for craniosynostosis: evidence for linkage of the Saethre-Chotzen syndrome to distal chromosome 7p. *J Med Genet* **29**:681–685.
Reardon W, Winter RM (1994). Syndrome of the month. Saethre-Chotzen syndrome. *J Med Genet* **31**:393–396.
Thompson EM, Baraitser M, Hayward RD (1984). Parietal foramina in Saethre-Chotzen syndrome. *J Med Genet* **21**:369–372.

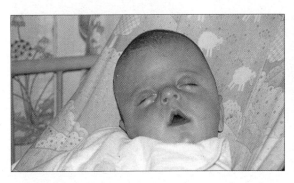 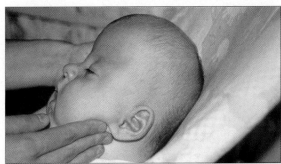

60A–60I Note the prominent forehead with facial asymmetry and ptosis. In the lateral pictures there is a reduced angle between forehead and nose and a prominent ear crus. Some patients (**60G**) have duplication of the hallux.

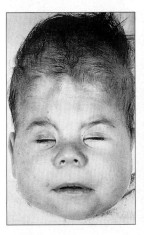 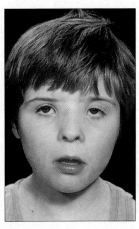 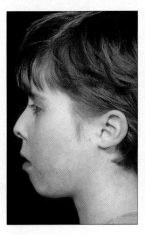 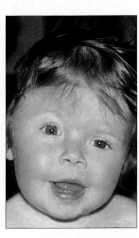

60C   60D   60E   60F

60G

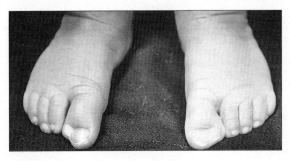

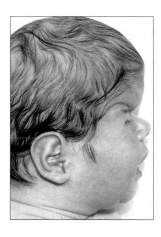

60H

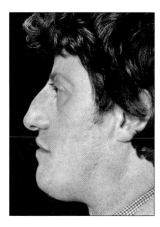

60I

TRIGONOCEPHALY, ISOLATED (AUTOSOMAL DOMINANT) 61A–61B

Isolated trigonocephaly can occasionally be inherited as an autosomal dominant condition.
Genetic aspects: Autosomal dominant in some families.

References
Frydman M, Kauschansky A, Elian E (1984). Trigonocephaly: a new familial syndrome. *Am J Med Genet* **18**:55–59.
Hennekam RCM, Van Den Boogaard M-J (1990). Autosomal dominant craniosynostosis of the sutura metopica. *Clin Genet* **38**:374–377.
Oi S, Matsumoto S (1987). Trigonocephaly (metopic synostosis). Clinical, surgical and anatomical concepts. *Child's Nerv Syst* **3**:259–265.

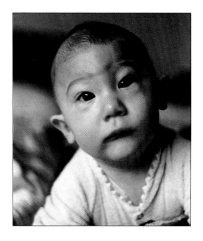

61A and 61B Note the prominent metopic ridge and the triangular shape of the skull.

BALLER–GEROLD SYNDROME 62A–62C

Individuals with this syndrome have coronal craniosynostosis and radial defects. The thumb can be absent and the ulna is usually short and curved. The ears are hypoplastic and malformed. Occasional findings include hypertelorism, epicanthic folds, a prominent nasal bridge, midline capillary haemangiomas, anal atresia and mental retardation. Short stature has been frequently observed. The differential diagnosis includes Roberts syndrome and 'premature chromosome separation' should be looked for (Huson *et al.*).
Genetic aspects: Autosomal recessive.

References

Boudreaux JM, Colon MA, Lorusso GD *et al.* (1990). Baller-Gerold syndrome: an eleventh case of craniosynostosis and radial aplasia. *Am J Med Genet* **37**:447–450.

Huson SM, Rodgers CS, Hall CM, Winter RM (1990). The Baller-Gerold syndrome: phenotypic and cytogenetic overlap with Roberts syndrome. *J Med Genet* **27**:371–375.

Lin AE, McPherson E, Nwokoro NA *et al.* (1993). Further delineation of the Baller-Gerold syndrome. *Am J Med Genet* **45**:519–524.

Van Maldergem L, Verloes A, Lejeune L, Gillerot Y (1992). The Baller-Gerold syndrome. *J Med Genet* **29**:266–268.

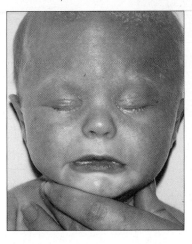

62A Note unusual head shape due to craniosynostosis.

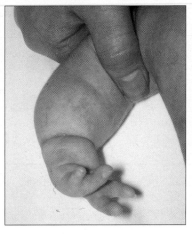

62B Note absent thumb and shortened forearm.

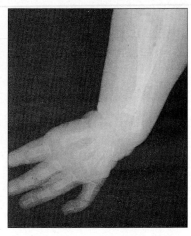

62C Note short dislocated radius and absent thumb.

GREIG CEPHALOPOLYSYNDACTYLY

63A–63F

In this syndrome there is the association of pre- and post-axial polydactyly with subtle craniofacial abnormalities. There is a high forehead with frontal bossing, macrocephaly, hypertelorism and a broad base to the nose. In the hands post-axial polydactyly is more common than pre-axial polydactyly, but both occur. The thumbs are often broad and the post-axial polydactyly is usually a post-minimus. The thumbnail may be bifid, as may the terminal phalanx. In the feet the hallux is very often duplicated with syndactyly of toes one, two and three, and post-axial polydactyly is less common. A few cases have had mild communicating hydrocephalus or craniosynostosis.

Genetic aspects: Autosomal dominant. The gene maps to 7p13. Interruption of the GLI3 gene has been demonstrated in two cases involving apparently balanced translocations.

References

Baraitser M, Winter RM, Brett EM (1983). Greig cephalopolysyndactyly: report of 13 affected individuals in three families. *Clin Genet* **24**:257–265.

Brueton L, Huson SM, Winter RM, Williamson R (1988). Chromosomal localisation of a developmental gene in man: direct DNA analysis demonstrates that Greig cephalopolysyndactyly maps to 7p13. *Am J Med Genet* **31**:799–804.

Gollop TR, Fontes LR (1985). The Greig cephalopolysyndactyly syndrome: report of a family and review of the literature. *Am J Med Genet* **22**:59–68.

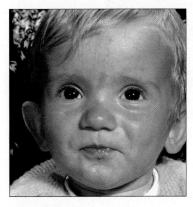

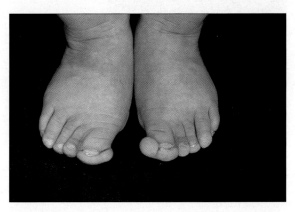

63A–63F Note broad forehead, post-axial polydactyly in the hands (post-minimus), pre-axial polydactyly in the feet (occasional post-axial polydactyly also occurs in the feet).

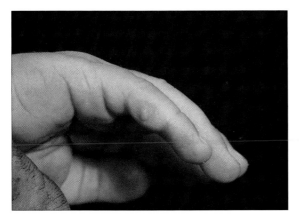

63C

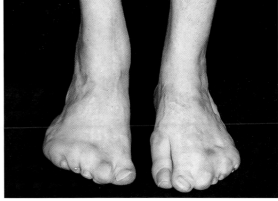

63D

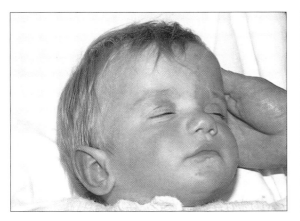

63E

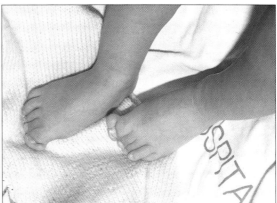

63F

CARPENTER SYNDROME – ACROCEPHALOPOLYSYNDACTYLY TYPE II 64A–64B

In this form of craniosynostosis polydactyly is common. The facial features consist of a high forehead, mid-facial hypoplasia giving a flat facial profile, bilateral ptosis, epicanthic folds, anteverted nostrils and occasionally proptosis. In the hands there is brachydactyly, soft tissue syndactyly and occasional post-axial polydactyly. Radiographs reveal aplasia or hypoplasia of the middle phalanges and two ossification centres of the proximal phalanx of the thumb. In the feet the most characteristic abnormality is pre-axial polydactyly. Other features include obesity, and dental problems arising because of the high, narrow palate. Occasionally, a mixed hearing loss can occur. Mental deficiency is not always present and IQs have ranged from 60 to 104 (Frias *et al.*).
Genetic aspects: Autosomal recessive.

References
Carpenter G (1909). Case of acrocephaly with other congenital malformations. *Proc R Soc Med* **2**:45–53, 199–201.
Cohen DM, Greem JG, Miller J et al. (1987). Acrocephalopolysyndactyly type II - Carpenter syndrome: clinical spectrum and an attempt at unification with Goodman and Summit syndromes. *Am J Med Genet* **28**:311–324.
Der Kaloustian VM, Sinno AA, Nassar SI (1972). Acrocephalopolysyndactyly type II (Carpenter syndrome). *Am J Dis Child* **124**:716–718.
Frias JL, Felman AH, Rosenbloom AL et al. (1978). Normal intelligence in two children with Carpenter syndrome. *Am J Med Genet* **2**:191–199.
Jamil MN, Bannister CM, Ward G (1992). Carpenter's syndrome (acrocephalopolysyndactyly type II) with normal intelligence. *Br J Neurosurg* **6**:243–247.
Robinson LK, James HE, Mubarak SJ et al. (1985). Carpenter syndrome: natural history and clinical spectrum. *Am J Med Genet* **20**:461–469.

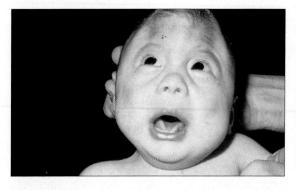

64A Note the facial dysmorphism due to craniosynostosis.

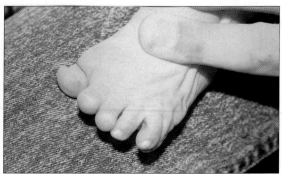

64B Note pre-axial polydactyly and acrocephaly.

BEARE–STEVENSON SYNDROME 65A–65E

This is a distinctive dysmorphic syndrome recognisable at birth by the presence of cutis gyrata involving the scalp, face, ears, lips and limbs. In addition, there is acanthosis nigricans of the skin, prominent eyes, acrocephaly, choanal atresia, a cleft palate or cleft uvula, and umbilical protrusion. Craniosynostosis is common and three cases have had a cloverleaf skull. In one of the patients there was a reflection of the skin for a considerable distance onto the umbilical stump. In males the scrotum may be bifid.

Genetic aspects: All cases have been isolated and there is a possible paternal age effect.

References

Beare JM, Dodge JA, Nevin NC (1969). Cutis gyratum, acanthosis nigricans and other congenital anomalies: a new syndrome. *Br J Dermatol* **81**:241–247.

Hall BD, Cadle RG, Golabi M et al. (1992). Beare-Stevenson cutis gyrata syndrome. *Am J Med Genet* **44**:82–89.

Stevenson RE, Ferlauto GJ, Taylor HA (1978). Cutis gyratum and acanthosis nigricans associated with other anomalies: a distinctive syndrome. *J Pediatr* **92**:950–952.

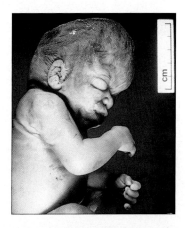
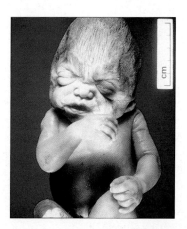
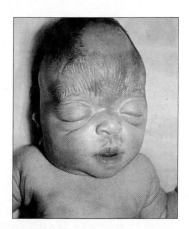

65A–65C Note tall skull, cutis gyratum of forehead, protruding eyes, mid-facial hypoplasia and flat nasal bridge.

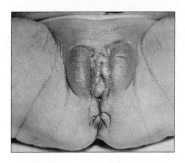

65D Anterior separation of the labia majora.

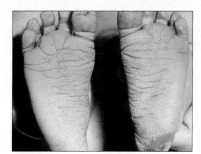

65E Deep furrows on the soles of the feet.

SYNDROMES DIAGNOSED THROUGH EYE ABNORMALITIES

KIVLIN SYNDROME 66

Vision is impaired by a sclerocornea, which is characterised by extension of opaque scleral tissue and fine vascular arcades into the peripheral cornea. If Peters' anomaly is present, the opacity tends to be more central and is associated with irido-corneal adhesions. The face is round with a long philtrum, a short nose and a long cupid's bow mouth. The eyes seem widely spaced and the forehead is prominent. In the limbs there is rhizomelic shortening, although in some reports the mesomelic and acromelic elements seem to be especially involved. Hypotonia, joint hyperextensibility, congenital heart defects, renal abnormalities, hypospadias, and cryptorchidism, are additional features in some cases. Mental retardation in some is part of the spectrum. The cases described by Van Schooneveld *et al.*, may well have had the same condition.

Genetic aspects: Autosomal recessive.

References

Frydman M, Weinstock AL, Cohen HA *et al.* (1991). Autosomal recessive Peters anomaly, typical facial appearance, failure to thrive, hydrocephalus, and other anomalies: further delineation of the Krause-Kivlin syndrome. *Am J Med Genet* **40**:34–40.
Hennekam RCM, Van Schooneveld MJ, Ardinger HH *et al.* (1993). The Peters'-Plus syndrome: description of 16 patients and review of the literature. *Clin Dysmorphol* **2**:283–300.
Kivlin JD, Fineman RM, Crandall AS *et al.* (1986). Peters' anomaly as a consequence of genetic and nongenetic syndromes. *Arch Ophthalmol* **104**:61–64.
Thompson EM, Winter RM, Baraitser M (1993). Kivlin syndrome and Peters'-Plus syndrome: are they the same disorder? *Clin Dysmorphol* **2**:301–316.
Van Schooneveld MJ, Delleman JW *et al.* (1984). Peters'-plus: a new syndrome. *Ophthal Paed Genet* **4**:141–146.

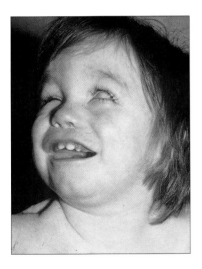

66 Note the sclerocornea, wide mouth and thin upper lip.

FRASER–CRYPTOPHTHALMOS SYNDROME 67A–67F

The main features are cryptophthalmos (covering of the globe by fused palpebral fissures), syndactyly and abnormal genitalia. The cryptophthalmos might be bilateral or unilateral, or in some cases may not be present at all. It is frequently accompanied by an absence of eyebrows and eyelashes and a tongue of hair can extend from the anterior hairline to the outer margin of the orbit. The nose is broad, with a flat bridge, and may have a groove at the tip or a coloboma of the nares. The external ear may be malformed or low-set. Stenosis of the external auditory meatus should be sought. Laryngeal stenosis, renal agenesis, and genital abnormalities (hypospadias, clitoromegaly) are common. The syndactyly is cutaneous and involves variable digits without a fixed pattern. Mental retardation occurs in 80% of survivors.

Genetic aspects: Autosomal recessive.

References

Boyd PA, Keeling JW, Lindenbaum RH (1988). Fraser syndrome (cryptophthalmos-syndactyly syndrome): a review of eleven cases with postmortem findings. *Am J Med Genet* **31**:159–168.

Koenig R, Spranger J (1986). Cryptophthalmos-syndactyly syndrome without cryptophthalmos. *Clin Genet* **29**:413–416.

Schauer GM, Dunn LK, Godmilow L *et al.* (1990). Prenatal diagnosis of Fraser syndrome at 18.5 weeks gestation, with autopsy findings at 19 weeks. *Am J Med Genet* **37**:583–591.

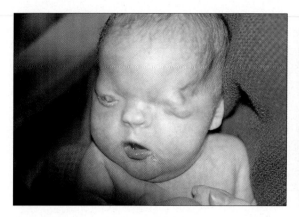 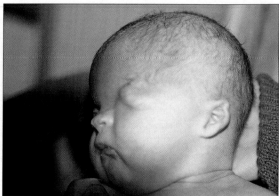

67A and 67B Note the covered eyes and the reflection of the hair onto the upper eyelid.

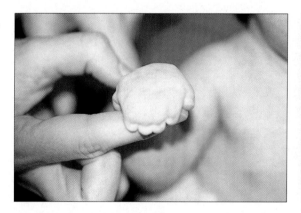

67C Cutaneous syndactyly in the same patient.

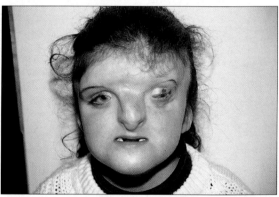

67D Another patient post-operatively. Note the unusual shape to the nose and broad nasal bridge.

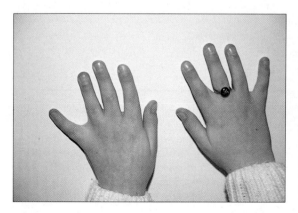

67E Cutaneous syndactyly in the previous patient.

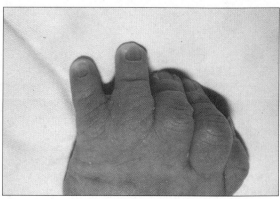

67F Similar features in a further case.

FRONTO-FACIO-NASAL DYSPLASIA 68A–68B

There are severe facial abnormalities in this condition. There is hypertelorism, a widow's peak, cranium bifidum occultum, a bifid nose and a cleft lip and palate. The nasal alae are hypoplastic or cleft and there is often mid-facial hypoplasia. There are often eyelid colobomas, S-shaped palpebral fissures, and a limbic dermoid of the eye. Other ocular features include small eyes, iris colobomas and cataracts. A frontally situated lipoma, causing a swelling at the nasion, was reported in one patient and an encephalocele has been described. Reardon et al. provide a good review.

Genetic aspects: Autosomal recessive.

References

Gollop TR (1981). Fronto-facio-nasal dysostosis - a new autosomal recessive syndrome (Letter). *Am J Med Genet* **10**:409–412.
Reardon W, Winter RM, Taylor D, Baraitser M (1994). Frontofacionasal dysplasia: a new case and review of the phenotype. *Clin Dysmorphol* **3**:70–74.

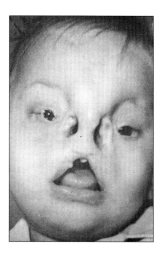
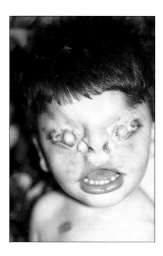

68A and 68B Note clefting of upper lip, severe deficiency of the alae nasi and severely disorganised development of the globes.

ANOPHTHALMIA (AUTOSOMAL RECESSIVE) 69A–69B

Clinically, it may be difficult to distinguish between severe microphthalmos and anophthalmos. Although there is an association with many syndromes, isolated anophthalmos can occur without other apparent abnormalities.

Genetic aspects: Many cases are autosomal recessive.

References

da Silva EO, De Sousa SS (1981). Clinical anophthalmia. *Hum Genet* **57**:115–116.
Kohn G, El Shawwa R, El Rayyes E (1988). Isolated "clinical anophthalmia" in an extensively affected Arab kindred. *Clin Genet* **33**:321–324.
Pearce WG, Nigam S, Rootman J (1974). Primary anophthalmos: histological and genetic features. *Can J Ophthalmol* **9**:141–145.

69A and 69B The eyes are absent.

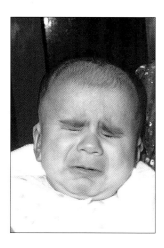
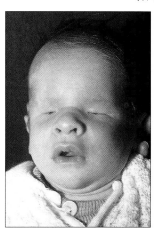

RIEGER SYNDROME

Rieger syndrome consists of Rieger anomaly associated with hypodontia, peg-shaped teeth, mid-face hypoplasia, a short philtrum and relative prognathism. The peri-umbilical skin may be redundant and anal stenosis and Meckel diverticulum have been reported. Mental retardation is rarely present. Rieger anomaly is a consequence of abnormal cleavage of the anterior chamber. This results in iris hypoplasia, and strands running from the iris to the posterior surface of the cornea (synechiae). Posterior embryotoxon is usually present and glaucoma may be a complication.

Genetic aspects: Autosomal dominant. The locus may be at 4q25 or 4q27 (see review by Vaux et al.).

References

Motegi T, Nakamura K, Terakawa T *et al.* (1988). Deletion of a single chromosome band 4q26 in a malformed girl: exclusion of Rieger syndrome associated gene(s) from the 4q26 segment. *J Med Genet* **25**:628–630.

Tewari S, Govila CP, Garg AP (1991). Rieger's syndrome. *J Oral Pathol Med* **20**.514–515.

Vaux C, Sheffield L, Keith CG, Voullaire L (1992). Evidence that Rieger syndrome maps to 4q25 or 4q27. *J Med Genet* **29**:256–258.

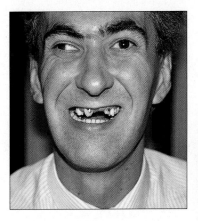

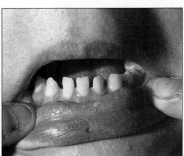

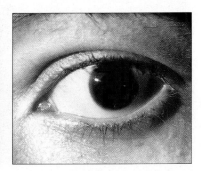

70A Note the hypodontia.

70B Note hypoplastic and missing teeth.

70C Note the iris dysplasia.

NORRIE DISEASE

The main features are a pseudoglioma of the eyes which progresses to phthisis bulbi with opaque corneae and cataract, mental retardation (severe in one-third, mild in a further third, normal intelligence in the remainder), and sensorineural deafness in one-third. The clinical features can be quite variable.

Genetic aspects: X-linked recessive. The locus is situated on the proximal short arm of the X chromosome. Berger *et al.* and Chen *et al.* reported the cloning of a candidate gene.

References

Berger W, van de Pol D, Warburg M *et al.* (1992). Mutations in the candidate gene for Norrie disease. *Hum Molec Genet* **1**:461–466.

Chen Z-Y, Hendriks RW, Jobling MA *et al.* (1992). Isolation and characterization of a candidate gene for Norrie disease. *Nature Genetics* **1**:204–208.

Goodyear HM, Sonksen PM, McConachie H (1989). Norrie's disease: a prospective study of development. *Arch Dis Child* **64**:1587–1592.

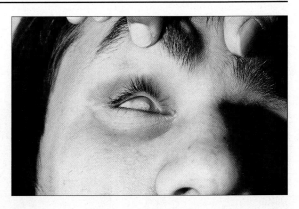

71 Note the small shrunken eye.

MEGALOCORNEA – SKELETAL ABNORMALITIES 72A–72B

In this syndrome there is megalocornea and multiple skeletal anomalies. All growth parameters are below the third centile. The head is brachycephalic with a prominent forehead and a frontal cowlick. There is hypertelorism, a saddle nose and micrognathia. There are mild flexion deformities of the fingers, talipes equinovarus and kyphoscoliosis. Developmental delay is part of the clinical picture.

Genetic aspects: Uncertain. Megalocornea alone can be inherited as either an X-linked recessive, autosomal dominant or recessive condition but those with skeletal abnormalities have been to date sporadic. Frank *et al.* reported a child who was the offspring of Arab first cousins.

References

Chen JD, Mackey D, Fuller H *et al.* (1989). X-linked megalocornea: close linkage to DXS87 and DXS94. *Hum Genet* **83**:292–294.

Frank Y, Ziprkowski M, Romano A *et al.* (1973). Megalocornea associated with multiple skeletal anomalies: a new genetic syndrome. *J Genet Hum* **21**:67–72.

Neuhauser G, Kaveggia EG, France TD, *et al.* (1975). Syndrome of mental retardation, seizures, hypotonic cerebral palsy and megalocorneae, recessively inherited. *Z Kinderheilkd* **120**:1–18.

Temtamy SA, Abdel-Hamid J, Hussein F *et al.* (1991). Megalocornea mental retardation syndrome (MMR): delineation of a new entity (MMR-2) (Abstract). *Am J Hum Genet* **49(Suppl.)**:125.

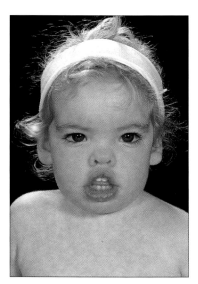 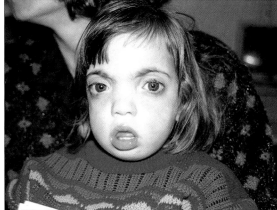

72A and 72B
Note the bossed forehead, bushy eyebrows, large eyes with megalocornea, a flat nasal bridge with a broad, slightly grooved nasal tip, and carp-shaped mouth with prominent lips.

LENZ MICROPHTHALMIA 73A–73B

Affected individuals have mild to severe microphthalmos, with colobomas in about 75% of cases. Other ocular features include blepharoptosis (75%), epicanthic folds, short palpebral fissures, lens subluxation and retinal detachment. Ear abnormalities include simple helices and antihelices, and protruding lobes. Orofacial abnormalities include cleft lip/palate (33%) and crowded or wide-spaced teeth (67%). The shoulders may be sloping due to hypoplasia of the lateral third of the clavicles, the chest may be barrel-shaped and there may be kyphoscoliosis or a gibbus. Digital abnormalities include syndactyly, clinodactyly, camptodactyly and duplication of the thumbs. All cases have mental retardation.

Genetic aspects: X-linked recessive.

References

Baraitser M, Winter RM, Taylor DSI (1982). Lenz microphthalmia - a case report. *Clin Genet* **22**:99–101.

Goldberg MF, McKusick VA (1971). X-linked colobomatous microphthalmos and other congenital anomalies. A disorder resembling Lenz's dysmorphogenetic syndrome. *Am J Ophthalmol* **71**:1128–1133.

Pallota R (1983). The Lenz microphthalmia syndrome: a case report. *Ophthal Paed Genet* **3**:103.

Traboulsi EI, Lenz W *et al.* (1988). The Lenz microphthalmia syndrome. *Am J Ophthalmol* **105**:40–45.

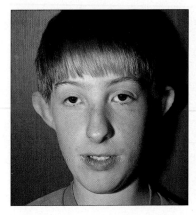
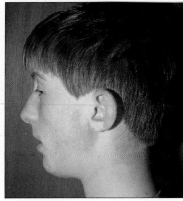

73A and 73B Note the small eyes and prominent ears. This boy has mild learning difficulties.

NANCE–HORAN – MESIODENS; CATARACT 74A–74D

This form of X-linked cataract is associated with characteristic tooth abnormalities. The latter consist of supernumerary incisors (mesiodens), anteverted pinnae and shortened metacarpals in males. Carrier females can have posterior sutural lens opacities, shaped like an inverted 'Y'. Obligate carriers have wide-spaced teeth that are either cone-shaped, or shaped like the blade of a screwdriver. A small proportion of affected males are mentally retarded.
Genetic aspects: X-linked. The gene has been mapped to Xp22 (Lewis *et al.*, Zhu *et al.*).

References
Bixler D, Higgins M, Hartsfield J Jr (1984). The Nance-Horan syndrome: a rare X-linked ocular-dental trait with expression in heterozygous females. *Clin Genet* **26**:30–35.
Lewis RA, Nussbaum RL, Stambolian D (1990). Mapping X-linked ophthalmic diseases: IV. Provisional assignment of the locus for X-linked congenital cataracts and microcornea (the Nance-Horan syndrome) to Xp22.2-p22.3. *Ophthalmology* **97**:110–121.
Walpole IR, Hockey A, Nicoll A (1990). Syndrome of the month. The Nance-Horan syndrome. *J Med Genet* **27**:632–634.

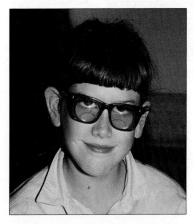

74A Note the patient in this slide is wearing glasses post cataract removal.

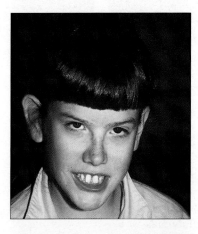

74B–74D Note the screwdriver-shaped incisors.

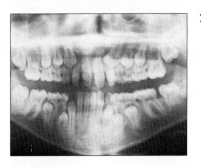

74C

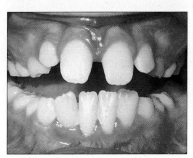

74D

SYNDROMES WITH CRANIOFACIAL AND LIMB ABNORMALITIES

NAGER ACROFACIAL DYSOSTOSIS   75A–75D

The facial defects resemble those seen in Treacher Collins syndrome and include down-slanting palpebral fissures, malar and mandibular hypoplasia and small, malformed or low-set ears. The thumbs may be absent or hypoplastic and there may be hypoplasia of the radius with radioulnar synostosis. Some cases have been reported with more severe limb defects and facial clefts.

Genetic aspects: There is evidence for both autosomal dominant and recessive inheritance in different families. In general, those with a severe phenotype (especially severe limb defects and facial clefts) are more likely to be recessive.

References
Aylsworth AS, Lin AE, Friedman PA (1991). Nager acrofacial dysostosis: male-to-male transmission in two families. *Am J Med Genet* **41**:83–88.

Chemke J, Mogilner BM *et al.* (1988). Autosomal recessive inheritance of Nager acrofacial dysostosis. *J Med Genet* **25**:230–232.

Hall BD (1989). Nager acrofacial dysostosis: autosomal dominant inheritance in mild to moderately affected mother and lethally affected phocomelic son. *Am J Med Genet* **33**:394–397.

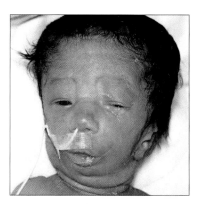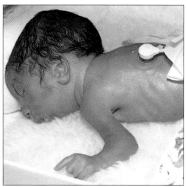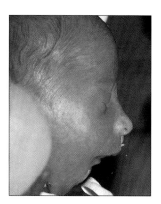

75A–75C Note the small jaw, malar hypoplasia (Treacher Collins-like appearance). **75C**

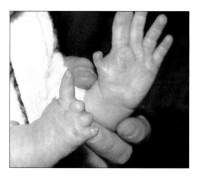

75D Note small thumbs and digital anomalies.

ACROFACIAL DYSOSTOSIS WITH POST-AXIAL DEFECTS (MILLER SYNDROME)   76A–76C

This condition must be differentiated from Treacher Collins and Nager syndromes. Similar features to Treacher Collins syndrome include malar hypoplasia, a small jaw, a cleft lip and/or palate, prominent eyes with down-slanting palpebral fissures and an ectro- pion. However, the face is usually more rounded, with a small jaw and cupped ears. There may be colobomata of the eyelids (supra- or infra-orbital). The limb defects consist of an absence or incomplete development of the fifth digital ray of all four limbs, and, frequently, forearm abnormalities (the ulna and radius can be short with occasional radioulnar synostosis). Intelligence is usually normal.

Genetic aspects: Apparently autosomal recessive pedigrees have been described (Fineman *et al.*, Giannotti *et al*)., but Robinow *et al.* and Robinow and Chen reported a mother and son with features of the condition.

References

Donnai D, Hughes HE, Winter RM (1987). Postaxial acrofacial dysostosis (Miller) syndrome. *J Med Genet* **24**:422–425.

Fineman RM (1981). Recurrence of the post-axial acrofacial dysostosis syndrome in a siblingship: implications for genetic counselling. *J Pediatr* **98**:87–88.

Giannotti A, Digilio MC, Virgili Q et al. (1992). Familial post-axial acrofacial dysostosis syndrome. *J Med Genet* **29**:752.

Ogilvy-Stuart AL, Parsons AC (1991). Miller syndrome (post-axial acrofacial dysostosis): further evidence for autosomal recessive inheritance and expansion of the phenotype. *J Med Genet* **28**:695–700.

Robinow M, Johnson GF, Apesos J (1986). Robin sequence and oligodactyly in mother and son. *Am J Med Genet* **25**:293–297.

Robinow M, Chen H (1990). Genee-Wiedemann syndrome in a family (Letter). *Am J Med Genet* **37**:293.

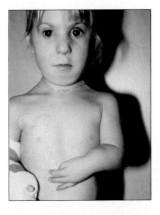

76A Note ulnar ray deficiency.

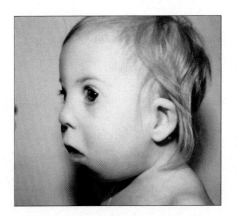

76B Note small jaw, ectropion and malar hypoplasia.

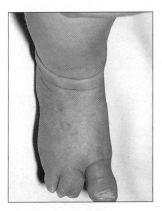

76C Deficiency of lateral ray digits and syndactyly of toes.

ACROFACIAL DYSOSTOSIS WITH SEVERE LIMB DEFECTS 77

There is a severe form of acrofacial dysostosis with post-axial defects. Rodriguez and Palacios described a stillborn female with maxillary, malar and mandibular hypoplasia, low-set, malformed ears and a coloboma of the left lower lid. The tongue was bilobed and there was a cleft of the soft palate. There was bilateral syndactyly of the fourth and fifth fingers, synostosis of the fourth and fifth metacarpals and absent ulnae. The scapulae were hypoplastic with absence of the lower half. The clavicles were broad and short. There was humero-radial synostosis. The femurs were hypoplastic and fused to the tibiae and the fibulae were separated into proximal and distal parts. The fourth and fifth toes were fused. There were hemivertebrae in the sacrum and absent ischial and pubic bones. Poissonnier et al. described a similar case. Stephan reported an even more severely affected case.

Genetic aspects: Autosomal recessive.

References

Poissonnier M et al. (1983). Lethal mandibulofacial and ulno-fibular dysostosis. *Ann Pediatr (Paris)* **30**:713–717.

Rodriguez JI, Palacios J (1990). Severe post-axial acrofacial dysostosis: an anatomic and angiographic study. *Am J Med Genet* **35**:490–492.

Stephan MJ (1990). Autosomal recessive form of mandibular dysostosis (Letter). *Am J Med Genet* **35**:493–495.

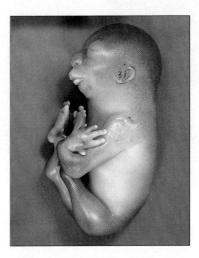

77 Note small jaw and severe limb defects.

ADAMS–OLIVER – SCALP DEFECTS; TERMINAL TRANSVERSE DEFECTS 78A–78D

In this syndrome terminal transverse limb defects are associated with aplasia cutis of the scalp ('scalp defects'). Occasionally, the scalp defects can be extensive, affecting the cranial vault and underlying vessels and leading to life-threatening haemorrhage. Chitayat *et al.* reported a case with acrania. At other times the scalp lesions are subtle and need to be looked for. The limb defects usually consist of terminal reductions of the fingers and toes, although most affected individuals have relatively minor limb defects.

Congenital heart defects may be part of the condition. There might be evidence of vascular lesions elsewhere, i.e. cutis marmorata telangiectasia or intracranial vascular anomalies.

Genetic aspects: Autosomal dominant inheritance is found in most families.

References

Bork K, Pfeifle J (1992). Multifocal aplasia cutis congenita, distal limb hemimelia, and cutis marmorata telangiectatica in a patient with Adams-Oliver syndrome. *Br J Dermatol* **127**:160–163.

Chitayat D, Meunier C, Hodgkinson KA *et al.* (1992). Acrania: a manifestation of the Adams-Oliver syndrome. *Am J Med Genet* **44**:562–566.

Fryns JP (1987). Syndrome of the month: congenital scalp defects with distal limb reduction anomalies. *J Med Genet* **24**:493–496.

Kuster W, Lenz W *et al.* (1988). Congenital scalp defects with distal limb anomalies (Adams-Oliver syndrome): report of ten cases and review of the literature. *Am J Med Genet* **31**:99–116.

Whitley CB, Gorlin RJ (1991). Adams-Oliver syndrome revisited. *Am J Med Genet* **40**:319–326.

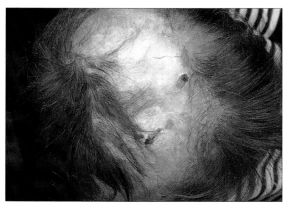 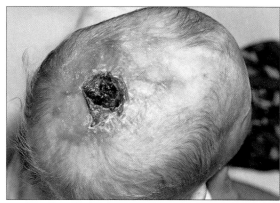

78A and 78B Note aplasia cutis congenita.   **78B**

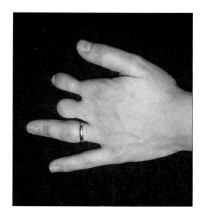 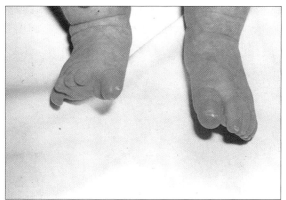

78C and 78D Note terminal transverse deficiency of the fingers and toes.

DEAFNESS-ONYCHODYSTROPHY-ONYCHOLYSIS-RETARDATION (DOOR SYNDROME) 79A–79C

The features of this condition are contained in the acronym, 'DOOR'. This stands for Deafness-Onycho-dystrophy-Onycholysis-Retardation.

Sometimes this is expanded to DOORS where 'S' is for seizures. The diagnosis is suggested by looking at the hands and feet. The great toes and thumbs are long, and often have three segments (triphalangy), while the other fingers and toes are short due to an absent or hypoplastic distal phalanx. The nails are absent or poorly formed. The facial features contribute to the diagnosis, especially bilateral ptosis, a short broad nose, a broad nasal tip and large nostrils. In severe cases, where seizures begin in the neonatal period, the prognosis is poor and status epilepticus can be a problem. In these cases the deafness can often be identified only on brain-stem evoked responses. Patton *et al.* noted elevated plasma and urinary 2-oxoglutarate in three unrelated patients. Other patients have been less severely affected.

Genetic aspects: Autosomal recessive. Note that there may also be an autosomal dominant condition with deafness and similar hand abnormalities, but without seizures or retardation.

References

Cantwell RJ (1975). Congenital sensori-neural deafness associated with onycho-osteo dystrophy and mental retardation. *Humangenetik* **26**:261–265.

Eronen M, Somer M, Gustafsson B, Holmberg C (1985). New syndrome: a digito-reno-cerebral syndrome. *Am J Med Genet* **22**:281–285.

Nevin NC, Thomas PS, Calvert J et al. (1982). Deafness, onycho-osteodystrophy, mental retardation (DOOR) syndrome. *Am J Med Genet* **13**:325–332.

Patton MA, Krywawych S, Winter RM et al. (1987). DOOR syndrome (deafness, onycho-, osteodystrophy, and mental retardation): elevated plasma and urinary 2-oxoglutarate in three unrelated patients. *Am J Med Genet* **26**:207–215.

Qazi QH, Nangia BS (1984). Abnormal distal phalanges and nails, deafness, mental retardation, and seizure disorder: a new familial syndrome. *J Pediatr* **104**:391–394.

Sanchez O, Mazas JJM, Ortiz De Dematos I (1981). The deafness, onycho-osteo-dystrophy, mental retardation syndrome – two new cases. *Hum Genet* **58**:228–230.

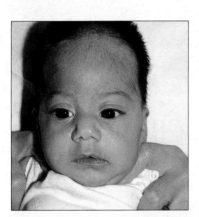
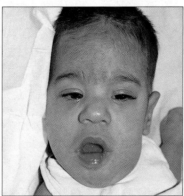

79A and 79B Note the high forehead, bilateral ptosis and short broad nasal tip.

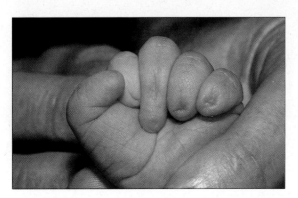

79C Note absent/hyoplastic nails.

COFFIN–SIRIS SYNDROME 80A–80D

There is characteristically hypoplasia of the nails, especially involving the fifth finger and toenails, associated with mental retardation. The other clinical features are sparse scalp hair in conjunction with hirsutism elsewhere, especially on the face, where the eyebrows might be conjoined, but also over the back. Facial features tend to be coarse, the lips are often thick, the nasal bridge flat and the mouth large. This rare mental retardation syndrome is easy to over-diagnose. Some cases have turned out to have small chromosomal deletions, as happened to the case published in the previous edition of this atlas (Baraitser and Winter).

Genetic aspects: Autosomal recessive.

References

Baraitser M, Winter RM (1993). *A Colour Atlas of Clinical Genetics*, Wolfe, London.
Carey JC, Hall BD (1978). The Coffin-Siris syndrome: five new cases including two siblings. *Am J Dis Child* **132**:667–671.
Coffin GS, Siris E (1970). Mental retardation with absent fifth finger-nail and terminal phalanx. *Am J Dis Child* **119**:433–439.
Haspeslagh M, Fryns JP, Van den Berghe H (1984). The Coffin-Siris syndrome: report of a family and further delineation. *Clin Genet* **26**:374–378.
Levy P, Baraitser M (1991). Syndrome of the month. Coffin-Siris syndrome. *J Med Genet* **28**:338–341.
Rabe P, Haverkamp F, Emons D *et al.* (1991). Syndrome of developmental retardation, facial and skeletal anomalies, and hyperphosphatasia in two sisters: nosology and genetics of the Coffin-Siris syndrome. *Am J Med Genet* **41**:350–354.
Richieri-Costa A *et al.* (1986). Coffin-Siris syndrome in a Brazilian child with consanguineous parents. *Rev Brasil Genet* **9**:169–177.

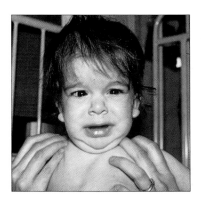 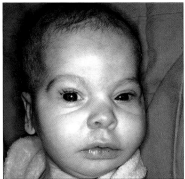 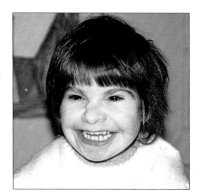

80A–80C Note the thick lips, hairy forehead, and sparse scalp hair.

SMITH-LEMLI-OPITZ SYNDROME TYPE I 81A–81D

The combination of microcephaly, 2–3 syndactyly of the toes, small proximally placed thumbs, and occasional post-axial polydactyly and cataracts should suggest the diagnosis at term. Males have hypospadias and a hypoplastic scrotum. The facial features consist of bi-temporal narrowing, ptosis, anteverted nostrils, a broad nasal tip, prominent lateral palatine ridges and micrognathia. Various internal malformations have been reported including pyloric stenosis, cleft palate, pancreatic anomalies and lung segmentation defects. Plasma levels of cholesterol are low and 7-dehydrocholesterol are raised. This is proving to be a useful diagnostic test. A defect in the enzyme that reduces the C-7,8 double bond of the latter intermediate has been postulated.

Genetic aspects: Autosomal recessive.

References

de Die-Smulders C, Fryns JP (1992). Smith-Lemli-Opitz syndrome: the changing phenotype with age. *Genetic Counseling* **3**:77–82.

Irons M, Elias ER, Tint GS *et al.* (1994). Abnormal cholesterol metabolism in the Smith-Lemli-Opitz syndrome: report of clinical and biochemical findings in four patients and treatment in one patient. *Am J Med Genet* **50**:347–352.

Opitz JM, Penchaszadeh VB *et al.* (1987). Smith-Lemli-Opitz (RSH) syndrome bibliography. *Am J Med Genet* **28**:745–750.

Penchaszadeh VB (1987). Invited editorial comment: the nosology of the Smith-Lemli-Opitz syndrome. *Am J Med Genet* **28**:719–722.

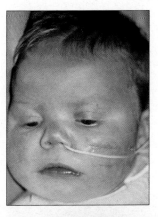

81A–81C Note the bi-temporal narrowing, and short nose with anteverted nostrils.

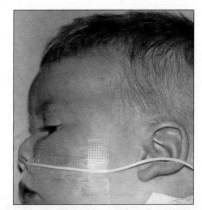

81B

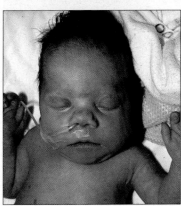

81C

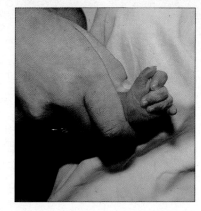

81D The thumbs are small.

SMITH–LEMLI–OPITZ SYNDROME TYPE II (SEVERE LETHAL FORM)   82A–82B

Some infants have a severe lethal form of the Smith-Lemli-Opitz (SLO) syndrome. In males the external genitalia can be ambiguous or female. Post-axial poly-dactyly in the hands, and a valgus deformity of the feet with syndactyly of several toes, are more common than in type 1 SLO. A cleft palate and hypoplasia of the anterior portion of the tongue are common. Other additional findings are unilobar lungs, hypoplastic kidneys, agenesis of the gall-bladder, cerebellar hypoplasia, cardiac defects and enlarged pancreatic islets with giant cells. The condition has similar biochemical changes to SLO type 1.

Genetic aspects: Autosomal recessive.

References

Curry CJR, Carey JC, Holland JS *et al.* (1987). Smith-Lemli-Opitz syndrome – type II: multiple congenital anomalies with male pseudohermaphroditism and frequent early lethality. *Am J Med Genet* **26**:45–57.

Donnai D, Young ID, Owen WG *et al.* (1986). The lethal multiple congenital anomaly syndrome of polydactyly, sex reversal, renal hypoplasia, and unilobular lungs. *J Med Genet* **23**:64–71.

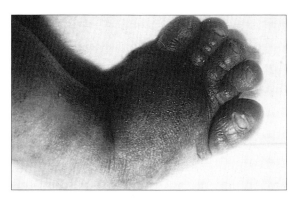

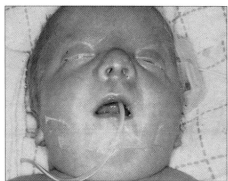

82A There is a calcaneovalgus deformity with 2–3 toe syndactyly and a short dorsiflexed hallux.

82B The face is round and the nostrils anteverted.

HYDROLETHALUS SYNDROME 83A–83D

The name was given because of hydramnios, hydrocephalus and the lethality in almost all cases. Post-axial polydactyly occurs in the majority and pre-axial polydactyly of the toes, with a markedly angulated extra hallux can be a striking and characteristic feature. The face is striking, with a small mandible and hypertelorism, and the tongue can be malformed, small or absent. A VSD is found in over 50% of cases and stenosis or atresia of the trachea or bronchi is common. As well as hydrocephalus, a posterior encephalocele can be present. At post-mortem a small cerebrum, absent corpus callosum and pituitary and occipitoschisis are seen. The foramen magnum is said to have a keyhole shape. The condition can be differentiated from Meckel syndrome in that the kidneys are normal.

Genetic aspects: Autosomal recessive.

References

Anyane-Yeboa K, Collins M, Kupsky W *et al.* (1987). Hydrolethalus (Salonen-Herva-Norio) syndrome: further clinicopathological delineation. *Am J Med Genet* **26**:899–907.

Aughton DJ, Cassidy SB (1987). Hydrolethalus syndrome: report of an apparent mild case, literature review and differential diagnosis. *Am J Med Genet* **27**:935–942.

Salonen R, Herva R, Reijo N (1981). The hydrolethalus syndrome: delineation of a 'new' lethal malformation syndrome based on 28 patients. *Clin Genet* **19**:321–330.

Salonen R, Herva R (1990). Syndrome of the month: hydrolethalus syndrome. *J Med Genet* **27**:756–759.

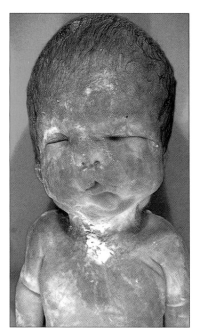

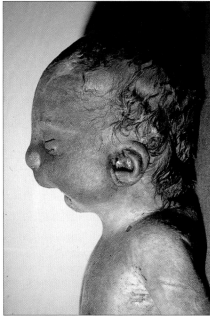

83A–83C Note hydrocephalus, cleft lip and small chin.

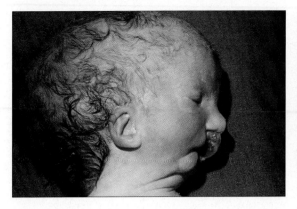

83C

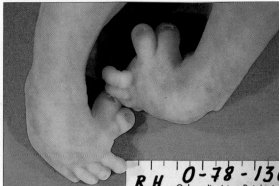

83D Note pre-axial polydactyly of the feet.

MECKEL–GRUBER SYNDROME (DYSENCEPHALIA SPLANCHNOCYSTICA)   84A–84C

The main features are occipital encephalocele associated with microcephaly, hydrocephaly or anencephaly, anophthalmia or microphthalmia, polymicrogyria, cleft lip and palate, polycystic kidneys, hepatic fibrosis and cysts, ambiguous genitalia, congenital heart defect and post-axial polydactyly. The most consistent features are the hepatic and renal lesions.

Genetic aspects: Autosomal recessive.

References

Farag TI, Usha R, Uma R *et al.* (1990). Phenotypic variability in Meckel-Gruber syndrome. *Clin Genet* **38**:176–179.

Fraser FC, Lytwyn A (1981). Spectrum of anomalies in the Meckel syndrome, or: 'maybe there is a malformation syndrome with at least one constant anomaly'. *Am J Med Genet* **9**:67–73.

Herriot R, Hallam LA, Gray ES (1991). Dandy-Walker malformation in the Meckel syndrome. *Am J Med Genet* **39**:207–210.

Lowry RB, Hill RH, Tischler B (1983). Survival and spectrum of anomalies in the Meckel syndrome. *Am J Med Genet* **14**:417–421.

Salonen R (1984). The Meckel syndrome: clinicopathological findings in 67 patients. *Am J Med Genet* **18**:671–689.

Various Authors (1984). The Meckel symposium. *Am J Med Genet* **18**:649–711.

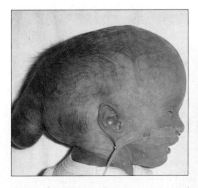
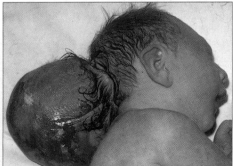
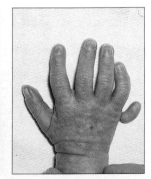

84A and 84B Note the posterior encephalocele.

84C Note post-axial polydactyly.

RUBINSTEIN–TAYBI SYNDROME   85A–85H

The facial features are characterised by microcephaly, down-slanting palpebral fissures, hypertelorism, long eyelashes, mild ptosis, posteriorly rotated ears and a convex nose with the columella protruding below the alae nasi on lateral view. The thumbs and halluces are broad, or occasionally bifid, with medial deviation. The tips of the other fingers may be spatulate. The facial features become more marked with age.

Genetic aspects: Most cases are sporadic. Several sets of concordant monozygotic twins and the occasional siblings have been reported and Hennekam *et* *al.* (1990) reported an affected mother and son, suggesting dominant inheritance. Microdeletions of 16p13 have been demonstrated by FISH techniques in 10–20% of cases (Breuning *et al.*).

References

Allanson JE (1990). Rubinstein-Taybi syndrome: the changing face. *Am J Med Genet* **Suppl.6**:38–41.

Breuning MH, Dauwerse HG, Fugazza G et al. (1993). Rubinstein-Taybi syndrome caused by submicroscopic deletions within 16p13.3. *Am J Hum Genet* **52**:249–254.

Hennekam RCM (1993). Rubinstein-Taybi syndrome: a history in pictures. *Clin Dysmorphol* **2**:87–92.

Hennekam RCM, Van Den Boogaard M-J, Sibbles BJ, Van Spijker HG (1990). Rubinstein-Taybi syndrome in the Netherlands. *Am J Med Genet* **Suppl.6**:17–29.

Hennekam RCM, Stevens CA, van De Kamp JJP (1990). Etiology and recurrence risk in Rubinstein-Taybi syndrome. *Am J Med Genet* **Suppl.6**:56–64.

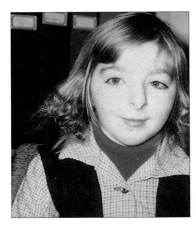
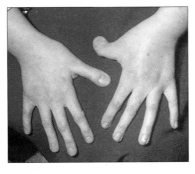
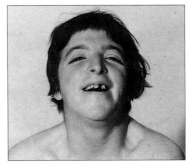

85A–85G A series of patients showing down-slanting palpebral fissures, ptosis, a hooked nose with prominent columella, broad deviated thumbs and broad big toes.

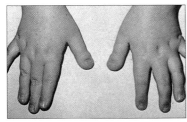

85D

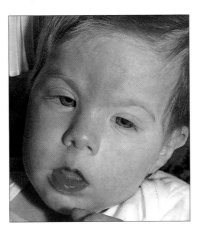

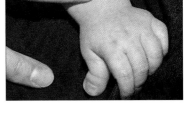

85F

85E

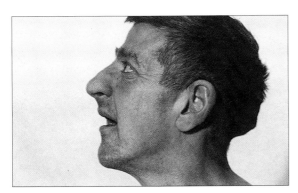

85G

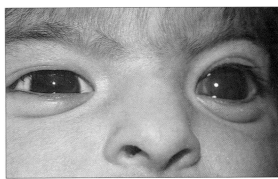

85H Shows glaucoma in the left eye, which can occur.

OTO-PALATO-DIGITAL (TAYBI) SYNDROME 86A–86B

The overall impression is said to be of 'pugilistic' facies and this may become more marked with age. The palate is cleft and the face is characteristic with hypertelorism, prominent supra-orbital ridges, poorly modelled pinnae, a broad nasal bridge with a small nose and mouth, and an anti-mongoloid eye-slant. Conductive deafness is caused by abnormalities of the auditory ossicles. The ends of the thumbs, halluces and sometimes the other digits are flattened and skin syndactyly, clinodactyly and short square nails are usually seen. The appearance in the feet is particularly characteristic with a large gap between the first and second toes, a short hallux and lateral curvature of the toes (a 'tree-frog' appearance).

Genetic aspects: X-linked recessive. The gene maps to Xq28 (Biancalana *et al.*). Females may show mild manifestations.

References

Biancalana V, Le Marec B, Odent S et al. (1991). Oto-palato-digital syndrome type I: further evidence for assignment of the locus to Xq28. *Hum Genet* **88**:228–230.

Dudding BA, Gorlin RJ, Langer LO (1967). The oto-palato-digital syndrome. A new symptom-complex consisting of deafness, dwarfism, cleft palate, characteristic facies, and a generalized bone dysplasia. *Am J Dis Child* **113**:214–221.

Gorlin RJ, Poznanski AK, Hendon I (1973). The oto-palato-digital (OPD) syndrome in females. Heterozygote expression of an X-linked trait. *Oral Surg* **35**:218–224.

Langer LO Jr (1967). The roentgenographic features of the oto-palato-digital (OPD) syndrome. *Am J Roentgenol* **100**:63–70.

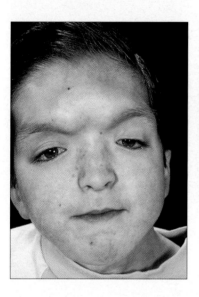
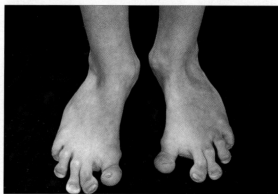

86A and 86B
Note pugilistic face and 'tree-frog' feet.

OTO-PALATO-DIGITAL SYNDROME TYPE II 87A–87D

The face is characterised by hypertelorism, down-slanting palpebral fissures, micrognathia, posteriorly rotated ears, a prominent forehead, microstomia and a cleft palate. The fingers are flexed and overlapping with syndactyly, notched or bifid terminal phalanges and there is post-axial polydactyly with short halluces and thumbs. Radiographs of affected individuals reveal dense, curved or wavy long bones, wavy short ribs, sloping clavicles and spread-out ilia, tall thickened ischia and flat acetabulae. In many cases the condition has been lethal in the neonatal period but in those who survive the facial features become less severe, the bone curvature improves and the osteosclerosis of the long bones lessens.

Genetic aspects: X-linked recessive.

References

Andre M, Vigneron J, Didier F (1981). Abnormal facies, cleft palate, and generalized dysostosis: a lethal X-linked syndrome. *J Pediatr* **98**:747–752.

Fitch N, Jequier S, Gorlin RJ (1983). The oto-palato-digital syndrome, proposed type II. *Am J Med Genet* **15**:655–664.

Holder SE, Winter RM (1993). Syndrome of the month. Otopalatodigital syndrome type II. *J Med Genet* **30**:310–313.

Stratton RF, Bluestone DL (1991). Oto-palato-digital syndrome type II with X-linked cerebellar hypoplasia/hydrocephalus. *Am J Med Genet* **41**:169–172.

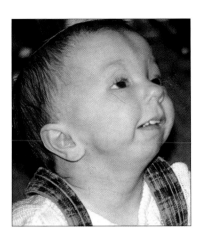

87A Note small jaw and mouth and posteriorly rotated ears.

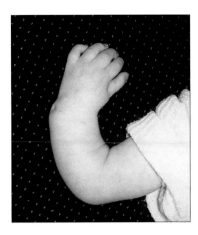

87B Note bowed radius and skin dimple.

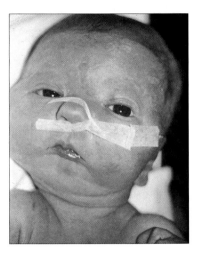

87C Note hypertelorism, down-slanting palpebral fissures, and small jaw and mouth.

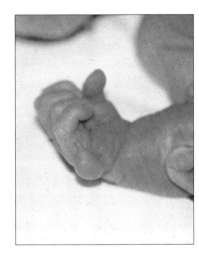

87D Note post-axial polydactyly of the fingers.

ORAL-FACIAL-DIGITAL SYNDROME TYPE I

88A–88E

The facial features are prominent milia in infancy, a broad nasal root, dystopia canthorum, hypoplasia of the alar cartilages and narrow nares. There is a midline cleft or notch of the upper lip, multiple hyperplastic oral frenulae, an asymmetrical cleft palate, clefting of the maxillary alveolar ridge and a lobulated tongue with hamartomata. The digital features are brachydactyly and skin syndactyly of the hands, clinodactyly, polydactyly of the hallux, and brachydactyly of the toes. Other abnormalities include polycystic kidneys, partial alopecia and CNS abnormalities leading to mental retardation (these include hydrocephaly, porencephaly and agenesis of the corpus callosum).

Genetic aspects: X-linked dominant. The gene is lethal in males, who are thought to die *in utero*.

References

Baraitser M (1986). Syndrome of the month: the orofaciodigital (OFD) syndromes. *J Med Genet* **23**:116–119.

Donnai D, Kerzin-Storrar L, Harris R (1987). Familial orofaciodigital syndrome type I presenting as adult polycystic kidney disease. *J Med Genet* **24**:84–87.

Salinas CF, Pai GS, Vera CL et al. (1991). Variability of expression of the orofaciodigital syndrome type I in black females: six cases. *Am J Med Genet* **38**:574–582.

Toriello HV (1993). Review. Oral-facial-digital syndromes, 1992. *Clin Dysmorphol* **2**:95–105.

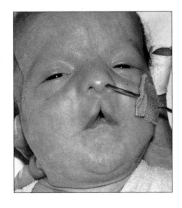

88A Note the midline cleft, facial milia and the hypoplastic alae nasi.

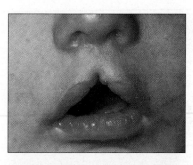

88B Close-up of midline cleft.

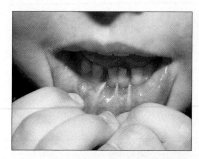

88C Multiple frenulae.

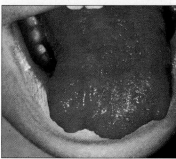

88D Tongue indentations are common.

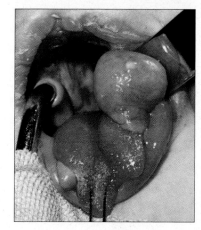

88E Note the tongue tumours and clefting.

ORAL-FACIAL-DIGITAL SYNDROME TYPE II

89

The facial and oral features are similar to OFD-I but the tip of the nose may be bifid and milia are not pronounced in infancy. Another distinguishing feature is conductive hearing loss in OFD-II. In the limbs there may be post-axial polydactyly and skin syndactyly of the fingers, and bilateral duplication of the hallux is characteristic. Pseudoarthrosis of the tibia can be a feature.

Genetic aspects: Autosomal recessive.

References

Reardon W, Harbord MG, Hall-Craggs MA *et al.* (1989). Central nervous system malformations in Mohr's syndrome. *J Med Genet* **26**:659–663.

Rimoin DL, Edgerton MT (1967). Genetic and clinical heterogeneity in the oral-facial-digital syndromes. *J Pediatr* **71**:94.

Toriello HV (1988). Heterogeneity and variability in the oral-facial-digital syndromes. *Am J Med Genet* **Suppl.4**:149–159.

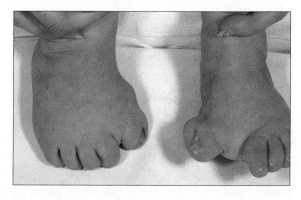

89 Symmetrical pre-axial polydactyly is characteristic.

MOHR–MAJEWSKI SYNDROME

90A–90F

Cases have been reported with clinical features transitional between Mohr syndrome (OFD II) and Majewski syndrome (short rib-polydactyly II). Affected individuals have a midline cleft or notch of the upper lip, multiple oral frenulae, fleshy nodules or hamartomas of the tongue, and a high or cleft palate. In the hands, post-axial polydactyly is common and in the feet, pre- and post-axial polydactyly. The tibia is severely hypoplastic, but is not ovoid in shape, as seen in Majewski syndrome. The ribs are relatively normal, allowing survival, but in some cases rib shortening is seen.

Genetic aspects: Autosomal recessive.

References

Burn J, Dezateux C, Hall CM *et al.* (1984). Orofaciodigital syndrome with mesomelic limb shortening. *J Med Genet* **21**:189–192.

Meinecke P, Hayek H (1990). Orofaciodigital syndrome type IV (Mohr-Majewski syndrome) with severe expression expanding the known spectrum of anomalies. *J Med Genet* **27**:200–202.

Silengo MC, Bell GL, Biagioli M *et al.* (1987). Oro-facial-digital syndrome II. Transitional type between the Mohr and the Majewski syndromes: report of two new cases. *Clin Genet* **31**:331–336.

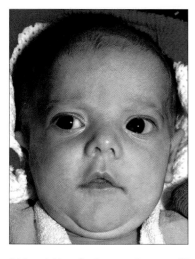
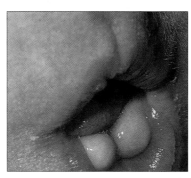
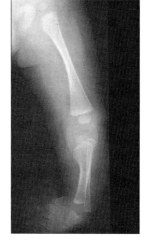

90A and 90B The face can be normal but in **90B** there can be seen sublingual nodules.

90C There is hypoplasia of the tibia.

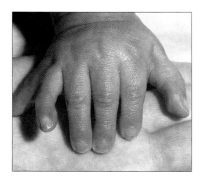

90D Note post-axial polydactyly in the hands.

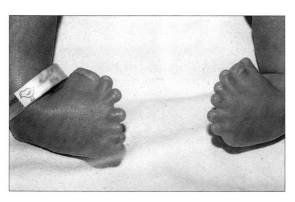
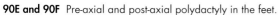
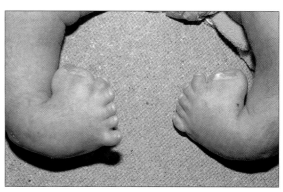

90E and 90F Pre-axial and post-axial polydactyly in the feet.   **90F**

TRICHO-RHINO-PHALANGEAL (TRP) SYNDROME

The hair is sparse, the nose bulbous and pear-shaped with notched alae nasi, the philtrum long and the ears protruding. The hands have prominent joints and the fingers are tapering with clinodactyly. Cone-shaped epiphyses of the phalanges are apparent on X-ray.

Genetic aspects: Autosomal dominant. There are considerable similarities to the Langer-Giedion syndrome. Both conditions may be caused by small deletions of the long arm of chromosome 8.

References

Beals RK (1973). Tricho-rhino-phalangeal dysplasia. Report of a kindred. *J Bone Joint Surg A* **55**:821–826.

Buhler EM, Malik NJ (1973). The tricho-rhino-phalangeal syndrome(s): chromosome 8 long arm deletion: is there shortest region of overlap between reported cases? TRP I and TRP II syndromes: are they separate entities? *Am J Med Genet* **19**:113–119.

Cope R, Beals RK, Bennett RM (1986). The trichorhinophalangeal dysplasia syndrome: report of eight kindreds, with emphasis on hip complications, late presentations, and premature osteoarthritis. *J Pediatr Orthop* **6**:133–138.

Giedion A, Burdea M, Fruchter Z et al. (1973). Autosomal dominant transmission of the tricho-rhino-phalangeal syndrome – report of four unrelated families, review of 60 cases. *Helv Paediatr Acta* **28**:249–259.

Goldblatt J, Smart RD (1986). Tricho-rhino-phalangeal syndrome without exostoses, with an interstitial deletion of 8q23. *Clin Genet* **29**:434–438.

Haan EA, Hull YJ, White S et al. (1989). Tricho-rhino-phalangeal and branchio-oto syndromes in a family with an inherited rearrangement of chromosome 8q. *Am J Med Genet* **32**:490–494.

Langer LO, Krassikoff N, Laxova R et al. (1984). The tricho-rhino-phalangeal syndrome with exostoses (or Langer Giedion syndrome): four additional patients without mental retardation and review of the literature. *Am J Med Genet* **19**:81–111.

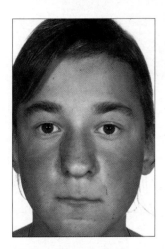 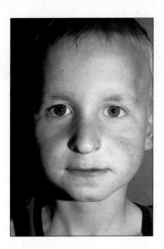 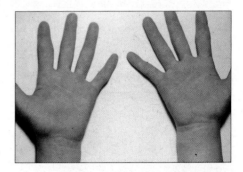

91A and 91B Note the pear-shaped nose, hypoplasia of the alar nasi, sparse scalp hair and thin upper lip.

91C Note abnormal angulation of the phalanges and broadening of the proximal phalangeal joints.

ROBERTS (PSEUDOTHALIDOMIDE) SYNDROME

The main clinical features are severe shortening of the limbs, with radial defects and oligodactyly or syndactyly, and a characteristic face with hypertelorism, severe cleft lip, a prominent premaxilla, a mid-face capillary haemangioma, cloudy corneae or cataracts and dysplastic or small ears. Other defects may be seen such as large genitalia, congenital heart defects and cystic kidneys. Many affected infants die in the newborn period, and survivors may have mental retardation (although intelligence can also be normal). Centromeric staining of chromosomes shows premature centromere separation ('chromosome puffs') and this test has been used for prenatal diagnosis. The syndrome is probably the same as SC-phocomelia in view of the fact that in both conditions chromosome analysis shows premature centromere separation.

Genetic aspects: Autosomal recessive.

References
Hirschhorn K, Kaffe S (1992). Prenatal diagnosis of Roberts
syndrome (Letter). *Prenatal Diagn* **12**:976.
Holden KR, Jabs EW, Sponseller PD (1992).
Roberts/pseudothalidomide syndrome and normal intelligence:
approaches to diagnosis and management. *Dev Med Child
Neurol* **34**:534–538.
Keppen LD, Gollin SM, Seibert JJ, Sisken JE (1991). Roberts
syndrome with normal cell division. *Am J Med Genet*
38:21–24.

Robins DB, Ladda RL, Thieme GA *et al*. (1989). Prenatal detection
of Roberts-SC phocomelia syndrome: report of two siblings with
characteristic manifestations. *Am J Med Genet* **32**:390–394.
Romke C, Froster-Iskenius U, Heyne K *et al*. (1987). Roberts
syndrome and SC phocomelia. A single genetic entity. *Clin
Genet* **31**:170–177.
Stioui S, Privitera O, Brambati B *et al*. (1992). First-trimester prenatal
diagnosis of Roberts syndrome. *Prenatal Diagn* **12**:145–149.

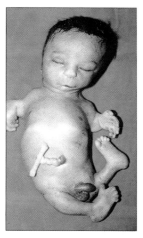
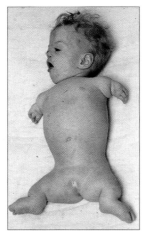
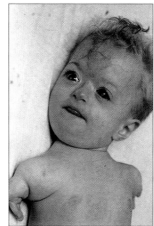

92A–92D Note severe phocomelia involving all four limbs. The facial features consist of hypertelorism, cleft lip and palate and facial haemangiomas.

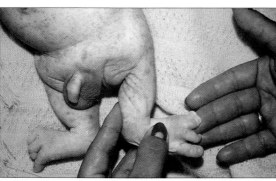

92D

OCULO-DENTO-DIGITAL SYNDROME

The nose is pinched with hypoplastic alae nasi and thin nares. Microphthalmia, microcornea, glaucoma and a persistent pupillary membrane have all been noted. Enamel hypoplasia of the teeth is common. Syndactyly of the third, fourth and fifth digits is characteristic. Commonly, this is skin syndactyly, but the terminal phalanges can be fused. Radiographs show hyperplasia of the body of the mandible and alveolar ridges, and broadening of the tubular bones. Brueton *et al.* have suggested that syndactyly type III has overlapping features. Spasticity and hyperreflexia have been reported.

Genetic aspects: Autosomal dominant.

References
Brueton LA, Huson SM, Farren B, Winter RM (1990).
Oculodentodigital dysplasia and type III syndactyly: separate
genetic entities or disease spectrum? *J Med Genet*
27:169–175.
Gutmann DH, Zackai EH, McDonald-McGinn DM *et al.* (1991).
Oculodentodigital dysplasia syndrome associated with
abnormal cerebral white matter. *Am J Med Genet* **41**:18–20.
Judisch GF, Martin-Casals A, Hanson JW, Olin WH (1979).
Oculodentodigital dysplasia: four new reports and a literature
review. *Arch Ophthalmol* **97**:878–884.
Traboulsi EI, Parks MM (1990). Glaucoma in oculo-dento-osseous
dysplasia. *Am J Ophthalmol* **109**:310–313.

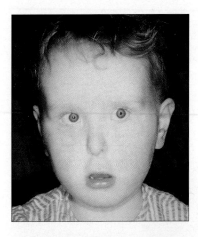

93A Note the hypoplasia of the alae nasi and the small eyes.

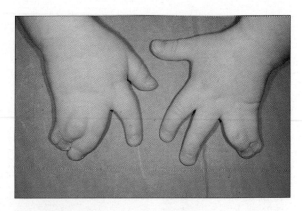

93B Note the 4–5 syndactyly.

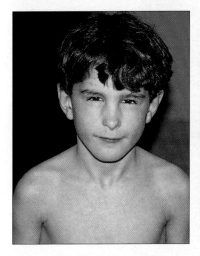

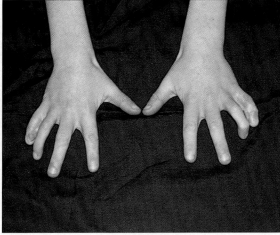

93C and 93D Note similar abnormalities in another child.

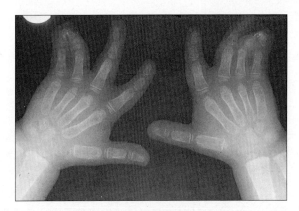

93E Note bony syndactyly often only of the terminal phalanges.

LACRIMO-AURICULO-DENTO-DIGITAL (LADD) SYNDROME   94A–94C

Characteristic features are absence or atresia of the lacrimal puncta or canaliculi, leading to epiphora and chronic eye infections, cup-shaped or malformed ears, sensorineural or conductive deafness, and abnor-malities of the hands. The latter consist of hypoplas-tic, bifid or finger-like thumbs, clinodactyly of the fifth finger and other minor abnormalities. The teeth are hypoplastic with marked caries; the lateral incisors may be peg-shaped. Renal anomalies may be a rare feature of the condition (Roodhooft *et al.*).

Genetic aspects: Autosomal dominant with variable expression.

References
Bamforth JS, Kaurah P (1992). Lacrimo-auriculo-dento-digital syndrome: evidence for lower limb involvement and severe congenital renal anomalies. *Am J Med Genet* **43**:932–937.

Heinz GW, Bateman JB, Barrett DJ et al. (1993). Ocular manifestations of the lacrimo-auriculo-dento-digital syndrome. *Am J Ophthalmol* **115**:243–248.

Hollister DW, Klein SH, De Jager HJ et al. (1973). The lacrimo-auriculo-dento-digital syndrome. *J Pediatr* **83**:438–444.

Kreutz JM, Hoyme HE. Levy-Hollister syndrome (1988). *Pediatrics* **82**:96–99.

Roodhooft AM, Brussaard CC, Elst E, Van Acker KJ (1990). Lacrimo-auriculo-dento-digital (LADD) syndrome with renal and foot anomalies (Case report). *Clin Genet* **38**:228–232.

Thompson E, Pembrey M, Graham JM (1985). Phenotypic variation in LADD syndrome. *J Med Genet* **22**:382–385.

Wiedemann H-R, Drescher J (1986). LADD syndrome: report of new cases and review of the clinical spectrum. *Eur J Pediatr* **144**:579–582.

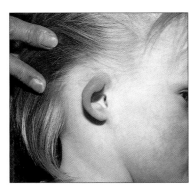 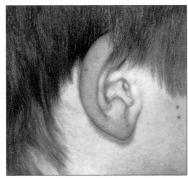 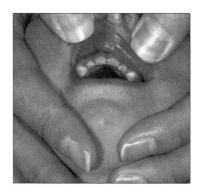

94A and 94B Note the cup-shaped, malformed ears.

94C Note small, abnormally shaped teeth.

TOWNES–BROCKS SYNDROME

The main features are triphalangeal thumbs, an imperforate anus, overfolded helices to the ears, sensorineural deafness and pes planus. Pre-auricular pits or tags may be present, as may a conductive component to the deafness. Partial trisomy 22 must be ruled out.

Genetic aspects: Autosomal dominant with very variable expression.

References
De vries-Van der Weerd M-AC et al. (1988). A new family with Townes–Brocks syndrome. *Clin Genet* **34**:195–200.

Koenig R, Schick U, Fuchs S. Townes–Brocks syndrome. *Eur J Pediatr* 1990;**150**:100–103.

O'Callaghan M, Young ID (1990). Syndrome of the month. Townes–Brocks syndrome. *J Med Genet* **27**:457–461.

Walpole IR, Hockey A (1982). Syndrome of imperforate anus, abnormalities of hands and feet, satyr ears and sensorineural defects. *J Pediatr* **100**:250–252.

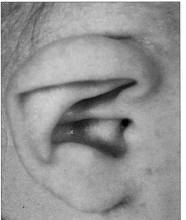 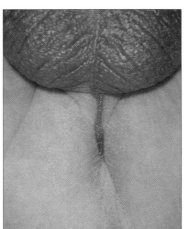

95A Note the overfolded helix.

95B Note the imperforate anus.

OKIHIRO SYNDROME (DUANE ANOMALY WITH RADIAL DEFECTS)   96A–96B

The Duane anomaly is characterised by limitation of abduction of the eye in association with retraction and narrowing of the palpebral fissure on adduction. It often presents as a strabismus. It can occur within families combined with radial defects of variable severity. These range from thenar eminence hypoplasia to an inability to flex the interphalangeal joint of the thumb and, at their severest, to radial club hand. Spinal abnormalities, deafness, and occasionally renal anomalies, may occur. Chromosomes should be examined carefully as mosaic trisomy for the proximal part of the long arm of chromosome 22 can cause similar clinical features.

Genetic aspects: Autosomal dominant with variable expression.

References
Ferrell RL, Jones B, Lucas RV (1966). Simultaneous occurrence of Holt–Oram and the Duane syndromes. *J Pediatr* **69**:630–634.

Hayes A, Costa T, Polomeno RC (1985). The Okihiro syndrome of Duane anomaly, radial ray abnormalities, and deafness. *Am J Med Genet* **22**:273–280.

MacDermot KD, Winter RM (1987). Radial ray defect and Duane anomaly: report of a family with autosomal dominant transmission. *Am J Med Genet* **27**:313–319.

Okihiro MM, Tasaki T, Nakano KK, Bennett BK (1977). Duane syndrome and congenital upper-limb anomalies. *Arch Neurol* **34**:174–179.

96A There is bilateral radial aplasia.

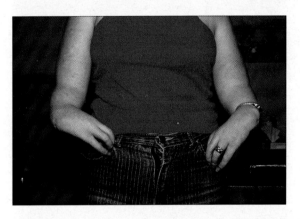

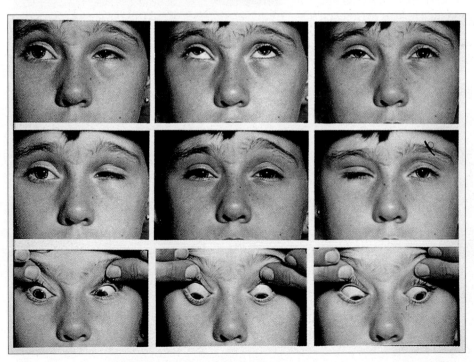

96B Note the Duane phenomenon.

FEMORAL HYPOPLASIA – UNUSUAL FACIES SYNDROME

97A–97F

The typical facial features include a short upturned nose, a long philtrum, a thin upper lip, a small jaw and a cleft palate. There might be an upward slant of the palpebral fissures. The femora are mostly bilaterally affected and they are short with lateral bowing. The femoral defects may be asymmetrical. Pre-axial polydactyly of the feet has been reported.

Genetic aspects: Most cases are sporadic. There has been only one report in which a father and daughter were affected. There is also an association with maternal diabetes.

References

Burn J, Winter RM, Baraitser M *et al.* (1984). The femoral hypoplasia-unusual facies syndrome. *J Med Genet* **21**:331–340.

Daentl DL, Smith DW, Scott CI *et al.* (1975). Femoral hypoplasia-unusual facies syndrome. *J Pediatr* **86**:107–111.

Gleiser S *et al.* (1978). Femoral hypoplasia-unusual facies syndrome, from another viewpoint. *Eur J Pediatr* **128**:1–5.

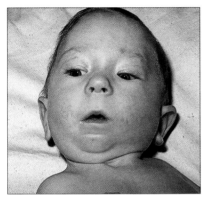 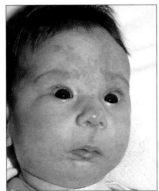 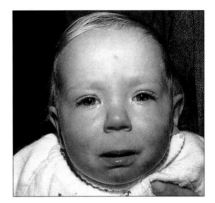

97A–C Note short stubby nose, anteverted nostrils, long philtrum, thin upper lip and micrognathia.

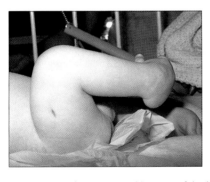 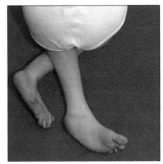 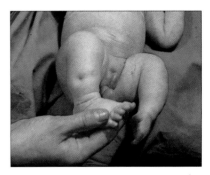

97D–F Note shortening and bowing of the legs.

POPLITEAL PTERYGIUM SYNDROME

98A–98E

There is cleft lip/palate, lower lip pits, popliteal webs (pterygia), syndactyly or absence of fingers or toes, hypoplastic toenails, and genital anomalies consisting of a small penis and hypoplastic scrotum in males, and hypoplastic labia majora and clitoromegaly in females. A pyramid of skin overlying the nail of the great toe is characteristic. The edge of the pterygium in the knee contains the neurovascular bundle and care must be taken when releasing the web. Occasionally, pterygia are seen elsewhere, for example in the groin.

Genetic aspects: Autosomal dominant. There is also a severe lethal form of the condition which may be autosomal recessive.

References

Bixler D, Poland C, Nance WE (1973). Phenotypic variation in the popliteal pterygium syndrome. *Clin Genet* **4**:220–228.

Froster-Iskenius UG (1990). Syndrome of the month. Popliteal pterygium syndrome. *J Med Genet* **27**:320–326.

Gorlin RJ, Sedano HO, Cervenka J (1968). Popliteal pterygium syndrome: a syndrome comprising cleft lip-palate, popliteal and intercrural pterygia, digital and genital anomalies. *Pediatrics* **41**:503–509.

Hunter A (1990). The popliteal pterygium syndrome: report of a new family and review of the literature. *Am J Med Genet* **36**:196–208.

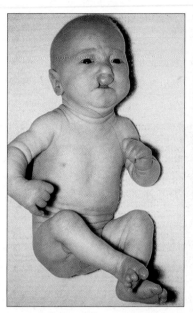

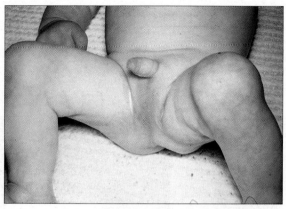

98A and 98B
Note the web of skin in the popliteal region, hypoplastic scrotum, and bilateral cleft lip and palate.

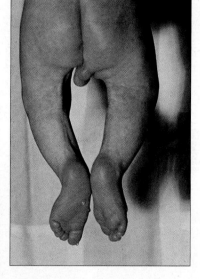

98C and 98D
Note the webs behind the knee.

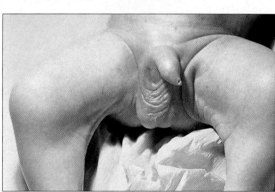

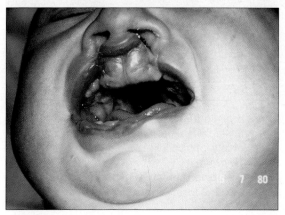

98E Note bilateral cleft lip and palate, and lower lip pits in newborn boy.

SCHINZEL–GIEDION SYNDROME

Generalised hirsutism, talipes equinovarus and hypospadias in males are common. The head has been described as a 'figure 8' shape: viewed from the front the forehead is tall and prominent, there is severe temporal narrowing, and the cheeks are rather chubby. A groove under the eyes is characteristic and the earlobes are fleshy and anteriorly displaced. Choanal atresia may be a feature. The nails are narrow and deep-set, and post-axial polydactyly has been reported in some cases. At post-mortem examination hydronephrosis and hydroureter, and congenital heart defects, are all seen. Radiology reveals sclerosis of the base of the skull, a gap in the occipital bone, broad ribs, curved long bones and hypoplastic phalanges.

Genetic aspects: Autosomal recessive.

References

Al-Gazali Ll, Farndon P, Burn J *et al.* (1990). Syndrome of the month. The Schinzel-Giedion syndrome. *J Med Genet* **27**:42–47.

Donnai D, Harris R (1979). A further case of a new syndrome including midface retraction, hypertrichosis, and skeletal anomalies. *J Med Genet* **16**:483–486.

Schinzel A, Giedion A (1978). A syndrome of severe midface retraction, multiple skull anomalies, clubfeet, and cardiac and renal malformations in siblings. *Am J Med Genet* **1**:361–375.

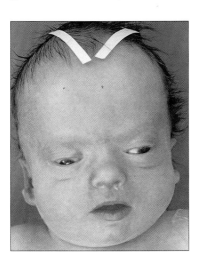
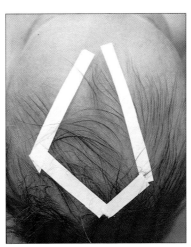

99A–99D Note the tall forehead, open anterior fontanelle and the coarse facial features with chubby cheeks giving the face an overall figure of eight shape. Note also the hypospadias in **99C**.

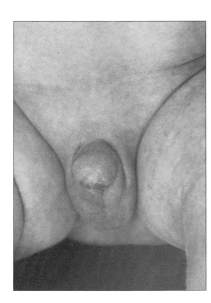

99C

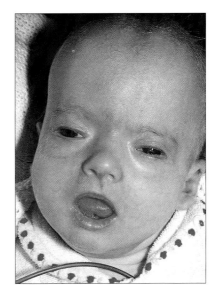

99D

SYNDROMES RECOGNISED THROUGH LIMB DEFECTS

HOLT–ORAM SYNDROME 100

This condition presents with heart abnormalities and skeletal malformations. The heart defect is most commonly an ASD, or more rarely a VSD, but other lesions have also occurred. 85% of affected individuals have heart lesions. The limb abnormalities are variable. The thumbs are most commonly involved and they might be digitalised, absent, hypoplastic, triphalangeal or, rarely, bifid. The other fingers might be absent, or have clinodactyly or syndactyly. Scaphoid abnormalities are common and include hypoplasia and bipartite ossification (supposedly due to delayed fusion of the os centrale). The other carpals may be hypoplastic, enlarged, irregular or fused. The first metacarpal may have both proximal and distal epiphyses. Radial, ulnar and humeral hypoplasia can also be seen, with the radius being preferentially involved.

Genetic aspects: Autosomal dominant. Expression is variable and care must be taken in assessing apparently normal family members. Hand X-rays and a careful cardiac assessment are essential. Linkage has been demonstrated to markers on 12q, but there is also definite locus heterogeneity.

References

Holt M, Oram S (1960). Familial heart disease with skeletal malformations. *Br Heart J* **22**:236–242.

Hurst JA, Hall CM, Baraitser M (1991). Syndrome of the month: the Holt–Oram syndrome. *J Med Genet* **28**:406–410.

Najjar H, Mardini M et al. (1988). Variability of the Holt–Oram syndrome in Saudi individuals. *Am J Med Genet* **29**:851–855.

Smith AT, Sack GH, Taylor GJ (1979). Holt–Oram syndrome. *J Pediatr* **95**:538–543.

100 Note the radial ray deficiency.

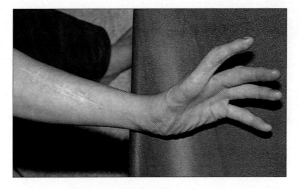

MARFAN SYNDROME 101A–101D

Patients with this well known syndrome have a combination of dolichostenomelia, arachnodactyly, pectus deformities of the chest, mitral or aortic regurgitation, ectopia lentis and mild joint laxity. Other evidence of a generalised connective tissue disorder may be present such as scoliosis and skin striae. A dilated aortic root can usually be demonstrated by echocardiography and aortic aneurysms can ensue. Average life expectancy is halved. 95% of deaths are due to a cardiovascular cause. All patients with this disorder should be followed up by a cardiologist with regular echocardiography to look for dilatation of the aortic root. Propranolol therapy reduces the incidence of this complication (Pyeritz *et al.*). The condition has been shown to be caused by mutations of the fibrillin gene on chromosome 15 (Sykes).

Genetic aspects: Autosomal dominant.

References

El Habbal MH (1992). Cardiovascular manifestations of Marfan syndrome in the young. *Am Heart J* **123**:752–757.

Hirata K, Triposkiadis F, Sparks E et al. (1992). The Marfan syndrome: cardiovascular physical findings and diagnostic correlates. *Am Heart J* **123**:743–752.

Joseph KN, Kane HA, Milner RS et al. (1992). Orthopedic aspects of the Marfan phenotype. *Clin Orthop* **277**:251–261.

McKusick VA (1991). The defect in Marfan syndrome. *Nature* **352**:279–281.

Pyeritz RE (1989). Effectiveness of beta-adrenergic blockade in the Marfan syndrome: experience over ten years. *Am J Med Genet* **32**:245–2250.

Sykes B (1993). Marfan gene dissected. *Nature Genetics* **3**:99–100.

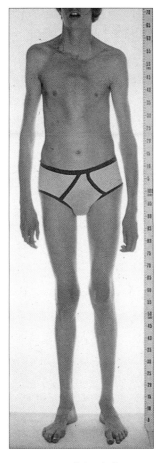

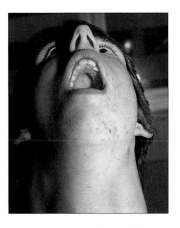

101B Note high arched palate.

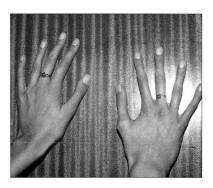

101C Note arachnodactyly.

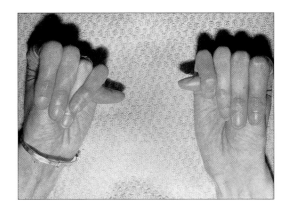

101A Note tall thin habitus with pectus excavatum.

101D Note positive thumb sign (Steinberg).

MARFAN SYNDROME, SEVERE NEONATAL

102A–102B

This is a severe neonatal form of Marfan syndrome. One of the hallmarks of the condition, apart from a marked marfanoid habitus, is severe cardiovascular problems in the neonatal period. These consist of marked cardiac valve insufficiency and aortic dilatation, frequently leading to early death. Many of the infants have congenital contractures of the large joints, hypermobility of the fingers, micrognathia, and an anterior chest deformity. The face has a crumpled appearance. Some cases have pulmonary emphysema and ocular abnormalities.

Genetic aspects: Most cases appear to be sporadic, some have had possible homozygosity for the Marfan gene and a few have had an affected parent. Morse *et al.* provide a good review. Kainulainen *et al.* reported mutations in the fibrillin gene on chromosome 15 (FBN1) in patients with the severe neonatal form of Marfan syndrome.

References

Buntinx IM, Willems PJ, Spitaels SE *et al.* (1991). Neonatal Marfan syndrome with congenital arachnodactyly, flexion contractures, and severe cardiac valve insufficiency. *J Med Genet* **28**:267–273.

Kainulainen K, Karttunen L, Puhakka L *et al.* (1994). Mutations in the fibrillin gene responsible for dominant ectopia lentis and neonatal Marfan syndrome. *Nature Genetics* **6**:64–69.

Morse RP, Graham JM Jr, Rockenmacher S, *et al.* (1989). Diagnosis and management of Marfan's syndrome during infancy. *Am J Med Genet* **32**:239–240.

Superti-Furga A, Raghunath M, Willems PJ (1992). Deficiencies of fibrillin and decorin in fibroblast cultures of a patient with neonatal Marfan syndrome. *J Med Genet* **29**:875–878.

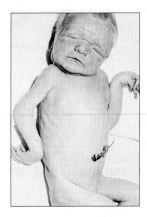

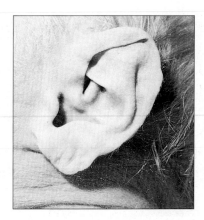

102A–B Note the joint contractures, long fingers and crumpled ears.

FEMUR-FIBULA-ULNA COMPLEX (FFU SYNDROME) 103A–103B

In this condition femoral defects are associated with fibular, ulnar and other limb abnormalities. Striking asymmetry of the limbs is common, often with abnormalities just being unilateral. Upper limbs are more often affected than lower limbs, and the right side and male individuals are preferentially affected. Common abnormalities of the arms include amelia, peromelia of the humerus, and humeroradial synostosis, as well as the ulnar ray defects. There may be bifurcation of the distal humerus.

Genetic aspects: Most cases are sporadic. In one series of 491 patients, there was only one set of affected siblings, with normal parents (Lenz *et al.*, 1993).

References

Hamanishi C (1980). Congenital short femur: clinical, genetic, and epidemiological comparison of the naturally occurring condition with that caused by thalidomide. *J Bone Joint Surg* **62**:307–320.

Lenz W, Feldmann U (1977). Unilateral and asymmetric limb defects in Man: delineation of the femur-fibula-ulna complex. *BDOAS* **13(1)**:269–285.

Lenz W, Zygulska M, Horst J (1993). FFU complex: an analysis of 491 cases. *Hum Genet* **91**:347–356.

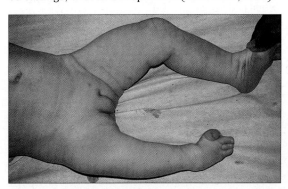

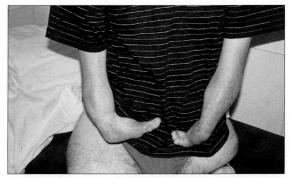

103A and 103B Note the severe limb defects involving femur, fibula and ulna.

LIMB/PELVIS-HYPOPLASIA/APLASIA SYNDROME 104A–104C

The malformations consist of hypoplasia and marked angulation of the proximal part of the femur, absence of the fibula and a malformed (usually hypoplastic) ulna. Multiple digits may be absent to give a split hand appearance or monodactyly. Both lower limbs are usually involved and may have the appearance of small stick-like projections with very hypoplastic or absent feet. The thorax is barrel shaped and the pelvis markedly malformed. One case, diagnosed prenatally, had an occipital meningocele and a hypoplastic cerebellum. The disorder differs from Femur-Fibula-Ulna (FFU) syndrome by virtue of its occurrence in siblings, and because of the more severe limb defects.

Genetic aspects: Autosomal recessive.

References

Al-Awadi SA, Teebi AS et al. (1985). Profound limb deficiency, thoracic dystrophy, unusual facies, and normal intelligence: a new syndrome. *J Med Genet* **22**:36–38.

Camera G, Ferraiolo G, Leo D et al. (1993). Limb/pelvis-hypopla-sia/aplasia syndrome (Al-Awadi/Raas-Rothschild syndrome): report of two Italian siblings and further confirmation of autosomal recessive inheritance. *J Med Genet* **30**:65–69.

Farag TI, Al-Awadi SA, Marafie MJ et al. (1993). The newly recognised limb/pelvis-hypoplasia/aplasia syndrome: report of a Bedouin patient and review. *J Med Genet* **30**:62–64.

Raas-Rothschild A, Goodman RM et al. (1988). Pathological features and prenatal diagnosis in the newly-recognised limb/pelvis-hypoplasia/aplasia syndrome. *J Med Genet* **25**:687–697.

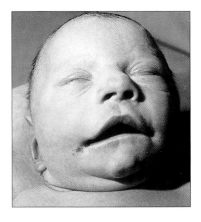
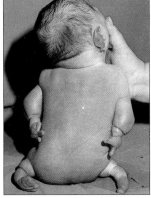
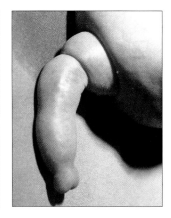

104A Note carp-shaped mouth, pointed chin and dysplastic ears.

104B and 104C There is severe limb hypoplasia involving all four limbs.

SPLIT HAND / FOOT-TIBIAL DEFECTS

105A–105C

Tibial aplasia and a split hand/foot deformity can be associated as part of an autosomal dominant condition. Expression is variable with some cases manifesting with only hypoplastic great toes and the most severe cases having transverse hemimelia of all four limbs. Some cases have hypoplastic ulnae, bifurcation of the femurs, absent patellae or post-axial polydactyly. Cup-shaped ears appear to be a further manifestation of the condition.

Genetic aspects: Autosomal dominant.

References

Hoyme HE, Jones KL et al. (1987). Autosomal dominant ectrodactyly and absence of long bones of upper or lower limbs: further clinical delineation. *J Pediatr* **111**:538–543.

Majewski F, Kuster W, ter Haar B et al. (1985). Aplasia of tibia with split-hand/split-foot deformity. Report of six families with 35 cases and considerations about variability and penetrance. *Hum Genet* **70**:136–147.

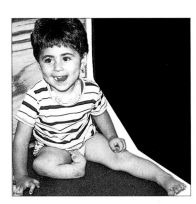
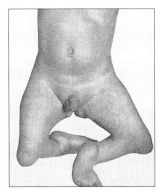
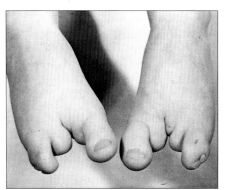

105A Young boy with unilateral tibial aplasia, and clefts of the hands.

105B Bilateral tibial aplasia.

105C Note the split feet.

GREBE SYNDROME

This condition is characterised by severe shortening of the upper and lower limbs. The hands and the fingers are particularly tiny, the digits resembling stubby toes. There might also be limitation of movement at various joints and polydactyly. Intelligence is normal.

Genetic aspects: Autosomal recessive.

References

Curtis D (1986). Heterozygote expression in Grebe chondrodysplasia. *Clin Genet* **29**:455–456.

Garcia-Castro JM, Perez-Comas A (1975). Nonlethal achondrogenesis in two Puerto Rican siblingships. *J Pediatr* **87**:948–952.

Kumar D, Curtis D, Blank CE (1984). Grebe chondrodysplasia and brachydactyly in a family. *Clin Genet* **25**:68–72.

Quelce-Salgado A (1964). A new type of dwarfism with various bone aplasias and hypoplasias of the extremities. *Acta Genet (Basel)* **14**:63.

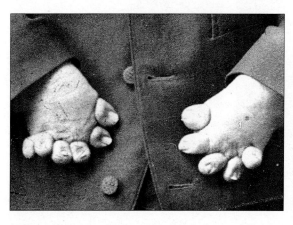

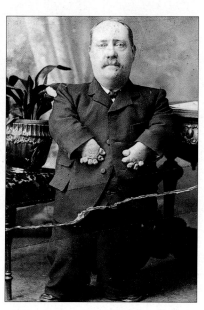

106A and 106B Note short stubby toe-like fingers and polydactyly on the right hand and the severe short stature.

DISORGANISATION-LIKE SYNDROME

Some infants may have a constellation of abnormalities similar to those caused by the mouse mutant 'Disorganisation' (Hummel). Affected infants have a combination of a high degree of polydactyly, usually unilateral, associated with ectopic digits or limbs arising from the trunk. Renal agenesis may also be a marker for the condition. Mice heterozygous for the Disorganisation gene have similar defects and may have complete limb duplication. Several human cases from the literature, reported with limb duplication, have also had skin papillae or hamartomatous lesions, suggesting that some of these may have a similar aetiology.

Donnai and Winter have also suggested that some cases classified as the result of amniotic bands or early amnion rupture may also fit into the 'Disorganisation-like' spectrum, raising the possibility of an intrinsic embryonic defect as a cause for the lesions in some of these cases.

Genetic aspects: Most cases are sporadic. The mouse mutant is autosomal dominant with reduced penetrance.

References

de Michelena MI, Stachurska A (1993). Multiple anomalies possibly caused by a human homologue to the mouse disorganization (Ds) gene. *Clin Dysmorphol* **2**:131–134.

Donnai D, Winter RM (1989). Disorganisation: a model for 'early amnion rupture'. *J Med Genet* **26**:421–425.

Hummel KP (1959). Developmental anomalies in mice resulting from action of the gene Disorganization, a semidominant lethal. *Pediatrics* **23**:212–221.

Petzel MA, Erickson RP (1991). Disorganisation: a possible cause of apparent conjoint twinning. *J Med Genet* **28**:712–714.

Wainwright H, Viljoen D (1993). Developmental anomalies in monozygous twins resembling the human homologue of the mouse mutant disorganization. *Clin Dysmorphol* **2**:135–139.

Winter RM, Donnai D (1989). A possible human homologue for the mouse mutant disorganisation. *J Med Genet* **26**:417–420.

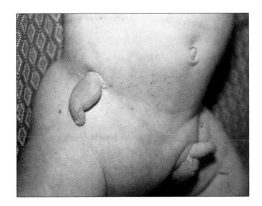

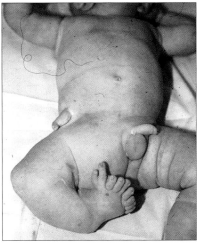

107A and 107B Note the digit-like appendage attached to the upper thigh and the high degree of polydactyly of the right foot.

AMNIOTIC BANDS / EARLY AMNION RUPTURE

Amputation defects of the limbs, craniofacial malformations and body wall defects can occur, apparently as the result of amniotic bands ('Streeter's bands') or early amnion rupture. Some authors have proposed a primary abnormality of development of the amniotic cavity and embryo whilst others have suggested that amnion rupture is the initiating event. The craniofacial abnormalities are often bizarre with unusual oblique facial clefts and severe cranial abnormalities resembling anencephaly. Cases have also been described with hydrocephaly due, for example, to aqueduct dysgenesis. Microcephaly, hydrocephaly, microphthalmia, and even anophthalmia have all been described in patients with the typical limb anomalies. Body wall defects are associated with a shortened cord. The condition has also been called the ADAM (Amniotic Deformity, Adhesions, Mutilations) complex.

Genetic aspects: The majority of cases are sporadic, although there have been rare familial recurrences (Lubinsky *et al.*).

References

Bamforth JS (1992). Amniotic band sequence: Streeter's hypothesis reexamined. *Am J Med Genet* **44**:280–287.

Donnai D, Read AP, Brandreth C *et al.* (1982). Prenatal detection of aberrant tissue bands and cord anomalies. *J Obstet Gynaecol* **2**:203–205.

Lubinsky M, Sujansky E, Sanger W *et al.* (1983). Familial amniotic bands. *Am J Med Genet* **14**:81–87.

Moerman P, Fryns J-P, Vandenberghe K, Lauweryns JM (1992). Constrictive amniotic bands, amniotic adhesions, and limb-body wall complex: discrete disruption sequences with pathogenetic overlap. *Am J Med Genet* **42**:470–479.

Van Allen MI, Siegel-Bartelt J, Dixon J *et al.* (1992). Constriction bands and limb reduction defects in two newborns with fetal ultrasound evidence for vascular disruption. *Am J Med Genet* **44**:598–604.

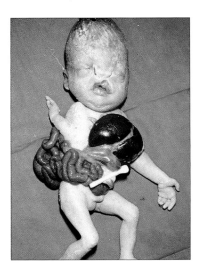

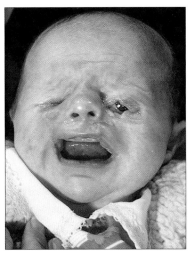

108A and 108B The result of bands involving the head and neck. In **108A** the abnormality is sometimes called the limb/body wall complex, which might represent early amnion rupture.

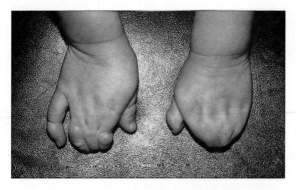

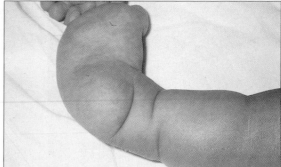

108C and 108D More typical limb defects due to amniotic bands.

AMYOPLASIA

This condition is part of the non-specific 'arthrogryposis' spectrum. All four limbs are affected in approximately two-thirds of patients, the upper limbs predominantly in a quarter, and the lower limbs predominantly in the remainder. The arms are extended and internally rotated at birth, with downward sloping shoulders ('waiter's tip' position). The hands and wrists are held in flexion. In the lower limbs there is usually severe talipes equinovarus, with flexion deformities of other joints associated with skin dimpling. A midline capillary haemangioma occurs in the glabellar region and congenital scoliosis is an occasional feature. Amyoplasia is occasionally associated with gastroschisis. Biopsy reveals extensive replacement of muscle by fibrous and adipose tissue.

Genetic aspects: The majority of cases are sporadic and recurrence risks are small.

References

Hageman G, Ippel EPF, Beemer FA *et al.* (1988). The diagnostic management of newborns with congenital contractures: a nosologic study of 75 cases. *Am J Med Genet* **30**:883–904.

Hall JG, Reed SD, Driscoll EP (1983). Amyoplasia: a common, sporadic condition with congenital contractures. *Am J Med Genet* **15**:571–590.

Reid COMV, Hall JG, Anderson C *et al.* (1986). Association of amyoplasia with gastroschisis, bowel atresia, and defects of the muscular layer of the trunk. *Am J Med Genet* **24**:701–710.

Sarwark JF, MacEwen GD, Scott Cl Jr (1990). Amyoplasia (a common form of arthrogryposis) (Review). *J Bone Joint Surg A* **72**:465–469.

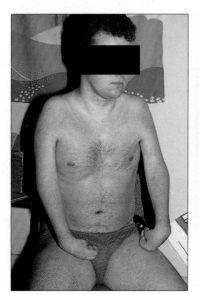

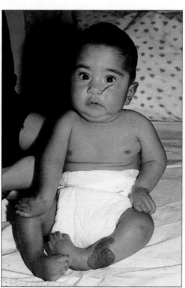

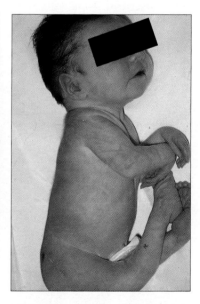

109A and 109B Note sloping shoulders and internally rotated upper limbs.

109C Joint contractures are a major feature.

CEREBRO-OCULO-FACIO-SKELETAL (COFS) SYNDROME

110A–110C

This diagnosis should be considered in infants presenting with microcephaly, microphthalmia, cataracts and joint contractures. There is often early death, and, in those who survive, severe failure to thrive. With increasing age the facial appearance becomes more characteristic, with deep-set eyes, a prominent nasal root and a sloping forehead. Both the jaw and the eyes are small. The condition is probably heterogeneous. Note the similarity with the Neu–Laxova syndrome (see separate entry). There is good evidence that some infants diagnosed initially as COFS subsequently develop Cockayne syndrome, including the sunken eye appearance, sensorineural deafness, photosensitivity, and basal ganglia calcification.

Genetic aspects: Autosomal recessive.

References

Casteels I, Wijnants A, Casaer P et al. (1991). Cerebro-oculo-facioskeletal (COFS) syndrome: the variability of presenting symptoms as a manifestation of two subtypes? *Genetic Counseling* **2**:43–46.

Gershoni-Baruch R, Ludatscher RM, Lichtig C et al. (1991). Cerebro-oculo-facio-skeletal syndrome: further delineation. *Am J Med Genet* **41**:74–77.

Insler MS (1987). Cerebro-oculo-facio-skeletal syndrome. *Ann Ophthalmol* **19**:54–55.

Lowry RB, MacLean R, McLean DM, Tischler B (1971). Cataracts, microcephaly, kyphosis and limited joint movements in two siblings: a new syndrome. *J Pediatr* **79**:282–284.

Patton MA, Giannelli F, Francis AJ et al. (1989). Early onset Cockayne's syndrome: case reports with neuropathological and fibroblast studies. *J Med Genet* **26**:154–159.

Winter RM, Donnai D, Crawfurd MD'A (1981). Syndromes of microcephaly, microphthalmia, cataracts, and joint contractures. *J Med Genet* **18**:129–133.

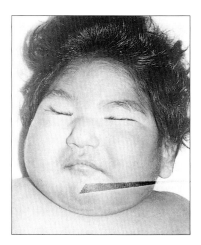
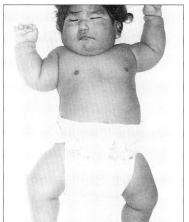
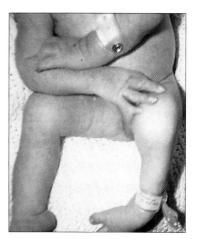

110A Note microcephaly and prominent nasal bridge.

110B and 110C There are multiple joint contractures.

PENA–SHOKEIR – MULTIPLE ANKYLOSES; PULMONARY HYPOPLASIA

111A–111F

Most cases with this condition are stillborn or have early demise. Multiple ankyloses, pulmonary hypoplasia, facial anomalies and polyhydramnios are the characteristic manifestations. Some cases have been found to display a congenital myopathy, some degeneration of the anterior horn cells, and some have had abnormalities of the cerebral cortex and cerebellum (including ischaemia and anoxic damage).

Thus, like the term arthrogryposis, Pena–Shokeir syndrome probably covers a number of separate entities all resulting in the same phenotype.

Genetic aspects: A recurrence risk of 10–15% seems appropriate because some, but not all, cases are autosomal recessive (Hall). The exception to these relatively high risks might be if a good autopsy reveals long-standing ischaemic/anoxic damage of the central nervous system. Maternal myasthenia gravis should always be ruled out by looking for fetal-specific anti-AChR antibodies.

References

Erdl R, Schmidtke K, Jakobeit M et al. (1989). Pena-Shokeir phenotype with major CNS-malformations: clinicopathological report of two siblings. *Clin Genet* **36**:127–135.

Hall JG (1986). Analysis of Pena Shokeir phenotype (Invited editorial comment). *Am J Med Genet* **25**:99–117.

Lavi E, Montone KT, Rorke LB, Kliman HJ (1991). Fetal akinesia deformation sequence (Pena-Shokeir phenotype) associated with acquired intrauterine brain damage. *Neurology* **41**:1467–1468.

Lindhout D et al. (1985). The Pena-Shokeir syndrome: report of nine Dutch cases. *Am J Med Genet* **21**:655–668.

Rodriguez JI, Palacios J (1991). Pathogenetic mechanisms of fetal akinesia deformation sequence and oligohydramnios sequence. *Am J Med Genet* **40**:284–289.

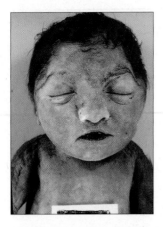 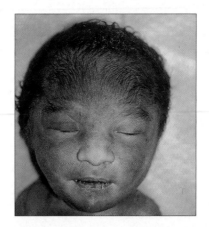 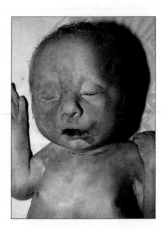

111A–111C Note the depressed nasal tip, prominent nasal bridge, hirsute forehead and facial haemangiomas.

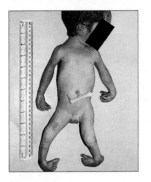 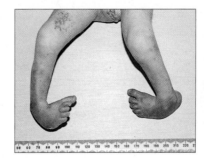 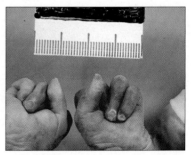

111D–111F Note multiple joint contractures.   **111F**

CAMPTODACTYLY TYPE TEL HASHOMER   111 2A–112D

The phenotype in this syndrome is relatively non-specific and it is likely that a number of mild myopathies could mimic the condition. The diagnosis should be considered in patients with distal arthrogryposis, a small mouth opening and a scoliosis.

The main features in the hands are camptodactyly and mild syndactyly with spindle-shaped fingers, and clinodactyly of the fifth fingers. Other limb abnormalities in some patients include radial dislocation, club feet, hallux valgus and overlapping toes. The face is asymmetrical, and there is ocular hypertelorism, a small mouth with dental crowding, and a high palate. The chest is long and narrow and the muscles, especially of the limbs and hands, appear to be atrophic. Short stature, brachycephaly, and winging of the scapulae are other features.

Genetic aspects: Autosomal recessive.

References

Franceschini P, Vardeu MP (1993). Inguinal hernia and atrial septal defect in Tel Hashomer camptodactyly syndrome: report of a new case expanding the phenotypic spectrum of the disease. *Am J Med Genet* **46**:341–344.

Gollop TR, Colletto GMDD (1984). The Tel Hashomer camptodactyly syndrome in a consanguineous Brazilian family. *Am J Med Genet* **17**:399–406.

Goodman RM, Katznelson B-M, Hertz M et al. (1974). Camptodactyly, with muscular hypoplasia, skeletal dysplasia, and abnormal palmar creases: Tel Hashomer camptodactyly syndrome. *J Med Genet* **13**:136–141.

Patton MA, MacDermot KD, Lake BD et al. (1986). Tel Hashomer camptodactyly syndrome: report of a case with myopathic features. *J Med Genet* **23**:268–271.

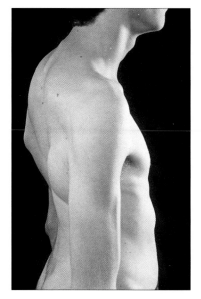
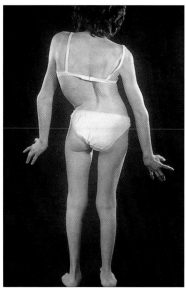

112A and 112B Note scoliosis.

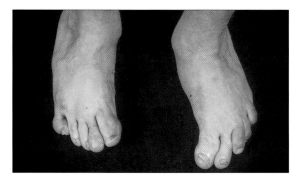
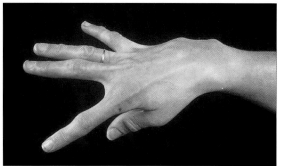

112C and 112D Note camptodactyly of fingers and toes and mild skin syndactyly.

BEAL CONTRACTURAL ARACHNODACTYLY

113A–113B

This syndrome has some features of Marfan syndrome, but joint problems can be more marked and cardiac abnormalities are less common. There is arachnodactyly of the fingers and toes associated with camptodactyly and contractures of the large joints. The latter features improve with age and physiotherapy. In contrast there may be a progressive scoliosis. The helix is flattened and crumpled with some loss of the architecture. Hypoplasia of skeletal muscle has been commented on. Bawle and Quigg reported a case with ectopia lentis and dilatation of the aortic root and pointed out that these features should be looked for.

Genetic aspects: Autosomal dominant. Bistritzer *et al.* reported two double second cousins from an inbred pedigree. They both had features of the condition, although parents were apparently normal. Cardiac examination and general development were normal. Lee *et al.* found linkage to a fibrillin-like gene located at 5q23-31 and this was confirmed by Tsipouras *et al.*

References

Anderson RA, Koch S, Camerino-Otero RD (1984). Cardiovascular findings in congenital contractural arachnodactyly: report of an affected kindred. *Am J Med Genet* **18**:265–271.

Bawle E, Quigg MH (1992). Ectopia lentis and aortic root dilatation in congenital contractural arachnodactyly. *Am J Med Genet* **42**:19–21.

Bistritzer T, Fried K, Lahat E *et al.* (1993). Congenital contractural arachnodactyly in two double second cousins: possible homozygosity. *Clin Genet* **44**:15–19.

Lee B, Godfrey M, Vitale E *et al.* (1991). Linkage of Marfan syndrome and a phenotypically related disorder to two different fibrillin genes (Letter). *Nature* **352**:330–334.

Macnab AJ, D'Orsogna L, Cole DEC *et al.* (1991). Cardiac anomalies complicating congenital contractural arachnodactyly. *Arch Dis Child* **66**:1143–1146.

Meire FM, Delleman WJ, Bleeker-Wagemakers EM (1991). Ocular manifestations of congenital Marfan syndrome with contractures – (CMC syndrome). *Ophthal Paed Genet* **12**:1–9.

Ramos Arroyo MA, Weaver DD, Beals RK (1985). Congenital contractural arachnodactyly. *Clin Genet* **27**:570–581.

Tsipouras P, Del Mastro R, Sarfarazi M *et al*. (1992). Genetic linkage of the Marfan syndrome, ectopia lentis, and congenital contractural arachnodactyly to the fibrillin genes on chromosome 15 and chromosome 5. *New Engl J Med* **326**:905–909.

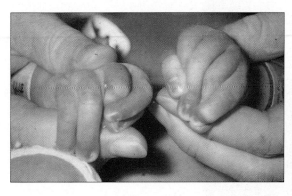
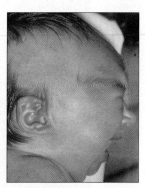

113A and 113B Crumpled helix of the ear, and long fingers with contractures.

LARSEN SYNDROME

There is joint hypermobility, multiple joint dislocations, especially of the knees, and talipes equinovarus. The mid-face is hypoplastic with a depressed nasal bridge. Cleft palate may be present. Radiographs reveal undermineralisation and overtubulation of the long bones, a bifid calcaneus and advanced bone age in the carpals, or extra carpal bones.

Genetic aspects: There is an autosomal dominant form and a more severe autosomal recessive form but in general it is difficult to tell the difference between them on clinical grounds.

References

Bowen JR, Otega K, Ray S, MacEwen GD (1985). Spinal deformities in Larsen's syndrome. *Clin Orthop* **197**:159–163.

Fryns JP, Lenaerts J, Van den Berghe H (1993). Larsen syndrome presenting as a familial syndrome of dwarfism, distinct oldish facial appearance and bilateral clubfeet in mother and daughter. *Genetic Counseling* **4**:43–46.

Larsen LJ, Schottstaedt ER, Bost FD (1950). Multiple congenital dislocations associated with characteristic facial abnormality. *J Pediatr* **37**:574–581.

Latta RJ, Graham CB, Aase JM *et al*. (1971). Larsen's syndrome: a skeletal dysplasia with multiple joint dislocations and unusual facies. *J Pediatr* **78**:291–298.

Stanley CS, Thelin JW, Miles JH (1988). Mixed hearing loss in Larsen syndrome. *Clin Genet* **33**:395–398.

Stanley D, Seymour N (1985). The Larsen syndrome occurring in four generations of one family. *Int Orthop* **8**:267–272.

Ventruto V *et al*. (1976). Larsen syndrome in two generations of an Italian family. *J Med Genet* **13**:538–539.

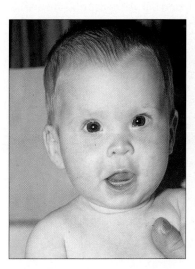
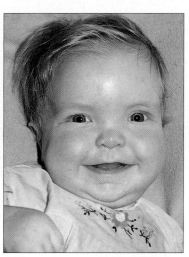

114A and 114B Note the flat mid-face and flat nasal bridge.

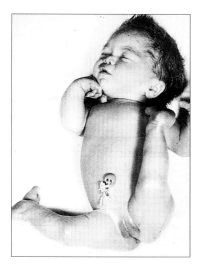

114C There are multiple joint dislocations.

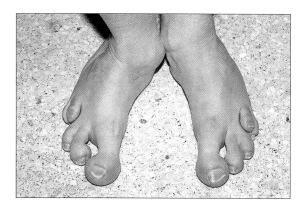

114D The ends of the toes are expanded and bulbous.

POLAND ANOMALY 115A–115B

McGillivray and Lowry estimated the incidence of Poland syndrome in British Columbia to be 1 in 32 000 and their review of the literature suggests a similar incidence from other studies. A hand abnormality is usually seen unilaterally in association with ipsilateral absence of one or more portions of the pectoralis major (usually the sternal head). There is shortening of phalanges and other elements of the digits in association with cutaneous syndactyly. The middle phalanges are relatively more severely affected and distal symphalangism can occur, giving the appearance of hypophalangia. The thumb is least severely affected. Ipsilateral rib defects and absence of the breast or nipple may also occur.

Genetic aspects: Familial recurrence of cases of Poland syndrome, as strictly defined above, are extremely rare, but there are occasional reports (David; Ten Kate *et al.*). Isolated absence of the pectoralis and shoulder girdle muscles without abnormalities of the limbs can be autosomal dominant (David and Winter). Bavinck and Weaver and others have suggested a vascular etiology for Poland syndrome, postulating vascular interruption around the sixth week of development.

References

Bavinck JNB, Weaver DD (1986). Subclavian artery supply disruption sequence: hypothesis of a vascular etiology for Poland, Klippel-Feil, and Moebius anomalies. *Am J Med Genet* **23**:903–918.

David TJ (1982). Familial Poland anomaly. *J Med Genet* **19**:293–296.

David TJ, Winter RM (1985). Familial absence of the pectoralis major, serratus anterior, and latissimus dorsi muscles. *J Med Genet* **22**:390–392.

Fraser FC, Ronen GM, O'Leary E (1989). Pectoralis major defect and Poland sequence in second cousins: extension of the Poland sequence spectrum. *Am J Med Genet* **33**:468–470.

McGillivray BC, Lowry RB (1977). Poland syndrome in British Columbia: incidence and reproductive experience of affected persons. *Am J Med Genet* **1**:65–74.

Ten Kate LP (1989). Poland anomaly in mother and daughter. *Am J Med Genet* **33**:519–521.

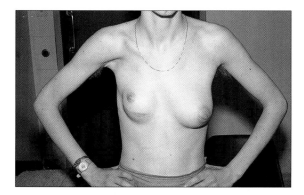

115A Note the aplasia of the pectoralis muscle on the right. The breast on that side is smaller.

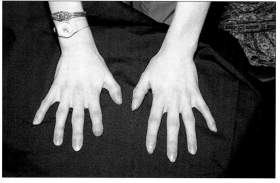

115B Note symbrachydactyly of the right hand.

NAIL – PATELLA SYNDROME (OSTEO-ONYCHODYSPLASIA)   116A–116E

The nails are abnormal from birth and are either absent or small and longitudinally ridged. Triangular lunules at the base of the nails are said to be particularly characteristic. Nails on the radial side of the hand are said to be more severely affected, so that the fourth and fifth fingernails may be relatively normal. Skeletal abnormalities include joint contractures and talipes equinovarus, posterior iliac spurs, a malformed capitellum of the radius, Madelung deformity and absent or hypoplastic patellae. Nephropathy may manifest with proteinuria or intermittent nephrotic syndrome and this will progress to renal failure in 10% of cases.

Genetic aspects: Autosomal dominant. The gene maps to 9q34, close to the COL5A1 collagen gene.

References

Greenspan DS, Byers MG, Eddy RL *et al.* (1992). Human collagen gene COL5A1 maps to the q34.2->q34.3 region of chromosome 9, near the locus for nail-patella syndrome. *Genomics* **12**:836–837.

Guidera KJ, Satter-White Y, Ogden JA *et al.* (1991). Nail patella syndrome: a review of 44 orthopedic patients. *J Pediatr Orthop* **11**:737–742.

Looij B Jr, Te Slaa RL *et al.* (1988). Genetic counselling in hereditary osteo-onychodysplasia (HOOD, nail-patella syndrome) with nephropathy. *J Med Genet* **25**:682–686.

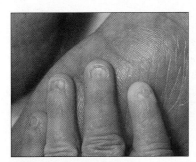
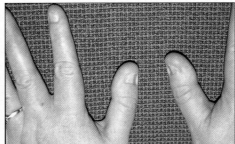

116A and 116B Note the hypoplastic and dystrophic nails.

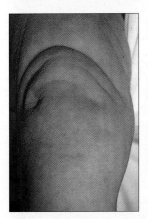
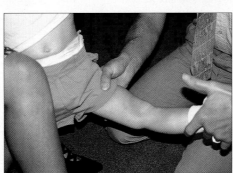
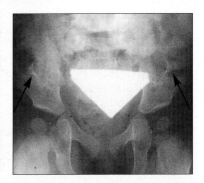

116C and 116D Note the knee deformity because of absence of the patella.

116E Note iliac spurs (arrows).

MULTIPLE PTERYGIUM SYNDROME   117A–117G

At birth there are usually multiple joint contractures with camptodactyly and talipes equinovarus or rocker-bottom feet. Sometimes the characteristic webbing of the joints (pterygia) does not develop until later in infancy. The neck is short and may be webbed. Webs also develop at the axillae and groin. Scoliosis and kyphosis may develop and the stance becomes crouched. The external genitalia can be hypoplastic in both males and females. The face is relatively immobile with downturned corners to the mouth, epicanthic folds and mild ptosis.

Genetic aspects: Autosomal recessive in most cases. Note also that there is a rare autosomal dominant form of multiple pterygium syndrome and severe lethal types, which are probably separate entities.

References

Chen H, Chang C-H, Misra RP *et al.* (1980). Multiple pterygium syndrome. *Am J Med Genet* **7**:91–102.

Hall JG, Reed SD, Rosenbaum KN *et al.* (1982). Limb pterygium syndromes: a review and report of eleven patients. *Am J Med Genet* **12**:377–409.

Thompson EM, Donnai D, Baraitser M *et al.* (1987). Multiple pterygium syndrome: evolution of the phenotype. *J Med Genet* **24**:733–749.

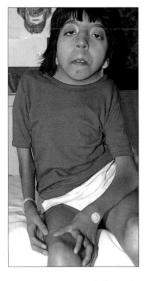 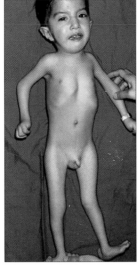 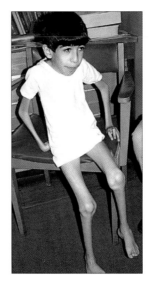 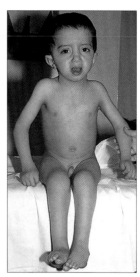

117A–117D Note bilateral ptosis, down-slanting palpebral fissures, and webbing at the elbows, neck and knees.

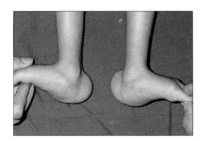 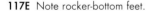 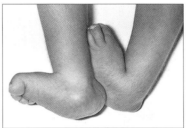 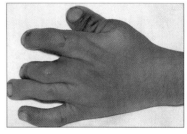

117E Note rocker-bottom feet. **117F** **117G** Note finger contractures often present at birth.

LETHAL MULTIPLE PTERYGIUM SYNDROME

Early in pregnancy multiple joint contractures with skin webs develop. Hypoplastic lungs, a history of polyhydramnios, oedema of the skin and cystic hygromas of the neck are also features of the condition. The face may be characterised by hypertelorism and downward-slanting palpebral fissures, and a cleft palate is common. The condition may be heterogeneous, but most cases appear to have a generalised neuromuscular defect with the other features being secondary.

Genetic aspects: Autosomal recessive.

References

Chen H, Immken L, Lachman R *et al.* (1984). Syndrome of multiple pterygia, camptodactyly, facial anomalies, hypoplastic lungs and heart, cystic hygroma, and skeletal anomalies: delineation of a new entity and review of lethal forms of multiple pterygium syndrome. *Am J Med Genet* **17**:809–826.

Moerman P, Fryns J-P, Cornelis A *et al.* (1990). Pathogenesis of the lethal multiple pterygium syndrome. *Am J Med Genet* **35**:415–421.

Ramer JC, Kilchevsky ES, Ladda RL (1991). Phenotypic variation of multiple pterygium syndrome in siblings, including identical twins. *Dysmorph Clin Genet* **5**:97–106.

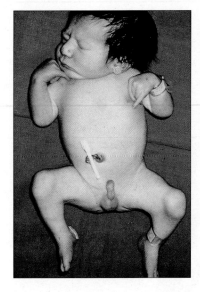
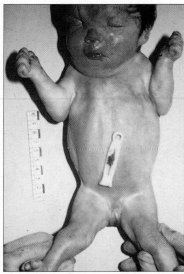

118A and 118B Note pterygia of knees and elbows, short neck, facial haemangioma, hypertelorism, epicanthic folds, flattened nose, talipes equinovarus, rocker-bottom feet, scoliosis and deformed chest.

NEU-LAXOVA SYNDROME

119A–119D

In this lethal syndrome, some infants look bizarre with staring eyes, limb contractures and grossly swollen hands and feet, in others, the phenotype may be less striking. Usually there is severe microcephaly, intrauterine growth retardation, absent eyelids, microphthalmia, cataracts, a hypoplastic nose, multiple joint contractures, skin syndactyly of the fingers, collodion skin and subcutaneous oedema. CNS abnormalities include lissencephaly, agenesis of the corpus callosum and a hypoplastic cerebellum.

Genetic aspects: Autosomal recessive.

References

Curry CJR (1982). Further comments on the Neu-Laxova syndrome. *Am J Med Genet* **13**:441–444.

Mueller RF, Winter RM, Naylor CPE (1983). Neu Laxova syndrome: two further case reports and comments on proposed subclassification. *Am J Med Genet* **16**:645–649.

Neu R, Kijii T, Gardner L, Nagyfy S, King S (1971). A lethal syndrome of microcephaly with multiple congenital anomalies in three siblings. *Pediatrics* **47**:610–612.

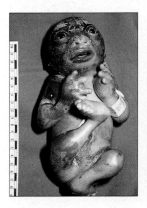
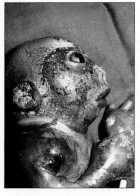
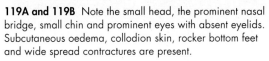
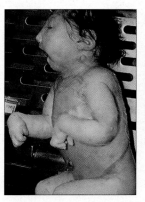
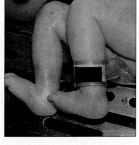

119A and 119B Note the small head, the prominent nasal bridge, small chin and prominent eyes with absent eyelids. Subcutaneous oedema, collodion skin, rocker bottom feet and wide spread contractures are present.

119C and 119D In some cases the facial features are less severe and there may be the appearance of 'collodion' skin.

MARDEN–WALKER SYNDROME
120A–120C

The features are blepharophimosis, microcephaly, micrognathia, multiple joint contractures, arachnodactyly, camptodactyly, kyphoscoliosis and delayed motor development. Associated features include low-set malformed ears, cleft palate, cerebral atrophy, and microcysts of the kidney. Congenital heart disease (dextrocardia and abnormal connections of the venae cavae) has also been seen. This syndrome is likely to consist more of a 'sequence' secondary to early neurological abnormalities and as such is probably genetically heterogeneous.

Genetic aspects: Autosomal recessive in definite cases.

References
Garcia-Alix A, Blanco D, Cabanas F *et al.* (1992). Early neurological manifestations and brain anomalies in Marden–Walker syndrome. *Am J Med Genet* **44**:41–45.
Giacoia GP, Pineda R (1990). Expanded spectrum of findings in Marden–Walker syndrome. *Am J Med Genet* **36**:495–499.
Linder N, Mathot I, Livoff A *et al.* (1991). Congenital myopathy with oculo-facial abnormalities (Marden–Walker syndrome). *Am J Med Genet* **39**:377–379.
Marden PM, Walker WA (1966). A new generalized connective tissue syndrome. *Am J Dis Child* **112**:225–228.
Ramer JC, Frankel CA, Ladda RL (1993). Marden–Walker phenotype: spectrum of variability in three infants. *Am J Med Genet* **45**:285–291.

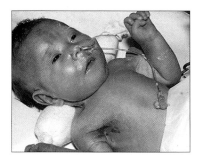 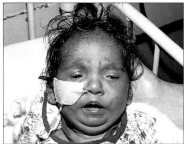 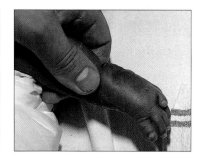

120A–120C Note the small mouth, short palpebral fissures, expressionless face, small nose with long philtrum, and long fingers and toes with joint contractures.

LIMB DEFECTS ASSOCIATED WITH HAEMATOLOGICAL ABNORMALITIES

AASE – TRIPHALANGEAL THUMB; CONGENITAL ANAEMIA
121A–121B

There is still controversy about the existence of this condition as an entity separate from Blackfan–Diamond congenital erythroid hypoplastic anaemia that may be steroid responsive. The main distinguishing features are hypoplastic or triphalangeal thumbs, cleft lip and palate and cardiac lesions. However, in a review of 200 cases of congenital erythroid hypoplastic anaemia, all thought to be the Blackfan–Diamond syndrome, 17 individuals had abnormal thumbs, nine had triphalangeal thumbs, three duplicated and three bifid thumbs. A flattened thenar eminence was found even when the thumbs appeared normal. This suggests that thumb abnormalities are an occasional feature of Blackfan–Diamond syndrome and may not represent a separate entity.

Genetic aspects: This is still uncertain. Aase and Smith originally reported affected siblings with normal parents, suggesting autosomal recessive inheritance. However, Hurst *et al.* reported a mother with congenital hypoplastic anaemia and normal limbs who had a son with absent thumbs and congenital hypoplastic anaemia.

The inheritance pattern of the Blackfan–Diamond syndrome has also not yet been clarified; most cases are thought to be sporadic, although dominant pedigrees have also been described (Hunter and Hakami; Voskochil *et al.*).

References

Aase JM, Smith DW (1969). Congenital anemia and triphalangeal thumbs: a new syndrome. *J Pediatr* **74**:417.

Alter BP (1978). Thumbs and anemia. *Pediatrics* **62**:613–614.

Hunter RE, Hakami N (1972). The occurrence of congenital hypoplastic anemia in half brothers. *J Pediatr* **81**:346–348.

Hurst JA, Baraitser M, Wonke B (1991). Autosomal dominant transmission of congenital erythroid hypoplastic anemia with radial abnormalities. *Am J Med Genet* **40**:482–484.

Muis N, Beemer FA, Van Dijken P et al. (1986). Aase syndrome. Case report and review of the literature. *Eur J Pediatr* **145**:153–157.

Viskochil DH, Carey JC, Glader BE et al. (1990). Congenital hypoplastic (Diamond–Blackfan) anemia in seven members of one kindred. *Am J Med Genet* **35**:251–256.

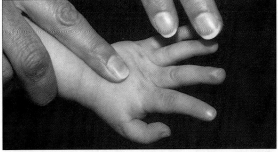

121A Note short thumb.

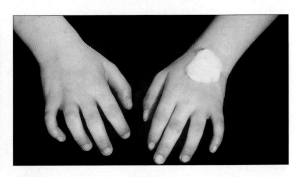

121B Note the triphalangeal thumbs.

THROMBOCYTOPENIA – ABSENT RADIUS (TAR) SYNDROME

121A-121B (labelled at right) **122A–122D**

Characteristically, there is radial aplasia, with preservation of the thumbs. Thrombocytopenia of early onset occurs. Megakaryocytes are reduced and anaemia, eosinophilia and a leukaemoid granulocytosis may be seen. If the infant survives, the haematological features become less severe. Lower limb malformations, congenital heart defect, and abnormalities of the ribs and cervical spine may also be seen.

Genetic aspects: Autosomal recessive.

References

Donnenfeld AE, Wiseman B, Lavi E, Weiner S (1990). Prenatal diagnosis of thrombocytopenia absent radius syndrome by ultrasound and cordocentesis. *Prenatal Diagn* **10**:29–35.

Hall JG. Syndrome of the month: thrombocytopenia and absent radius (TAR) syndrome (1987). *J Med Genet* **24**:79–83.

Hedberg VA, Lipton JM. Thrombocytopenia with absent radii: a review of 100 cases (1988). *Am J Ped Hemat Oncol* **10**:51–64.

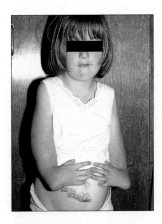

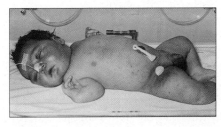

122B

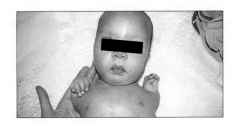

122D

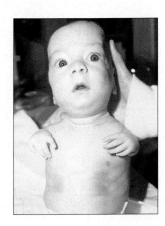

122C

122A–122D Note varying degrees of limb abnormalities with bilateral radial aplasia in **122A** and **122B**, and more severe upper limb defects in **122C** and **122D**. Note that the thumbs are present.

The initial signs of this condition may be radial defects at birth including hypoplasia of the thumbs, or occasionally supernumerary thumbs, and hypoplasia of the radius. The pancytopenia presents with mean age of onset of about 8 years and there is a tendency to leukaemia. Microcephaly, mental retardation and growth retardation are features, and bilateral mild hearing loss, with or without malformation of the ears, can occur. Patchy hyperpigmentation of the skin is a good clue to the diagnosis before the haematological abnormalities appear. Renal abnormalities, which occur in a quarter to a third of patients, are variable, and may include complete absence of one kidney, hypoplasia, or horseshoe kidney or double ureters. Chromosome breakage should be looked for. Auerbach *et al.*, (1985; 1989) have recommended the use of the DNA clastogen diepoxybutane for the investigation of possible Fanconi cases.

Note that some infants with hydrocephalus and VATER association have been shown to have Fanconi pancytopenia (Porteous *et al.*, Toriello *et al.*). There are also cases without skeletal or skin abnormalities who may just be mildly microcephalic.

Genetic aspects: Autosomal recessive. Linkage data are still confusing with both 9q and 20q being suggested as possible locations (Mann *et al.*).

References

Auerbach AD, Sagi M, Adler B (1985). Fanconi anemia: prenatal diagnosis in 30 fetuses at risk. *Pediatrics* **76**:794–800.

Auerbach AD, Rogatko A, Schroeder-Kurth TM (1989). International Fanconi Anemia Registry: relation of clinical symptoms to diepoxybutane sensitivity. *Blood* **73**:391–396.

Gordon-Smith EC, Rutherford TR (1991). Fanconi anemia – constitutional aplastic anemia (Review). *Semin Hematol* **28**:104–112.

Macdougall LG, Greeff MC, Rosendorff J, Bernstein R (1990). Fanconi anemia in black African children. *Am J Med Genet* **36**:408–413.

Mann WR, Venkatraj VS, Allen RG et al. (1991). Fanconi anemia: evidence for linkage heterogeneity on chromosome 20q. *Genomics* **9**:329–337.

Porteous MEM, Cross I, Burn J (1992). VACTERL with hydrocephalus: one end of the Fanconi anemia spectrum of anomalies? *Am J Med Genet* **43**:1032–1034.

Toriello HV, Pearson G, Sommer A (1993). Possible form of Fanconi pancytopenia as a phenocopy of the VACTERL association (Letter). *Clin Dysmorphol* **2**:183–185.

123 Note radial aplasia and pigmented macules.

BONE DYSPLASIAS

ACHONDROPLASIA 124A–124G

Achondroplasia can be diagnosed at birth. Clinically, there is rhizomelic limb shortening and a large head with a broad and prominent forehead. The fingers are short, tapered and splayed ('a trident hand'). Radiologically, the pelvis is abnormal with small square iliac wings, horizontal acetabular roofs and narrowing of the greater sciatic notch. Projecting medially from the acetabular roof there is a bony spike. The long bones are short and the metaphyses slope. There is a translucent area at the proximal ends of the femora in the neonatal period. Later, narrowing of the interpedicular distances in the lumbar region becomes evident. Because of the narrow chest, respiratory problems are not infrequent. A significant number of cases develop pyramidal signs in their lower limbs, because of an abnormal foramen magnum, resulting in either compression or hydrocephalus. Spinal cord stenosis might be an additional problem. Normal growth curves are provided by Horton *et al.*

Genetic aspects: Autosomal dominant. Most cases are fresh mutations and in these cases recurrence risks are small. However, there is a small risk to normal parents as germ-line mosaicism cannot be excluded. Where both parents are affected, homozygous cases can occur. These infants are much more severely affected and usual die early from compression of the foramen magnum and respiratory failure (Hall *et al.*). The gene maps to 4p and mutations have been demonstrated in the fibroblast growth factor receptor 3 (FGFR3) gene.

References

Dodinval P, Le Marec B (1987). Genetic counseling in unexpected familial recurrence of achondroplasia. *Am J Med Genet* **28**:949–955.

Hall JG, Dorst JP, Taybi H *et al.* (1969). Two probable cases of homozygosity for the achondroplasia gene. *BDOAS* **5(4)**:24–34.

Hecht JT, Butler IJ (1990). Neurologic morbidity associated with achondroplasia. *J Child Neurol* **5**:84–97.

Horton WA *et al.* (1978). Standard growth curves for achondroplasia. *J Pediatr* **93**:435–438.

Lavini F, Renzi-Brivio L, de Bastiani G (1990). Psychologic, vascular, and physiologic aspects of lower limb lengthening in achondroplastics. *Clin Orthop* **250**:138–142.

Pauli RM, Scott CI, Wassman ER *et al.* (1984). Apnea and sudden unexpected death in infants with achondroplasia. *J Pediatr* **104**:342–348.

Philip N, Auger M, Mattei JF, Giraud F (1988). Achondroplasia in siblings of normal parents. *J Med Genet* 1988;**25**:857–859.

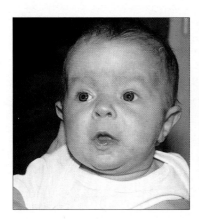
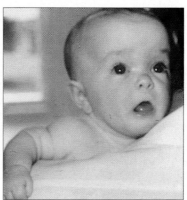

124A and 124B Note the large head with prominent forehead.

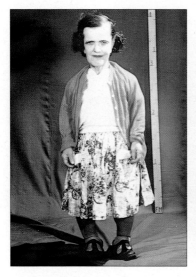
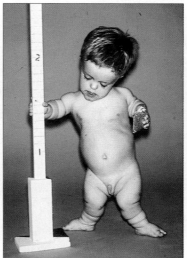
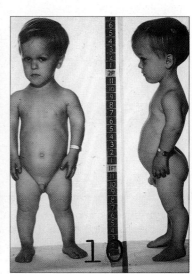

124C and 124D Note the rhizomelic limb shortening.

124E Note the lumbar lordosis.

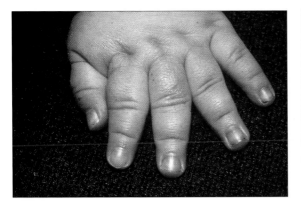

124F Note the trident-shaped hand.

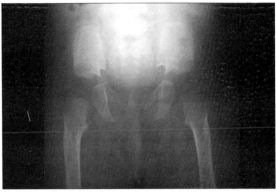

124G Note the short round iliac crests, narrow sacrosciatic notches, horizontal acetabular roof and oval translucency of proximal femora.

HYPOCHONDROPLASIA   125

The diagnosis might be difficult in the neonatal period, despite the presence of mild rhizomelic limb shortening and some bossing of the forehead. Limb shortening is less severe than in achondroplasia, and the two conditions breed true in families. Radiologically, the long bones are short with widened diaphyses and flared metaphyses. The fibulae seem to be disproportionately long. The interpedicular distance in the spine narrows caudally. These findings might not be clearly evident until the second or third year of life. Mild mental retardation has been suggested as a feature in 10–20% of cases. However, Wynne-Davies *et al.* found no evidence of this.

Genetic aspects: Autosomal dominant. FGFR3 mutations have been found.

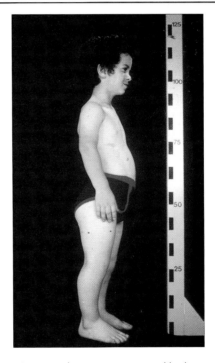

125 Note short stature, increased lumbar lordosis, rhizomelic shortening of the limbs and mild frontal bossing.

References
Appan S, Laurent S, Chapman M *et al.* (1990). Growth and growth hormone therapy in hypochondroplasia. *Acta Paediatr Scand* **79**:796–803.

Hall BD, Spranger J (1979). Hypochondroplasia: clinical and radiological aspects in 39 cases. *Radiology* **133**:95–100.

Maroteaux P, Falzon P (1988). Hypochondroplasia. Review of 80 cases. *Arch Fr Pediatr* **45**:105–110.

Sommer A, Young-Wee T, Frye T (1987). Achondroplasia-hypochondroplasia complex. *Am J Med Genet* **26**:949–958.

Wynne-Davies R, Patton MA (1991). The frequency of mental retardation in hypochondroplasia (Letter). *J Med Genet* **28**:644.

THANATOPHORIC DYSPLASIA   126A–126D

The limbs are very short and the chest is narrow. Most infants die within a few hours of birth from respiratory failure. The head is large with a prominent forehead and a depressed nasal bridge. Radiographs reveal shortening of the long bones with metaphyseal flaring and cupping, and characteristically curved femurs ('telephone receiver'). The iliac wings are hypoplastic and the sacrosciatic notches narrow.

Severe flattening of the vertebral bodies is seen which gives an 'H' or inverted 'U' shape when the lower thoracic and lumbar vertebrae are viewed on an AP radiograph. The incidence is about 1 in 20 000.

Genetic aspects: Most cases are sporadic. The condition is probably caused by a lethal autosomal dominant gene. Mutations of the Fibroblast Growth Factor 3 (FGFR3) gene have been demonstrated.

References

Elejalde BR, Mercedes de Elejalde M (1985). Thanatophoric dysplasia: fetal manifestations and prenatal diagnosis. *Am J Med Genet* **22**:669–683.

MacDonald IM, Hunter AGW *et al.* (1989). Growth and development in thanatophoric dysplasia. *Am J Med Genet* **33**:508–512.

Martinez-Frias ML *et al.* (1988). Thanatophoric dysplasia: an autosomal dominant condition? *Am J Med Genet* **31**:815–820.

Sillence DO, Rimoin DL, Lachman RS (1978). Neonatal dwarfism. *Pediatr Clin N Am* **25**:453–483.

Van Der Harten HJ, Brons JTJ, Dijkstra PF *et al.* (1993). Some variants of lethal neonatal short-limbed platyspondylic dysplasia: a radiological, ultrasonographic, neuropathological and histopathological study of 22 cases. *Clin Dysmorphol* **2**:1–19.

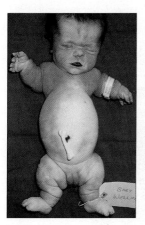 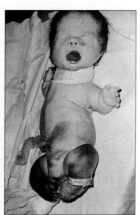 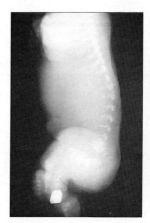 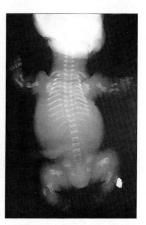

126A and 126B Note the short bowed limbs, small thorax, large head, and mid-facial hypoplasia.

126C and 126D Note the very short tubular bones with metaphyseal flaring and cupping, and the characteristic 'telephone receiver' femora. The vertebral bodies are flat, giving an inverted U- or H-shaped appearance in the AP projection.

THANATOPHORIC DYSPLASIA – CLOVER-LEAF SKULL 127

Thanatophoric dysplasia (TD) associated with a clover-leaf skull is a separate condition from isolated TD. In comparison with TD, the long bones are longer and may not be bowed; histological changes in the cartilage are similar but not so severe. The skull changes are very unusual in that the basal and occipital bones are underdeveloped so that the parietal bones form most of the back of the skull.

Genetic aspects: Mutations of the fibroblast growth factor 3 (FGFR3) gene have been demonstrated and most cases appear to represent new mutations, although affected siblings have been reported.

References

Corsello G, Maresi E, Rossi C *et al.* (1992). Thanatophoric dysplasia in monozygotic twins discordant for clover-leaf skull: prenatal diagnosis, clinical and pathological findings. *Am J Med Genet* **42**:122–126.

Kremens B, Kemperdick H, Borchard F *et al.* (1982). Thanatophoric dysplasia with clover-leaf skull. Case report and review of the literature. *Eur J Pediatr* **139**:298–303.

Machin GA (1992). Thanatophoric dysplasia in monozygotic twins discordant for clover-leaf skull: prenatal diagnosis, clinical and pathological findings. *Am J Med Genet* **44**:842.

Partington MW, Gonzales-Crussi F, Khakee SG, Wollin DG (1971). Clover-leaf skull and thanatophoric dwarfism. Report of four cases, two in the same siblingship. *Arch Dis Child* **46**:656–664.

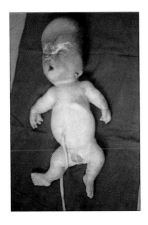

127 Note the clover-leaf skull appearance.

ACHONDROGENESIS TYPES 1 AND 2

128A–128B

Achondrogenesis type 1 (Parenti–Fraccaro type) and type 2 (Langer–Saldino type) are difficult to distinguish clinically. Both result in stillbirth or neonatal death and are characterised by severe micromelia, a relatively large head, a short neck, a short trunk and a protuberant abdomen. There is a flat nasal bridge and the nose is short with anteverted nostrils. Ossification of the skull, spine and pelvis is more deficient in type 1 than in type 2. The long bones are more severely micromelic in type 1 and there are spiky metaphyseal spurs in both, but more so in type 1. This group of conditions must be differentiated from hypochondrogenesis and lethal spondylo-epiphyseal dysplasia congenita – but this can be difficult (Borochowitz *et al.*). Indeed, the latter conditions and achondrogenesis type 2 appear to form a clinical spectrum of conditions caused by type 2 collagen defects (Spranger *et al.*).

Genetic aspects: Type 1 may be inherited as an autosomal recessive in some cases. Most cases of type 2 are sporadic and are likely to represent new autosomal dominant mutations.

References

Borochowitz Z, Lachman R *et al.* (1988). Achondrogenesis type I: delineation of further heterogeneity and identification of two distinct subgroups. *J Pediatr* **112**:23–31.
Borochowitz ZVI, Ornoy A, Lachman R *et al.* (1986). Achondrogenesis II-hypochondrogenesis: variability versus heterogeneity. *Am J Med Genet* **24**:273–288.
Spranger J, Winterpacht A, Zabel B (1994). The type II collagenopathies: a spectrum of chondrodysplasias. *Eur J Pediatr* **153**:56–65.
Whitley CB, Gorlin RJ (1983). Achondrogenesis: new nosology with evidence of genetic heterogeneity. *Radiology* **148**:693–698.

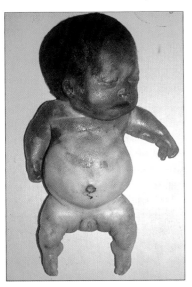

128A Note relatively large head, flat mid-face, short limbs and short trunk.

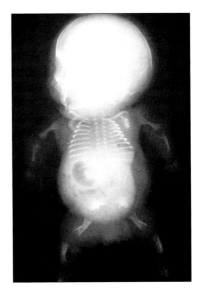

128B Achondrogeneis type 2. Note poor ossification of vertebral bodies and pelvis, and short long bones with metaphyseal widening.

HYPOCHONDROGENESIS

Clinically, the face is flat, with a depressed nasal bridge, a small thorax and a relatively large head. The limbs are short and the infant seems oedematous. Radiologically, the ribs are short, the iliac wings are hypoplastic, the acetabular roofs are flat, the femora are short and there are severe metaphyseal irregularities. The vertebral bodies are almost unossified, especially in the cervical region. Less severely affected infants might show some thoracolumbar ossification. This term was originally used by Stanescu *et al.* to denote a condition, lethal in the neonatal period, that radiologically resembles SED congenita and, morphologically, achondrogenesis type II, but with milder features. It seems likely that hypochondrogenesis and achondrogenesis type II are not distinct disorders, but are part of a disease spectrum.

Genetic aspects: All cases have been sporadic, and a new mutation for an autosomal dominant gene seems likely. Mutations in type II collagen genes have been demonstrated.

References

Borochowitz ZVI, Ornoy A, Lachman R *et al.* (1986). Achondrogenesis II-hypochondrogenesis: variability versus heterogeneity. *Am J Med Genet* **24**:273–288.

Horton WA, Machado MA, Ellard J *et al.* (1992). Characterization of a type II collagen gene (COL2A1) mutation identified in cultured chondrocytes from human hypochondrogenesis. *Proc Nat Acad Sci* **89**:4583–4587.

Maroteaux P, Stanescu V, Stanescu R (1983). Hypochondrogenesis. *Eur J Pediatr* **141**:14–22.

Stanescu V, Stanescu R, Maroteaux P (1977). Etude morphologique et biochemique du cartilage de croissance dans les osteochondrodysplasies. *Arch Fr Pediatr* **34**:Suppl.3.

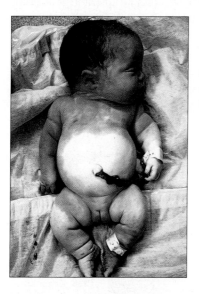

129A Note short rhizomelic limbs, short neck, large head and short thorax. The infant appears oedematous.

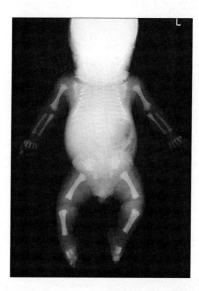

129B Note short ribs, hypoplastic iliac wings, flat acetabular roofs, and short tubular bones with metaphyseal widening. The vertebral bodies, especially in the cervical spine, are very poorly ossified.

ATELOSTEOGENESIS TYPE I

This is a form of short-limbed skeletal dysplasia where the diagnosis must be made from the radiological features. The face is characterised by micrognathia, a flat nasal bridge, mid-face hypoplasia, haemangiomas and cleft palate. There is rhizomelic shortening of the limbs, with talipes equinovarus and brachydactyly of the hands. Most cases die in the neonatal period, but note that there are sub-types with longer survival. The hallmark of the condition is a hypoplastic humerus that tapers distally. Other radiological features include a hypoplastic femur, platyspondyly, vertebral coronal clefts and absent or hypoplastic carpals, tarsals, metacarpals, metatarsals, and proximal and middle phalanges.

Genetic aspects: Uncertain.

References

Hunter AGW, Carpenter BF (1991). Atelosteogenesis I and boomerang dysplasia: a question of nosology. *Clin Genet* **39**:471–480.

Kozlowski K, Bateson EM (1984). Atelosteogenesis. *ROEFO* **140**:224–225.

Maroteaux P, Spranger J, Stanescu V (1982). Atelosteogenesis. *Am J Med Genet* **13**:15–25.

Stevenson RE, Wilkes G (1983). Atelosteogenesis with survival beyond the neonatal period. *Proc Gr Genet Center* **2**:32–38.

Temple K, Hall CA, Chitty L, Baraitser M (1990). A case of atelosteogenesis. *J Med Genet* **27**:194–197.

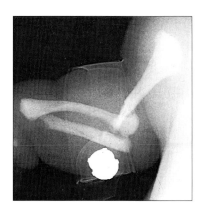

130 Note the tapering of the distal humerus

DIASTROPHIC DYSPLASIA

This severe bone dysplasia is characterised at birth by short limbs, severe talipes equinovarus, hitch-hiker (abducted) thumbs, a cleft palate in many, a characteristic swelling of the pinnae, which assumes the character of a cauliflower ear, and occasional dislocations of joints. Respiratory problems, due to a narrow chest and micrognathia, can be a cause of early death. Radiologically there is marked shortening of the first metacarpal, irregular lengths of the metacarpals, and bizarre ossification of the hand bones. Epiphyses and metaphyses are irregular and there is a 'V'-shaped or chevron deformity at the distal ends of the femora and tibiae. The vertebral bodies are irregular.

Genetic aspects: Autosomal recessive. Hastbacka *et al.* (1990) localised the gene to 5q and the same authors (Hastbacka *et al.* 1993) reported prenatal diagnosis using linked markers. Where linkage is not possible, ultrasound scanning looking at limb length is useful. Hastbacka *et al.* (1994) isolated the gene. It is a novel sulphate transporter gene.

References

Gustavson K-H, Holmgren G, Jagell S *et al.* (1985). Lethal and non-lethal diastrophic dysplasia. A study of 14 Swedish cases. *Clin Genet* **28**:321–334.

Hastbacka J, Kaitila I, Sistonen P, De la Chapelle A (1990). Diastrophic dysplasia gene maps to the distal long arm of chromosome 5. *Proc Nat Acad Sci* **87**:8056–8059.

Hastbacka J, Salonen R, Laurila P *et al.* (1993). Prenatal diagnosis of diastrophic dysplasia with polymorphic DNA markers. *J Med Genet* **30**:265–268.

Hastbacka J, De la Chapelle A, Mahtani MM *et al.* The diastrophic dysplasia gene encodes a novel sulfate transporter: positional cloning by fine-structure linkage disequilibrium mapping. *Cell* 1994;**78**:1073–1087.

Kaitila I, Ammala P, Karjalainen O *et al.* (1983). Early prenatal detection of diastrophic dysplasia. *Prenatal Diagn* **3**:237–244.

Poussa M, Merikanto J, Ryoppy S *et al.* (1991). The spine in diastrophic dysplasia. *Spine* **16**:881–887.

Richards BS (1991). Atlanto-axial instability in diastrophic dysplasia. A case report. *J Bone Joint Surg A* **73**:614–616.

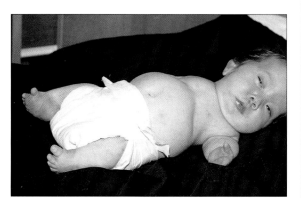

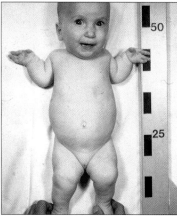

131A–131E Note the short limbs, club feet, small jaw, cystic swelling of the ears and short, proximally inserted, abducted thumbs (hitchhiker thumbs).

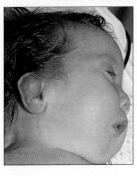

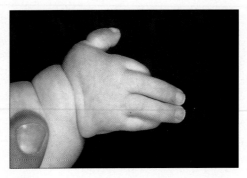

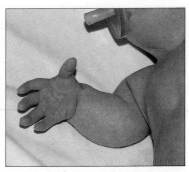

131C   **131D**   **131E**

CAMPTOMELIC DYSPLASIA

132A–132D

The hallmark of this condition is bowing of long bones, particularly the femur and tibia, sometimes with overlying skin dimples. Characteristically, the scapulae are hypoplastic. There is a large head, a small jaw, a cleft palate and a flat nasal bridge. The ears may be malformed and low-set. The chest is narrow and respiratory distress is common. Congenital dislocation of the hip occurs in the majority of patients, as does bilateral talipes equinovarus. A third of patients have cardiac defects (VSD, ASD, Fallot tetralogy) and a third of patients have hydronephrosis, mostly unilateral. Medullary cystic disease is a less common association. Ambiguous genitalia occur in the majority of patients with an XY karyotype. Other frequent malformations include laryngomalacia or tracheomalacia, hydrocephalus and arrhinencephaly.

Care should be taken in making the diagnosis – not all infants with bent long bones have this condition. Conversely, Friedrich *et al.* pointed out that the condition can occur without overt camptomelia.

Genetic aspects: Autosomal dominant. Cases have been reported with apparently balanced rearrangements in the 17q12-25 region (Tommerup *et al.*). Mutations in the Sox9 gene have been demonstrated (Foster *et al.*). Most cases are sporadic but occasional affected siblings have been reported.

References
Foster JW, Dominguez-Steglich MA, Guioli S *et al.* Campomelic dysplasia and autosomal sex reversal caused by mutations in an SRY-related gene. *Nature* 1994;**372**:525–530.

Friedrich U, Schaefer E, Meinecke P (1992). Campomelic dysplasia without overt campomelia (case report). *Clin Dysmorphol* **1**:172–178.

Houston CS, Opitz JM, Spranger JW *et al* (1983). The campomelic syndrome: review, report of 17 cases, and follow-up on the currently 17-year-old boy first reported by Maroteaux *et al* in 1971. *Am J Med Genet* **15**:3–28.

Tommerup N, Schempp W, Meinecke P *et al* (1993). Assignment of an autosomal sex reversal locus (SRA1) and campomelic dysplasia (CMPD1) to 17q24.3-q25.1. *Nature Genetics* **4**:170–174.

Young ID, Zuccollo JM, Maltby EL, Broderick NJ (1992). Campomelic dysplasia associated with a de novo 2q;17q reciprocal translocation. *J Med Genet* **29**:251–252.

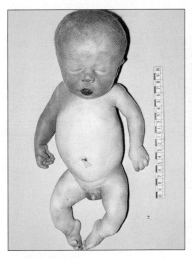

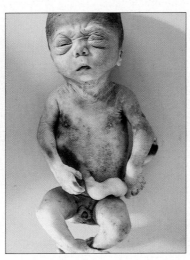

132A and 132B Note short bowed limbs, talipes equinovarus, flat midface, low nasal bridge and small jaw.

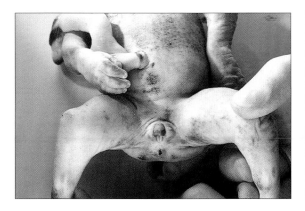

132C Note ambiguous genitalia.

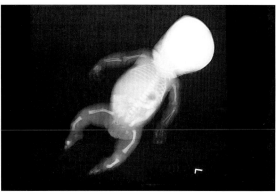

132D There is radiological evidence of radial and tibial bowing and hypoplastic scapulae.

KYPHOMELIC DYSPLASIA

133A–133B

In this condition there are short angulated femurs and bowing of other long bones. There are deep dimples over the angulation of the femurs. The face is characterised by micrognathia and a capillary haemangioma over the forehead and glabella. Associated features include mesomelic or rhizomelic shortening of the upper limbs, short ribs, flared irregular metaphyses and mid-face hypoplasia. In some cases the bowing improves with age. Intelligence is usually normal. This may well be a heterogeneous group. Pitt (1986) pointed out the similarities to femoral hypoplasia-unusual facies syndrome.

Genetic aspects: Inheritance is possibly autosomal recessive.

References

Maclean RN, Prater WK, Lozzio CB (1983). Skeletal dysplasia with short, angulated femora (kyphomelic dysplasia). *Am J Med Genet* **14**:373–380.

Pitt D (1986). Kyphomelic dysplasia versus femoral hypoplasia-unusual facies syndrome (Letter). *Am J Med Genet* **24**:365–366.

Temple IK, Thompson EM, Hall CM *et al* (1989). Kyphomelic dysplasia. *J Med Genet* **26**:457–460.

Turnpenny PD, Dakwar RA, Boulos FN (1990). Kyphomelic dysplasia: the first ten cases. *J Med Genet* **27**:269–272.

Viljoen D, Beighton P (1988). Kyphomelic dysplasia: further delineation of the phenotype. *Dysmorph Clin Genet* **1**:136–141.

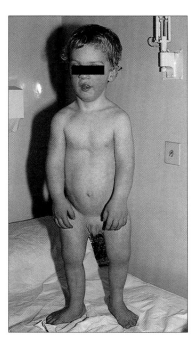

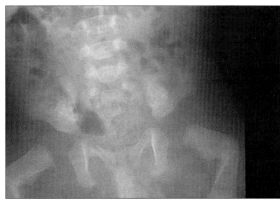

133A and 133B Note the rhizomelic shortening of the lower limbs and on X-ray the acute angulation of the femora.

OSTEOGENESIS IMPERFECTA TYPE I

This is the commonest form of osteogenesis imperfecta. Affected individuals may have blue sclerae with a tendency to fractures of the long bones, although healing occurs without deformity. In some families dentinogenesis imperfecta is a feature. Radiographs may reveal wormian bones of the skull and mild osteoporosis.

Genetic aspects: Autosomal dominant. Cells from individuals with type I OI secrete about half the normal amount of type I procollagen and the gene has been linked to one of the type I collagen loci, one at 7q21-22 and one at 17q21-22, in most families (Sykes).

References

Byers PH, Wallis GA, Willing MC (1991). Osteogenesis imperfecta: translation of mutation to phenotype (Review). *J Med Genet* **28**:433–442.

Cole DEC, Cohen MM Jr (1991). Osteogenesis imperfecta: an update (Editorial). *J Pediatr* **119**:73–74.

Prockop DJ (1992). Seminars in medicine of the Beth Israel Hospital, Boston. Mutations in collagen genes as a cause of connective tissue disease. *New Engl J Med* **326**:540–546.

Sykes B(1993). Linkage analysis in dominantly inherited osteogenesis imperfecta. *Am J Med Genet* **45**:212–216.

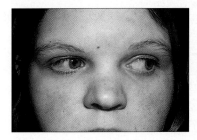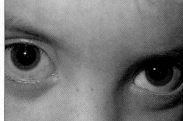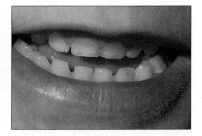

134A and 134B Note the blue sclerae.　　　　　　**134C** Note dentogenesis imperfecta.

OSTEOGENESIS IMPERFECTA TYPE II

This is the severe, usually lethal, form of osteogenesis imperfecta. The chest is narrow. The nose might be beaked and there are blue sclerae. There is a marked reduction of ossification of the cranial vault and facial bones. Beading of the ribs, indicating multiple fractures, is characteristic. The femora are broad and crumpled. The other long bones may have a similar appearance, or have multiple fractures. The vertebrae are flattened and hypoplastic, and the pelvis is hypoplastic with flattening of the acetabular roofs and iliac crests.

Genetic aspects: Sillence *et al.* have subdivided this condition into three separate subgroups according to radiological features. It is likely that most cases of OI type IIA are caused by new dominant mutations of one of the type I collagen genes, although recurrences have been reported which are thought to be caused by gonadal mosaicism in one parent. The overall recurrence risk is about 5%. Recurrence risks in types IIB and IIC are probably higher, as several affected siblings have been reported, as well as a higher incidence of parental consanguinity (Thompson *et al.*; Sillence *et al.*).

References

Edwards MJ, Wenstrup RJ, Byers PH, Cohn DH (1992). Recurrence of lethal osteogenesis imperfecta due to parental mosaicism for a mutation in the COL1A2 gene of type I collagen. The mosaic parent exhibits phenotypic features of a mild form of the disease. *Hum Mutat* **1**:47–54.

Sillence DO, Barlow KK, Garber AP *et al.* (1984). Osteogenesis imperfecta type II. Delineation of the phenotype with reference to genetic heterogeneity. *Am J Med Genet* **17**:407–423.

Thompson EM, Young ID, Hall CM, Pembrey ME (1987). Recurrence risks and prognosis in severe sporadic osteogenesis imperfecta. *J Med Genet* **24**:390–405.

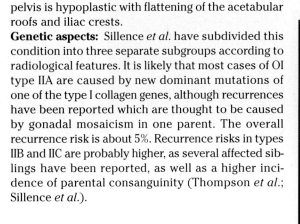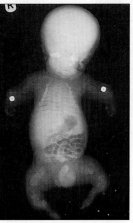

135A Note marked reduction of ossification of cranial vault, continuous beading of the ribs, and broad and crumpled femora with fine wavy margins.

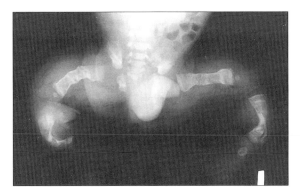

135B The long bones are short and crumpled.

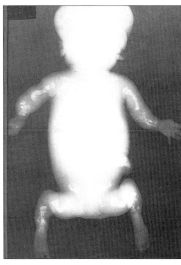

135C The radiological appearances are those of type IIC.

HYPOPHOSPHATASIA

136A–136E

There are at least two forms of this condition. One presents in the newborn period, whereas the other presents in childhood or in adulthood. Both have reduced chondro-osseous mineralisation with low levels of alkaline phosphatase in blood, cartilage and bone. In the infantile form stillbirth, or early death due to respiratory insufficiency, is not uncommon. The limb bones are deformed and sometimes fractured, and lethal osteogenesis imperfecta must be a diagnostic consideration. The bones are very poorly mineralised with irregular ossification of the metaphyses, which are widened and frayed. The skull is poorly ossified. The concentration of phosphoethanolamine is elevated in the urine. The tarda type presents with 'V'-shaped ossification defects of the metaphyses and with similar biochemical abnormalities.

Genetic aspects: The late onset form is mainly autosomal dominant whereas the severe type is autosomal recessive. The locus has been mapped to 1p34.36.

References

Brock DJH, Barron L (1991). First-trimester prenatal diagnosis of hypophosphatasia: experience with 16 cases. *Prenatal Diagn* **11**:387–391.

Fallon MD, Teitelbaum SL, Weinstein RS (1984). Hypophosphatasia: clinicopathologic comparison of the infantile, childhood, and adult forms. *Medicine* **63**:12–24.

Greenberg CR, Evans JA, McKendry-Smith S et al. (1990). Infantile hypophosphatasia: localization within chromosome region 1p36.1-34 and prenatal diagnosis using linked DNA markers. *Am J Hum Genet* **46**:286–292.

Macfarlane JD, Kroon HM, Van der Harten JJ (1992). Phenotypically dissimilar hypophosphatasia in two siblingships. *Am J Med Genet* **42**:117–121.

Moore CA, Ward JC, Rivas ML et al. (1990). Infantile hypophosphatasia: autosomal recessive transmission in two related siblingships. *Am J Med Genet* **36**:15–22.

Weiss MJ, Cole DEC, Ray K et al. (1988). A missense mutation in the human liver/bone/kidney alkaline phosphatase gene causing a lethal form of hypophosphatasia. *Proc Nat Acad Sci* **85**:7666–7669.

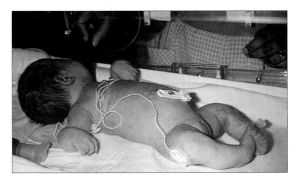

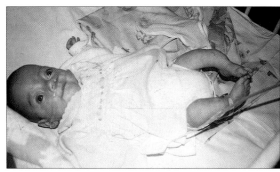

136A–136B Note the bent limbs and skin dimpling.

136B

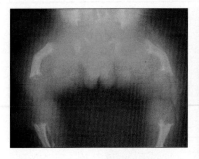

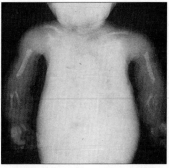

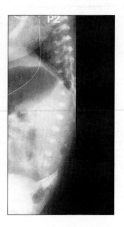

136E Poorly mineralised vertebral bodies.

136C Note under-mineralised bones and cupped and splayed metaphyses of the long bones.

136D Poorly ossified ribs and long bones.

JEUNE SYNDROME (ASPHYXIATING THORACIC DYSTROPHY)   137A–137E

The clinical picture is that of a neonate with a very small chest and variable rhizomelic shortening of the limbs. Half of all cases have a post-axial polydactyly. Patients often die in infancy because of respiratory insufficiency. Radiological confirmation of the diagnosis is essential. The ribs are short, and the ilia of the pelvis are small with irregularity of the acetabulum, from which a medial bony projection is visible, to give a trident appearance. Premature ossification of the capital femoral epiphyses is typically seen in the newborn. In those who survive, chronic renal failure is a common cause of death. Cystic changes are found in the kidney, but later there is peri-glomerular fibrosis. The picture can resemble juvenile nephronophthisis. Cirrhosis can also be a cause of early morbidity.

Genetic aspects: Autosomal recessive.

References
Cortina H, Beltran J, Olague R et al. (1979). The wide spectrum of the asphyxiating thoracic dysplasia. *Pediatr Radiol* **8**:93–99.
Hudgins L, Rosengren S, Treem W, Hyams J (1992). Early cirrhosis in survivors with Jeune thoracic dystrophy. *J Pediatr* **120**:754–756.
Langer LO Jr (1968). Thoracic-pelvic-phalangeal dystrophy. *Radiology* **91**:447–456.
Skiptunas SM, Weiner S (1987). Early prenatal diagnosis of asphyxiating thoracic dysplasia (Jeune's syndrome). Value of a fetal thoracic measurement. *J Ultrasound Med* **6**:41–43.
Wilson DJ, Weleber RG, Beals RK (1987). Retinal dystrophy in Jeune's syndrome. *Arch Ophthalmol* **105**:651–657.

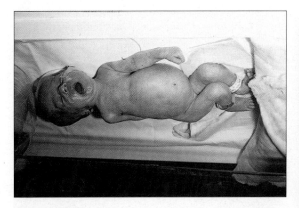

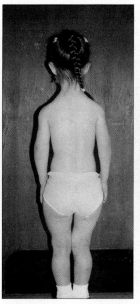

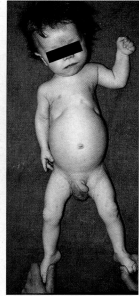

137A–137C Note the small, narrow thoracic cage and short limbs (mostly proximal). The protuberant abdomen in **137C** is secondary to the narrow thorax.

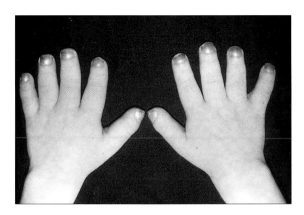

137D The fingers are short and stubby.

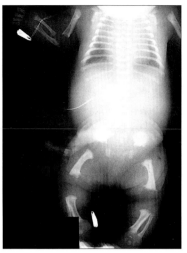

137E Note the narrow chest and trident configuration of the acetabular roof.

ELLIS–VAN CREVELD SYNDROME

138A–138D

The main features are post-axial polydactyly, mostly involving the hands but also occasionally the feet, meso/acromelic shortening of the limbs, small deep-set nails, multiple oral frenulae and a congenital heart defect, predominantly an ASD. There may be neonatal teeth and, later, malpositioning or late eruption. The ribs are short and the thorax is long and narrow. The radiological changes are difficult to distinguish from Jeune's syndrome, including the iliac bones in the pelvis being small and with a downward directed spike in the region of the triradiate cartilage. The long bones are short and the femora and humeri are thick and bowed.

Genetic aspects: Autosomal recessive.

References

da Silva EO, Janovitz D, de Albuquerque SC (1980). Ellis–van Creveld syndrome: report of 15 cases in an inbred kindred. *J Med Genet* **17**:349–356.

McKusick VA, Egeland JA, Eldridge R *et al.* (1964). Dwarfism in the Amish. I. The Ellis–van Creveld syndrome. *Bull Johns Hopk Hosp* **115**:306–336.

Prabhu SR, Dholakia HM (1978). Chondroectodermal dysplasia (Ellis–van Creveld syndrome): report of two cases. *J Oral Surg* **36**:631–637.

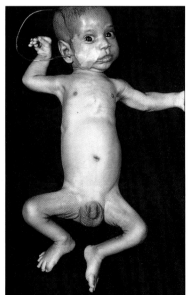

137E Note the trident configuration of the acetabular roof.

138A–138D Note the long, narrow thorax, post-axial polydactyly, natal teeth and multiple oral frenulae.

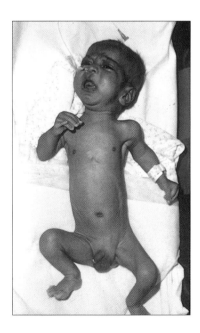

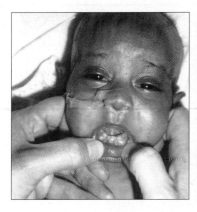

138C

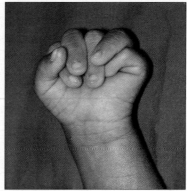

138D

SHORT RIB – POLYDACTYLY SYNDROME TYPE 1 (SALDINO–NOONAN)   139

Characteristics include a very narrow thorax, short limbs and post-axial polydactyly. The base of the ilium is hypoplastic and the vertebrae are rounded, sometimes with coronal clefts. The ends of the long bones are either pointed or have a convex central area of ossification with lateral metaphyseal spikes. Urogenital and anorectal abnormalities are common, including imperforate anus, vaginal atresia, ure-throvaginal fistula, persistent cloaca and ureteral atresia. Many cases have a congenital heart defect.

Genetic aspects: Autosomal recessive.

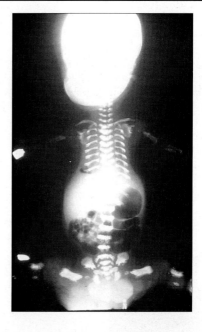

139 Note the severely shortened ribs, small pelvis and short tubular bones with jagged appearance of the metaphyses.

References
Grote W *et al.* (1983). Prenatal diagnosis of a short-rib-polydactylia syndrome type Saldino–Noonan at 17 weeks' gestation. *Eur J Pediatr* **140**:63–66.

Lowry RB, Wignall N (1975). Saldino–Noonan short rib-polydactyly dwarfism syndrome. *Pediatrics* (**56**):121–123.

Sillence D, Kozlowski K, Bar-Ziv J *et al.* (1987). Perinatally lethal short rib-polydactyly syndromes 1. Variability in known syndromes. *Pediatr Radiol* **17**:474–480.

Sillence DO (1980). Invited editorial comment: Non-Majewski short rib-polydactyly syndrome. *Am J Med Genet* **7**:223–229.

SHORT RIB – POLYDACTYLY SYNDROME TYPE 2 (MAJEWSKI)   140A–140C

The features which help to distinguish this form of short rib – polydactyly are a midline cleft of the upper lip and distinctive radiographic features. The pelvis and long bones are relatively normal, apart from the tibiae, which have a characteristic oval shape. Ambiguous genitalia are common.

Genetic aspects: Autosomal recessive.

References
Chen H, Yang SS, Gonzalez E *et al.* (1980). Short rib-polydactyly syndrome, Majewski type. *Am J Med Genet* **7**:215–222.

Cooper CP, Hall CM (1982). Lethal short-rib polydactyly syndrome of the Majewski type: a report of three cases. *Radiology* **144**:513–517.

Gembruch U, Hansmann M, Fodisch HJ (1985). Early prenatal diagnosis of short rib-polydactyly (SRP) syndrome type 1 (Majewski) by ultrasound in a case at risk. *Prenatal Diagn* **5**:375–362.

Walley VM, Coates CF, Gilbert JJ *et al.* (1983). Short rib-polydactyly syndrome, Majewski type. *Am J Med Genet* **14**:445–452.

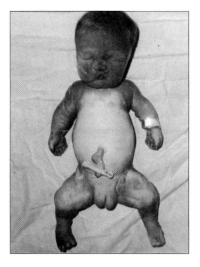

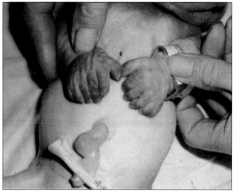

140B Note the polydactyly.

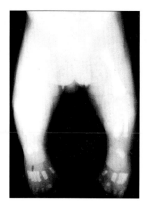

140C The pelvis is relatively normal, the tibiae are short and oval, and there is polydactyly of the toes.

140A Note the relatively large head, narrow chest and short limbs.

RHIZOMELIC CHONDRODYSPLASIA PUNCTATA   141A–141D

This is a severe form of chondrodysplasia punctata and affected individuals usually die in early infancy. There is asymmetrical rhizomelic shortening of the limbs with enlarged joints and contractures. The facial features are unusual with upslanting palpebral fissures, a depressed nasal bridge, hypertelorism, anteverted nostrils, full cheeks and cataracts. There may be ichthyosiform skin changes. At birth radiographs reveal flared metaphyses with epiphyseal stippling. There may also be stippling adjacent to the ischial and pubic bones and in the region of the larynx and sternum. Coronal clefts of the vertebrae are marked. In later infancy the bones become demineralised, the vertebrae become flattened and the epiphyseal stippling disappears. About two-thirds of patients die in the first year of life with others dying in late infancy; survival beyond 5 years is rare. Survivors develop microcephaly and mental retardation.

Pathological studies reveal abnormal peroxisomes in the liver. Reduced phytanic acid oxidation, defective plasmalogen synthesis and the presence of the unprocessed form of peroxisomal thiolase can be demonstrated. Acyl-CoA:dihydroxyacetone phosphate acyltransferase (DHAP-AT) levels are reduced. **Genetic aspects:** Autosomal recessive.

References
Gilbert EF, Opitz JM, Spranger JW et al. (1976). Chondrodysplasia punctata – rhizomelic form. *Eur J Pediatr* **123**:89–109.
Gray RG, Green A, Schutgens RBH et al. (1990). Antenatal diagnosis of rhizomelic chondrodysplasia punctata in the second trimester. *J Inherit Metab Dis* **13**:380–382.
Hoefler G, Hoefler S, Watkins PA et al. (1988). Biochemical abnormalities in rhizomelic chondrodysplasia punctata. *J Pediatr* **112**:726–733.
Hoefler S, Hoefler G, Moser AB et al. (1988). Prenatal diagnosis of rhizomelic chondrodysplasia punctata. *Prenatal Diagn* **8**:571–576.
Moser HW (1989). Rhizomelic chondrodysplasia punctata. *Adv Pediatr* **36**:21.
Spranger JW, Opitz JM, Bidder UB (1971). Heterogeneity of chondrodysplasia punctata. *Humangenetik* **11**:190–212.

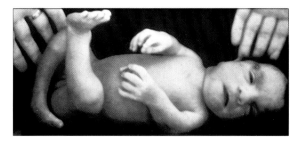

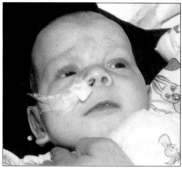

141B

141A–141C Note short limbs, most severe in the upper segments, and flat mid-face.

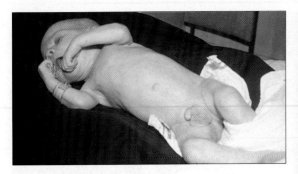

141C

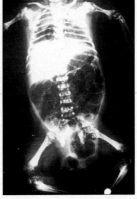

141D Note shortening of the humeri and femora and punctate calcification at knees, hips and upper limbs.

CHONDRODYSPLASIA PUNCTATA (X-LINKED RECESSIVE) 142A–142B

The most characteristic feature is the nasal configuration. The nose is flat with an absence of the normal nasofrontal angle. The philtrum is poorly developed and the maxilla is short. Because of this all patients have a relative prognathism. The nostrils have a semicircular shape when viewed from below. This abnormality of the nose has been called Binder syndrome. It is becoming apparent that many cases of 'Binder' syndrome have a mild form of chondrodysplasia punctata, so that a skeletal survey can be helpful (Sheffield *et al.*). This may reveal symmetrical stippling of multiple epiphyseal centres and of the larynx and trachea, although this disappears relatively rapidly with age. The terminal phalanges may be short.

Cataracts, ichthyosis, short stature and mental retardation are present in some cases. Ballabio *et al.* showed that short stature, chondrodysplasia punctata, mental retardation, steroid sulphatase deficiency, and Kallmann syndrome are all part of a contiguous gene syndrome.

The cases reported by Maroteaux under the title 'brachytelephalangic chondrodysplasia punctata' without mental retardation or ichthyosis may have a point mutation of a gene at Xpter.

Genetic aspects: Many cases are sporadic but X-linked inheritance has been reported. Heterozygous females may have mild short stature without radiological abnormalities.

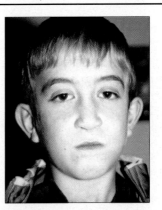

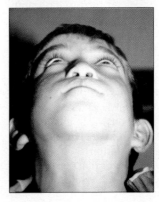

142A and 142B Note flattened nose with short columella and semi-circular nostrils.

References

Ballabio A, Bardoni B, Carrozzo R et al. (1989). Contiguous gene syndromes due to deletions in the distal short arm of the human X chromosome. *Proc Nat Acad Sci USA* **86**:10001–10005.

Curry CJR, Magenis RE, Brown M et al. (1984). Inherited chondrodysplasia punctata due to a deletion of the terminal short arm of an X chromosome. *New Engl J Med* **311**:1010–1015.

Maroteaux P (1989). Brachytelephalangic chondrodysplasia punctata: a possible X-linked recessive form. *Hum Genet* **82**:167–170.

Delaire J, Tessier P et al. (1980). Clinical and radiological aspects of maxillonasal dysostosis (Binder syndrome). *Head Neck Surg* **3**:105–122.

Ferguson JW, Thompson RPJ (1985). Maxillonasal dysostosis (Binder syndrome): a review of the literature and case reports. *Eur J Orthod* **7**:145–148.

Quarrell OWJ, Koch M, Hughes HE (1990). Syndrome of the month. Maxillonasal dysplasia (Binder's syndrome). *J Med Genet* **27**:384–387.

Sheffield LJ, Halliday JL, Jensen F (1991). Maxillonasal dysplasia (Binder's syndrome) and chondrodysplasia punctata (Letter). *J Med Genet* **28**:503–504.

CONRADI CHONDRODYSPLASIA PUNCTATA

There is asymmetric shortening of limbs and patchy skin abnormalities. The skin resembles the pitted skin of an orange, or there are patches of dry, scaly skin (follicular atrophoderma). On the scalp there are areas of alopecia and the hair is generally sparse and coarse. Cataracts may be present. Radiographs show multiple areas of punctate calcification at the epiphyseal centres but extra-cartilaginous areas might also be involved. Calcification in the cervical trachea has been noted. This chondrodysplasia punctata disappears with age.

Genetic aspects: Happle *et al.* have suggested that this condition is X-linked dominant with early fetal lethality in males. However, Traupe *et al.* failed to find linkage with any X-chromosome markers.

References

Edidin DV, Esterly NB, Bamzai AK, Fretzin DF (1977). Chondrodysplasia punctata (Conradi–Hunermann syndrome). *Arch Dermatol* **113**:1431–1434.

Happle R (1979). X-linked dominant chondrodysplasia punctata: review of literature and report of a case. *Hum Genet* **53**:65–73.

Happle R, Matthiass HH, Macher E (1977). Sex-linked chondrodysplasia punctata? *Clin Genet* **11**:73–76.

Kozlowski K, Bates EH, Young LW, Wood BP (1988). Radiological case of the month. Dominant X-linked chondrodysplasia punctata. *Am J Dis Child* **142**:1233–1234.

Mueller RF, Crowle PM, Jones RAK et al. (1985). X-linked dominant chondrodysplasia punctata: a case report and family studies. *Am J Med Genet* **20**:137–144.

Silengo MC, Luzzatti L, Silverman FN (1980). Clinical and genetic aspects of Conradi–Hunermann disease: a report of three familial cases and review of the literature. *J Pediatr* **97**:911–917.

Traupe H, Vetter U, Happle R et al. (1993). Exclusion of the biglycan (BGN) gene as a candidate gene for the Happle syndrome, employing an intragenic single-strand conformational polymorphism (Letter). *Hum Genet* **91**:89–90.

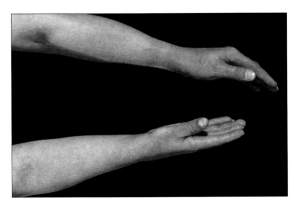

143A Note upper limb asymmetry.

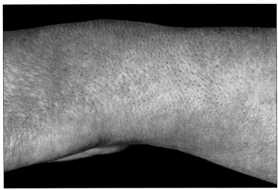

143B Note ichthyosis and pitted skin.

ACROMESOMELIC DYSPLASIA

The shortest segments are the forearms, lower legs, hands and feet. The short stature might be noted at birth but mostly becomes obvious during the first year of life. The forearms are bowed and the fingers and toes are very short. The head is relatively large with frontal bossing and a cleft palate is common. The radial head might be dislocated. Radiologically, there are short and broad proximal and middle phalanges, cone-shaped epiphyses and invaginated metaphyses. The vertebral bodies have a central anterior protrusion.

Genetic aspects: Ohba et al. reported an affected father and son, suggesting possible autosomal dominant inheritance but most cases are autosomal recessive.

References

Beighton P (1974). Autosomal recessive inheritance in the mesomelic dwarfism of Campailla and Martinelli. *Clin Genet* **5**:363–367.

Borelli P, Fassanelli S, Marini R (1983). Acromesomelic dwarfism in a child with an interesting family history. *Pediatr Radiol* **13**:165–168.

Del Moral RF, Jimenez JMS et al. (1989). Acromesomelic dysplasia: radiologic, clinical, and pathological study. *Am J Med Genet* **33**:415–419.

Hall CM, Stoker DJ, Robinson DC et al. (1980). Acromesomelic dwarfism. *Br J Radiol* **53**:999–1003.

Langer LO, Beals RK, Solomon IL et al. (1977). Acromesomelic dwarfism: manifestations in childhood. *Am J Med Genet* **1**:87–100.

Ohba K-I, Ohdo S, Sonoda T, Madokoro H (1989). Acromesomelic dysplasia in a father and son: autosomal dominant inheritance. *Acta Paediatr Japon* **31**:595–599.

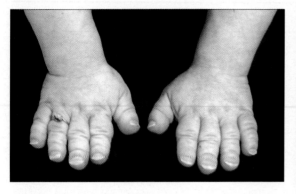

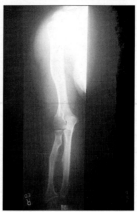

144B Note radius and short ulna.

144A Note short stubby digits.

JANSEN METAPHYSEAL DYSPLASIA 145A–145C

This condition presents with short stature and bowing of the radius, ulna, tibia and fibula. It is much more severe than the Schmid type. Joint mobility is often restricted and club feet might be a feature. Deafness in adulthood, sclerosis of the base of the skull, craniosynostosis and a narrow thorax can all occur. The radiological features consist of clubbing of the metaphyses, which are wide and irregularly calcified. The cupped and frayed appearance of the metaphyses can also be seen in the bones of the fingers. Hypercalcaemia may be present in infancy and the diagnosis of hyperparathyroidism is sometimes suggested.

Genetic aspects: Autosomal dominant.

References

Charrow J, Poznanski AK (1984). The Jansen type of metaphyseal chondrodysplasia: confirmation of a dominant inheritance and review of radiographic manifestations in the newborn and adult. *Am J Med Genet* **18**:321–327.

Kikuchi S, Hasue M et al. (1976). Metaphyseal dysostosis (Jansen type). Report of a case with long follow-up. *J Bone Joint Surg B* **58**:102–106.

Nazara Z, Hernandez A et al. (1981). Further clinical and radiological features in metaphyseal chondrodysplasia (Jansen type). *Radiology* **140**:697–700.

Silverthorn KG, Houston CS, Duncan BP (1987). Murk Jansen's metaphyseal chondrodysplasia with long-term follow-up. *Pediatr Radiol* **17**:119–123.

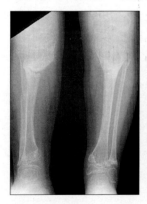

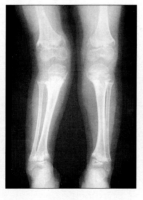

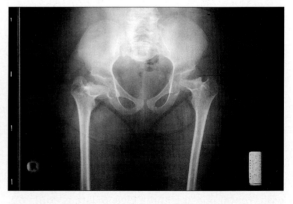

145A and 145B Note the severe metaphyseal changes.

145C Note absent femoral heads and deformed femoral necks.

SHWACHMAN SYNDROME 146

The metaphyseal changes consist of flaring and shortening of the ribs with changes at the proximal femora and around the knees. Slipping of the femoral head, coxa vara and progressive changes in the proximal femoral metaphyses cause walking difficulties. Valgus deformity of the elbows and knees and a narrow thorax due to short ribs can be seen. Pancreatic insufficiency, neutropenia, and short stature may be the

presenting clinical features. More severe haematological dysfunction may occur. An ichthyotic maculopapular rash is present in 60% of cases.
Genetic aspects: Autosomal recessive.

References

Aggett PJ, Cavanagh HPC, Matthew DJ *et al.* (1980). Shwachman's syndrome: a review of 21 cases. *Arch Dis Child* **55**:331–347.
Hill RE, Durie PR, Gaskin KJ *et al.* (1982). Steatorrhea and pancreatic insufficiency in Shwachman syndrome. *Gastroenterology* **83**:22–27.
Shwachman H, Diamond LK, Oski FA *et al.* (1964). The syndrome of pancreatic insufficiency and bone marrow dysfunction. *J Pediatr* **65**:645–663.

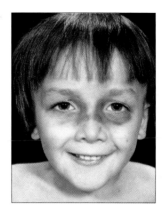

146 Note the wasted look with hyperpigmentation below the eyes. This child has severe failure to thrive.

SCHMID METAPHYSEAL DYSPLASIA   147A–147B

This is a relatively mild form of metaphyseal dysplasia resembling vitamin D deficiency rickets. Patients present in childhood with short bowed limbs, a pronounced lumbar lordosis and a waddling gait. Radiologically, the epiphyses are wide and the metaphyses flared, cupped and ragged. The course of the disease is relatively benign.
Genetic aspects: Inheritance is autosomal dominant. Mutations have been found in the type X collagen gene COL10A1 at 6q21 (Warman *et al.*).

References

Lachman RS, Rimoin DL, Spranger J (1988). Metaphyseal chondrodysplasia, Schmid type. Clinical and radiographic delineation with a review of the literature. *Pediatr Radiol* **18**:93–102.
Warman ML, Abbott M, Apte SS *et al.* (1993). A type X collagen mutation causes Schmid metaphyseal chondrodysplasia. *Nature Genetics* **5**:79–82.

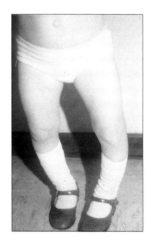

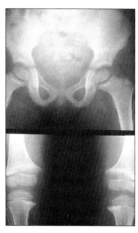

147A There is bowing of the knees.

147B Note the metaphyseal dysplasia of the hips and knees.

McKUSICK – CARTILAGE-HAIR HYPOPLASIA   148A–148D

The hallmarks of this condition are a form of metaphyseal dysplasia, short stature, fine, sparse, blond hair, a transient macrocytic anaemia (and an occasional hypoplastic anaemia) and an immunodeficiency. The median adult height in males is 131cm and in females 123cm (Makitie 1992). There is a particular susceptibility to varicella, indicating a defect of cellular immunity, but immunoglobulins are also deficient and neutropenia and lymphopenia can be seen. In the lower limbs the metaphyseal dysplasia is said to be more severe at the knee than at the proximal femur. Some cases have had aganglionic megacolon. In the study by Makitie (1992), seven out of 107 died in the first year of life.
Genetic aspects: Autosomal recessive. Sulisalo *et al.* assigned the gene to chromosome 9 by linkage analysis.

References

Le Merrer M, Maroteaux P (1991). Cartilage hair hypoplasia in infancy: a misleading chondrodysplasia. *Eur J Pediatr* **150**:847–851.

Makitie O (1992). Cartilage-hair hypoplasia in Finland: epidemiological and genetic aspects of 107 patients. *J Med Genet* **29**:652–655.

Makitie O, Kaitila I (1993). Cartilage-hair hypoplasia – clinical manifestations in 108 Finnish patients. *Eur J Pediatr* **152**:211–217.

McKusick VA, Eldridge R, Hostetler JA *et al.* (1965). Dwarfism in the Amish. II. Cartilage-hair hypoplasia. *Bull Johns Hopk Hosp* **116**:285–326.

Sulisalo T, Sistonen P, Hastbacka J *et al.* (1993). Cartilage-hair hypoplasia gene assigned to chromosome 9 by linkage analysis. *Nature Genetics* **3**:338–341.

van der Burgt I, Haraldsson A, Oosterwijk JC *et al.* (1991). Cartilage hair hypoplasia, metaphyseal chondrodysplasia type McKusick: description of seven patients and review of the literature. *Am J Med Genet* **41**:371–380.

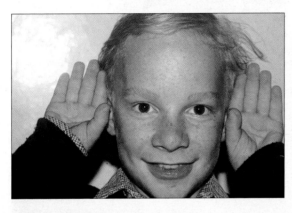

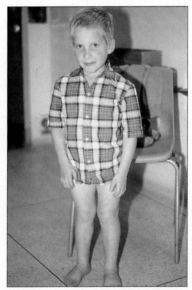

148A and 148B Note short stature, sparse depigmented hair and short fingers.

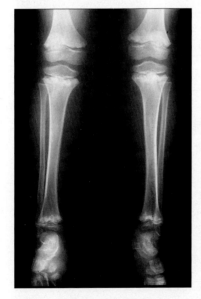

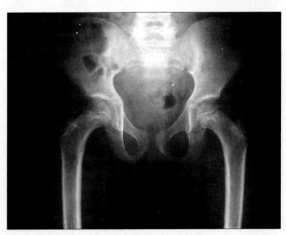

148C and 148D Note metaphyseal irregularities at the knee, ankle and hip.

RICKETS-ALOPECIA

This distinct form of rickets is associated with alopecia. The rickets becomes apparent in the first year of life and is usually refractory to large doses of vitamin D. End-organ unresponsiveness to vitamin D seems to be the likely cause.

Genetic aspects: Autosomal recessive.

References

Brooks M, Stern P, Bell N (1980). Vitamin-dependent rickets type II. *New Engl J Med* **302**:810.

Fraher LJ, Karmali R, Hinde FR *et al.* (1986). Vitamin D-dependent rickets type II: extreme end organ resistance to 1,25-dihydroxy vitamin D3 in a patient without alopecia. *Eur J Pediatr* **145**:389–395.

Rosen JF, Fleischman AR, Finberg L (1979). Rickets with alopecia: an inborn error of vitamin D metabolism. *J Pediatr* **94**:729–735.

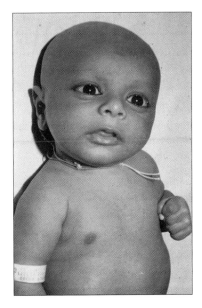

149 Note total alopecia in this child with rickets.

X-LINKED HYPOPHOSPHATAEMIC RICKETS

This condition is caused by a defect in renal tubular function leading to diminished reabsorption of phosphate with resulting hypophosphataemia. Affected individuals have short stature and vitamin D-resistant rickets. Radiographs may show ricketic changes at the metaphyses, pseudo-fractures and sometimes areas of osteosclerosis.

Genetic aspects: The condition is X-linked dominant. The gene maps to Xp11.2.

References

Balsan S, Tieder M (1990). Linear growth in patients with hypophosphatemic vitamin D-resistant rickets: influence of treatment regimen and parental height. *J Pediatr* **116**:365–371.

Bolino A, Devoto M, Enia G *et al.* (1993). Genetic mapping in the Xp11.2 region of a new form of X-linked hypophosphatemic rickets. *Eur J Hum Genet* **1**:269–279.

Hanna JD, Niimi K, Chan JCM (1991). X-linked hypophosphatemia: genetic and clinical correlates. *Am J Dis Child* **145**:865–870.

Reusz GS, Hoyer PF, Lucas M *et al.* (1990). X linked hypophosphataemia: treatment, height gain, and nephrocalcinosis. *Arch Dis Child* **65**:1125–1128.

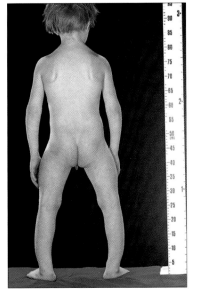

150A Note the bowed legs.

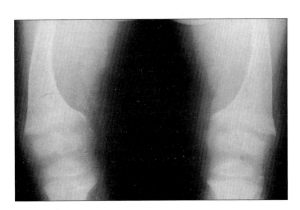

150B Note curvature of long bones, irregular cupped and splayed metaphyses, and coarse trabeculation of the femora.

SCHWARTZ–JAMPEL SYNDROME

This condition is a form of myotonic myopathy with an associated chondrodysplasia. Blepharophimosis, difficulty in opening the mouth, an expressionless face, ptosis, muscle wasting with myotonia and joint limitation all suggest an underlying abnormality of muscle. Radiographs show platyspondyly, coronal clefts of the vertebral bodies, and an epiphyseal dysplasia, especially around the hips. Skeletal abnormalities include kyphoscoliosis, lumbar lordosis, pectus carinatum, bowing of the long bones, pes planus, a valgus deformity of the ankles and wide metaphyses. Ocular abnormalities such as microphthalmia or cataract have been reported.

Genetic aspects: Most cases are autosomal recessive but a few dominant families have been reported.

References

Al Gazali LI (1993). The Schwartz–Jampel syndrome. *Clin Dysmorphol* **2**:47–54.

Edwards WC, Root AW (1982). Chondrodystrophic myotonia (Schwartz–Jampel syndrome): report of a new case and follow-up of patients initially reported in 1969. *Am J Med Genet* **13**:51–56.

Ferrannini E, Perniola T, Krajewska G et al. (1982). Schwartz–Jampel syndrome with autosomal dominant inheritance. *Eur Neurol* **21**:137–146.

Pascuzzi RM, Gratianne R, Azzarelli B, Kincaid JC (1990). Schwartz–Jampel syndrome with dominant inheritance. *Muscle Nerve* **13**:1152–1163.

Viljoen D, Beighton P (1992). Syndrome of the month: Schwartz–Jampel syndrome (chondrodystrophic myotonia). *J Med Genet* **29**:58–62.

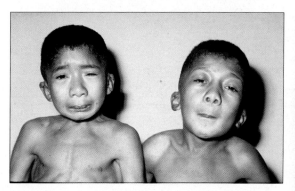

151A Note the blepharophimosis, expressionless face and pursed lips.

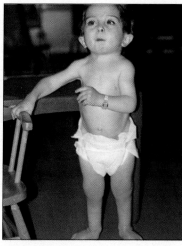

151B Note the posture due to underlying skeletal changes.

SPONDYLOEPIPHYSEAL DYSPLASIA CONGENITA

Onset is at birth, but severe short stature may not be obvious until 2–3 years. Clinically, there is a short trunk, short limbs and marked lordosis. Myopia, cleft palate and deafness can occur. Bone age is markedly delayed and the epiphyses are flattened and fragmented. The capital femoral epiphysis is severely affected. Delay in ossification of the pubic rami is characteristic. In infancy radiographs show ovoid vertebral bodies but later platyspondyly with irregular endplates develops. Odontoid hypoplasia may be a problem. The condition may be separated into two types according to the presence of severe coxa vara or not. In the former case, short stature is severe with a final height of between three and four feet. In the latter case final height might be between four and five feet.

Genetic aspects: Autosomal dominant. Mutations in the type II collagen gene COL2A1 have been demonstrated in some families.

References

Anderson IJ, Goldberg RB, Marion RW et al. (1990). Spondyloepiphyseal dysplasia congenita: genetic linkage to type II collagen (COL2A1). *Am J Hum Genet* **46**:896–901.

Cole WG, Hall RK, Rogers JG (1993). The clinical features of spondyloepiphyseal dysplasia congenita resulting from the substitution of glycine 997 by serine in the alpha1(II) chain of type II collagen. *J Med Genet* **30**:27–35.

Lee B, Vissing H, Ramirez F et al. (1989). Identification of the molecular defect in a family with spondyloepiphyseal dysplasia. *Science* **244**:978–979.

Ramesar R, Beighton P (1992). Spondyloepiphyseal dysplasia in a Cape Town family: linkage with the gene for type II collagen (COL2A1). *Am J Med Genet* **43**:833–838.

Tiller GE, Rimoin DL, Murray LW, Cohn DH (1990). Tandem duplication within a type II collagen gene (COL2A1) exon in an individual with spondyloepiphyseal dysplasia. *Proc Nat Acad Sci* **87**:3889–3893.

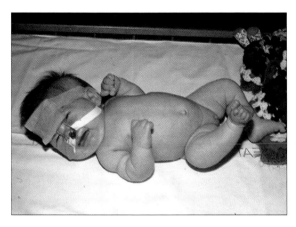

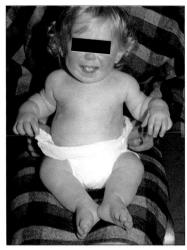

152A and 152B Note the short trunk, abnormal chest shape and short limbs.

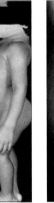

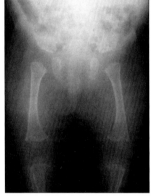

152D Note the abnormal ossification of the epiphyses, the short iliac bones and the horizontal acetabular roofs.

152C The older child develops joint contractures and an exaggerated lumbar lordosis.

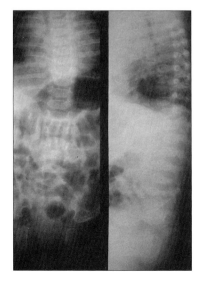

152E Note the oval or pear-shaped vertebral bodies and anterior pointing.

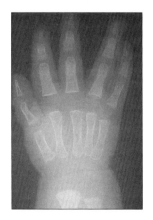

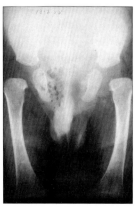

152F The ossification centres are retarded in their formation.

152G Absence of epiphyses, horizontal acetabular roofs and poor iliac ossification.

SPONDYLOEPIPHYSEAL DYSPLASIA TARDA (X-LINKED) 153A–153B

Presentation is between 5 and 10 years with back or hip pain. Characteristically, the vertebrae show a posterior hump of bone on their superior and inferior aspects when viewed laterally. Mild epiphyseal dysplasia is seen in the hips and shoulders, but rarely in other joints. This form of spondyloepiphyseal dysplasia is milder than the congenita type.

Genetic aspects: Most cases with the characteristic radiographic appearance of the spine are X-linked recessive. The gene maps to Xp22.

References

Bannerman RM, Ingall GB, Mohn JF (1971). X-linked spondyloepiphyseal dysplasia tarda: clinical and linkage data. *J Med Genet* **8**:291–301.

Iceton JA, Horne G (1986). Spondylo-epiphyseal dysplasia tarda: the X-linked variety in three brothers. *J Bone Joint Surg B* **68**:616–619.

Langer LO Jr (1964). Spondyloepiphyseal dysplasia tarda. Hereditary chondrodysplasia with characteristic vertebral configuration in the adult. *Radiology* **82**:833–839.

Szpiro-Tapia S, Sefiani A *et al.* (1988). Spondyloopiphyseal dysplasia tarda: linkage with genetic markers from the distal short arm of the X chromosome. *Hum Genet* **81**:61–63.

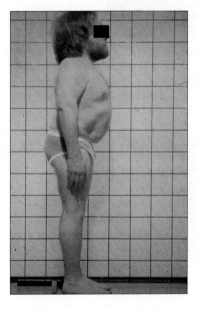

153A Note the short trunk.

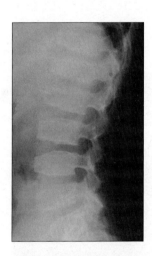

153B Note the characteristic hump of bone on the superior and inferior surfaces of the vertebral bodies.

STICKLER SYNDROME (HEREDITARY ARTHRO-OPHTHALMOPATHY) 154A–154D

At birth the features may be those of Pierre Robin association (cleft palate, micrognathia and glossoptosis). Radiological examination at this time may reveal coronal clefts of the vertebrae, mild platyspondyly and flaring of the metaphyses of the long bones. Later the outline of the bones becomes more normal but a mild epiphyseal dysplasia may develop, leading to early osteoarthritis. The main clinical problem after the neonatal period is a severe myopia with the risk of retinal detachment. Thus any child with Pierre Robin association should have careful ophthalmic follow-up.

Genetic aspects: Autosomal dominant with variable expression. Mutations in the type II collagen gene COL2A1 at 12q13 have been demonstrated in some families. In other families the gene maps to 6p22.

References

Ahmad NN, Ala-Kokko L, Knowlton RG *et al.* (1991). Stop codon in the procollagen II gene (COL2A1) in a family with the Stickler syndrome (arthro-ophthalmopathy). *Proc Nat Acad Sci* **88**:6624–6627.

Lewkonia RM (1992). The arthropathy of hereditary arthroophthalmopathy (Stickler syndrome). *J Rheumatol* **19**:1271–1275.

Spallone A (1987). Stickler's syndrome: a study of 12 families. *Br J Ophthalmol* **71**:501–509.

Temple IK (1989). Syndrome of the month. Stickler's syndrome. *J Med Genet* **26**:119–126.

Zlotogora J, Sagi M, Schuper A *et al.* (1992). Variability of Stickler syndrome. *Am J Med Genet* **42**:337–339.

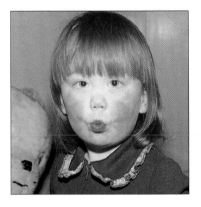
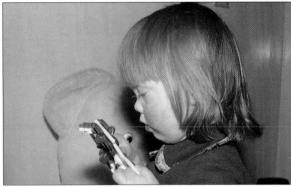

154A–154D Note the flat nasal bridge, small nose, prominent eyes, and (in some) small chin.

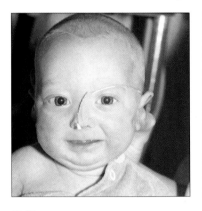
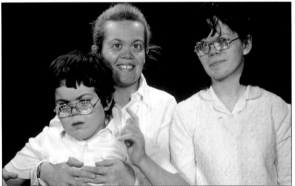

154C

154D

KNIEST SYNDROME

155A–155F

Severe short stature is present from birth and the face is usually flat with the head disproportionately large. The eyes might be prominent and there is often a cleft palate. Many infants will have respiratory problems in the neonatal period. Scoliosis is a frequent complication and the joints are often stiff and prominent. Other problems include myopia, which might lead to a detached retina, and sensorineural deafness. Radiographs show broad metaphyses and irregular epiphyses especially around the knees. There is platyspondyly and coronal clefts of the vertebrae and an additional ossification centre at the distal end of the middle phalanx. There is a lethal neonatal form that may represent the severe end of the clinical spectrum (Spranger and Maroteaux). Histologically, the cartilage has a characteristic 'Swiss-cheese' appearance.

Genetic aspects: Autosomal dominant. Mutations of the COL2A1 (type II collagen) gene have been demonstrated.

References

Chen H, Yang SS, Gonzalez E (1980). Kniest dysplasia: neonatal death with necropsy. *Am J Med Genet* **6**:171–178.

Lachman RS *et al.* (1975). The Kniest syndrome. *Am J Roentgenol* **123**:805–814.

Maumenee IH, Traboulsi EI (1985). The ocular findings in Kniest dysplasia. *Am J Ophthalmol* **100**:155–160.

Merrill KD, Schmidt TL (1989). Occipitoatlantal instability in a child with Kniest syndrome. *J Pediatr Orthop* **9**:338–340.

Spranger J, Maroteaux P (1991). Lethal Kniest disease. *Adv Hum Genet* **19**:65–67.

Winterpacht A, Hilbert M, Schwarze U *et al.* (1993). Kniest and Stickler dysplasia phenotypes caused by collagen type II gene (COL2A1) defect. *Nature Genetics* **3**:323–326.

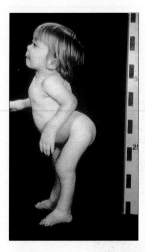
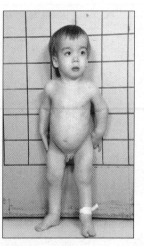
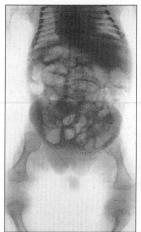
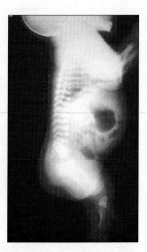

155A and 155B Note the short trunk, prominent joints and severe lordotic posture. The face shows mid-facial flattening with a flat nasal bridge.

155C–155E Note the expanded metaphyses, poor ossification of the epiphyses and, in the lateral X-ray of the spine, coronal clefts and platyspondyly.

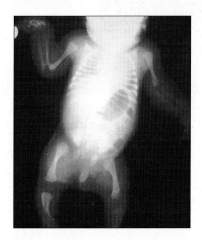

155E

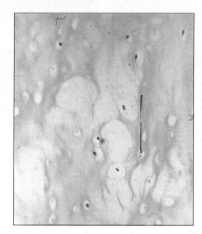

155F Histopathology of the cartilage shows a 'Swiss-cheese' appearance.

METATROPIC DYSPLASIA

156A–156F

This condition gets its name from the Greek for changing pattern; short-limbed dwarfism is present at birth but the back gradually becomes shorter with age. The joints are prominent, the chest narrow and there may be a caudal appendage overlying the sacrum. Radiographs reveal flaring of the metaphyses with flattened deformed epiphyses. The ribs are short with flaring and cupping of the anterior borders. The vertebrae become flattened with age with a characteristic anterior tongue of bone on lateral view. The fingers and toes may be very long. Severe kyphosis develops.

Genetic aspects: It has been suggested that inheritance is autosomal recessive (Beck *et al.*), but a dominant form seems to exist and 'recessive' cases could be caused by parental mosaicism. There is a variation in severity and a neonatal lethal form has been described.

References
Beck M, Roubicek M, Rogers JG (1983). Heterogeneity of metatropic dysplasia. *Eur J Pediatr* **140**:231–237.
Belik J, Anday EK, Kaplan F, Zackai E (1985). Respiratory complications of metatropic dwarfism. *Clin Pediatr* **24**:504–511.
Boden SD, Kaplan FS, Fallon MD *et al.* (1987). Metatropic dwarfism. Uncoupling of endochondral and perichondral growth. *J Bone Joint Surg A* **69**:174–184.
Kozlowski K, Campbell J *et al.* (1988). Metatropic dysplasia and its variants. (Analysis of 14 cases). *Australas Radiol* **32**:325–337.
Larose JH, Gay BG (1969). Metatropic dwarfism. *Am J Roentgenol* **106**:156–161.
Shohat M, Lachman R, Rimoin DL (1989). Odontoid hypoplasia with vertebral cervical subluxation and ventriculomegaly in metatropic dysplasia. *J Pediatr* **114**:239–243.

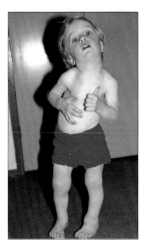
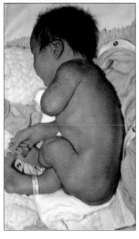
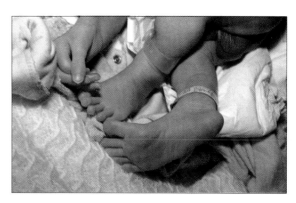

156A–156C Note the narrow chest, short limbs, prominent joints, and long hands and feet.

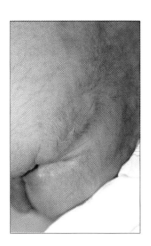
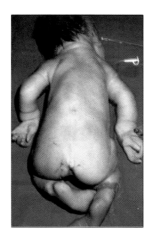
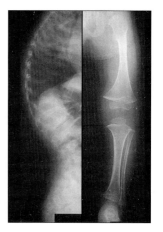

156D and 156E Note the caudal appendage.

156F Note the metaphyseal flaring and the platyspondyly.

MULTIPLE EPIPHYSEAL DYSPLASIA

157A–157B

Presentation may be with short stature, a waddling gait or painful joints. There is short stature and shortened digits and abnormal epiphyses. Radiographs reveal fragmented epiphyseal ossification centres of the long bones with relative sparing of the vertebrae. Secondary osteoarthritic changes can occur. The differential diagnosis includes spondylo-epiphyseal dysplasia and pseudoachondroplasia.

Genetic aspects: Autosomal dominant. Oehlmann *et al.* mapped the gene to 19q13 in a single large pedigree.

References

Amir D, Mogle P, Weinberg H (1985). Multiple epiphyseal dysplasia in one family. A further review of seven generations. *J Bone Joint Surg B* **67**:809–813.

Ingram RR (1992). Early diagnosis of multiple epiphyseal dysplasia. *J Pediatr Orthop* **12**:241–244.

Oehlmann R, Summerville GP, Yeh G *et al.* (1994). Genetic linkage mapping of multiple epiphyseal dysplasia to the pericentromeric region of chromosome 19. *Am J Hum Genet* **54**:3–10.

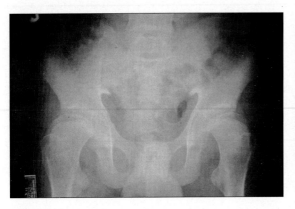

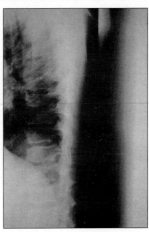

157B The vertebral end-plates are mildly flattened.

157A Note the arthritic changes at the hip joint.

PSEUDOACHONDROPLASIA

158A–158E

Short stature becomes apparent by 2–3 years. The limbs are short and the joints lax; arthritis develops later. Abnormal spinal curvature is common, but seldom severe. Genu varum or valgum can be a problem. Radiographs reveal biconvex vertebral bodies in infancy, with an anterior tongue later on. In adult life the vertebrae can show platyspondyly, or be of normal height, but they have the normal rectangular shape. Long pedicles, irregular upper and lower endplates and odontoid hypoplasia may be noted. A characteristic sign is slow development of the triradiate cartilage of the pelvis. Epiphyses are flat and delayed in development. The craniofacial appearance is normal. Adult height is usually between 90 and 145 cm.

Genetic aspects: There are autosomal dominant and recessive forms of this condition, not easily distinguished by clinical or radiological features.

References

Hall JG, Dorst JP, Rotta J, McKusick VA (1987). Gonadal mosaicisms in pseudoachondroplasia. *Am J Med Genet* **28**:143–152.

Maroteaux P, Stanescu R, Stanescu V et al. (1980). The mild form of pseudoachondroplasia. *Eur J Pediatr* **133**:227–231.

Wynne-Davies R, Hall CM, Young ID (1986). Pseudoachondroplasia: clinical diagnosis at different ages and comparison of autosomal dominant and recessive types. A review of 32 patients (26 kindreds). *J Med Genet* **23**:425–434.

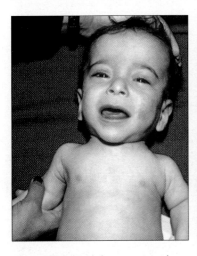

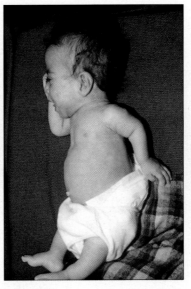

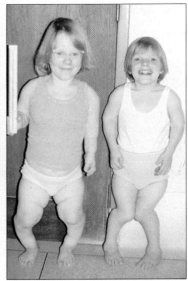

158A–158C Note short stature with short, bowed limbs and relatively normal cranio-facial appearance.

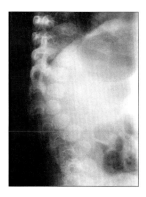

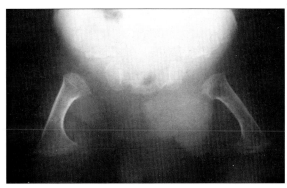

158D and 158E Note flattening of vertebral bodies with biconvex appearance, horizontal acetabulae with irregularity of articular surfaces, shortened femora with expanded metaphyses, and delayed ossification of femoral and capital epiphysis.

DYGGVE–MELCHIOR–CLAUSEN SYNDROME

159A–159C

This is a form of bone dysplasia. The main clinical features are mental retardation, short stature and progressive pectus carinatum. The skeletal changes are present by the age of 4 years when a delayed bone age, flattening of the vertebral bodies, with a radiolucent depression in their mid-portion, can be detected. Within a few years, the vertebral bodies become flatter and the iliac crests assume a characteristic lacy appearance. The femoral heads are delayed in their ossification and they might be fragmented. Progressive hip dislocation might occur. The head circumference is often below the third centile and, although many cases are severely retarded, the degree of retardation is variable.

Genetic aspects: The condition is probably heterogeneous with both autosomal recessive and X-linked recessive forms (Smith–McCort syndrome). The condition appears to be more common in the Lebanon than elsewhere.

References

Beighton P (1990). Syndrome of the month: Dyggve–Melchior–Clausen syndrome. *J Med Genet* **27**:512–515.

Dyggve HV, Melchior JC, Clausen J, Rastogi SC (1977). The Dyggve–Melchior–Clausen (DMC) syndrome: a 15-year follow-up and a survey of the present clinical and chemical findings. *Neuropaediatrie* **8**:429–442.

Spranger JW, Der Kaloustian VM (1975). The Dyggve–Melchior–Clausen syndrome. *Radiology* **114**:415–422.

Toledo SPA, Saldanha PH, Lamego C *et al.* (1979). Dyggve–Melchior–Clausen syndrome: genetic studies and report of affected sibs. *Am J Med Genet* **4**:255–261.

Winship WS, Rubin DL (1992). The Dyggve–Melchior–Clausen syndrome in Indian siblings. *Clin Genet* **42**:240–245.

Yunis E, Fontalvo J, Quintero L (1980). X-linked Dyggve–Melchior–Clausen syndrome. *Clin Genet* **18**:284–290.

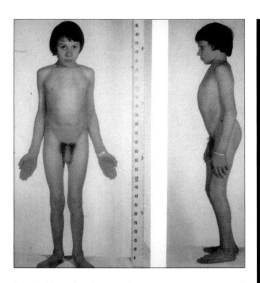

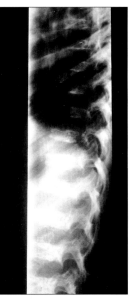

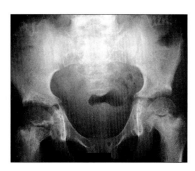

159A Note the short trunk, prominent sternum and lumbar lordosis.

159B and 159C Note lace-like appearance of iliac crests, hypoplastic basal portion of ilia and platyspondyly and irregular endplates of the vertebrae.

OSTEOLYSIS – NEPHROPATHY

160A–160C

There is progressive osteolysis of the carpal and tarsal bones together with nephropathy, resulting in hypertension and renal failure in early adult life. The tubular bones involved in foci of osteolysis are said to have a 'sucked candy' appearance. Corneal clouding can be a feature.

Genetic aspects: Autosomal dominant.

References

Carnevale A, Canun S, Mendoza L *et al.* (1987). Idiopathic multicentric osteolysis with facial anomalies and nephropathy. *Am J Med Genet* **26**:877–886.

Shinohara O, Kubota C, Kimura M *et al.* (1991). Essential osteolysis associated with nephropathy, corneal opacity, and pulmonary stenosis. *Am J Med Genet* **41**:482–486.

Warady BA, Haug SJ, Lindsley CB (1991). Multicentric osteolysis: an infrequently recognised renal-rheumatologic syndrome. *J Rheumatol* **18**:142–145.

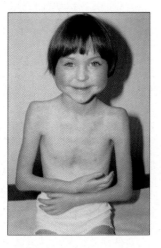

160A Note peculiar chubby cheeks, and doll-like facial appearance in spite of cachexia.

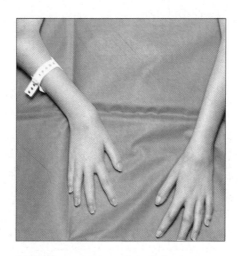

160B Note asymmetry of the limbs due to bone absorption.

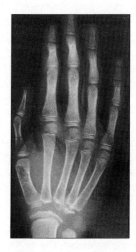

160C The proximal row of carpal bones is absent, fragments of the distal row remain and the end of the ulna has been reabsorbed.

WINCHESTER SYNDROME

161A–160B

Onset of the condition is towards the end of the first year of life with symmetrical painful swelling of the hands, fingers, wrists and ankles. Intermittent polyarthralgia results in progressive joint contractures. Oval or linear raised areas of thickened skin may appear over the back, flanks and lateral aspects of the arm. These lesions spread to cause leathery, thickened, hypertrichotic, pigmented skin. Other features are corneal opacities appearing in mid-childhood, retarded growth, carpal and tarsal osteolysis, and rheumatoid-like destruction of the small joints. Histology reveals replacement of bone with dense fibrous tissue and abnormal fibroblasts.

Genetic aspects: Autosomal recessive.

References

Brown SI, Kuwabara T (1970). Peripheral corneal opacification and skeletal deformities: a newly recognized acid mucopolysaccharidosis simulating rheumatoid arthritis. *Arch Ophthalmol* **83**:667–677.

Hollister DW, Rimoin DL, Lachman RS *et al.* (1974). The Winchester syndrome: a non-lysosomal connective tissue disease. *J Pediatr* **84**:701–709.

Winchester P, Grossman H, Lim WN, Danes BS (1969). A new acid mucopolysaccharidosis with skeletal deformities simulating rheumatoid arthritis. *Am J Roentgenol* **106**:121–128.

Winter RM (1989). Syndrome of the month. Winchester's syndrome. *J Med Genet* **26**:772–775.

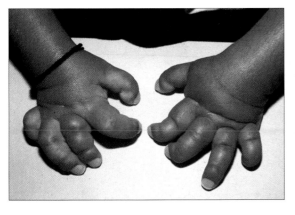

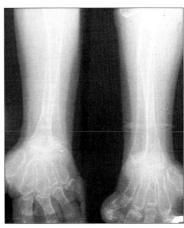

161B Note cortical thinning of radii and ulnae, carpal osteolysis, broad irregular metacarpals and phalanges, and severe osteoporosis.

161A Note the swelling and deformity of the fingers.

OLLIER ENCHONDROMATOSIS   162A–162C

The enchondromas appear as translucencies primarily in the metaphyses, but also in the diaphyses and epiphyses. Fractures may occur through these lesions, and asymmetry of the limbs may be a problem. Schwartz *et al.* suggest that the incidence of low-grade osteosarcoma is 25% by the age of 40 years. Other associated tumours include granulosa-cell ovarian tumours.

Genetic aspects: Most cases are sporadic, although occasional familial recurrences have been reported.

References
Mainzer F, Minagi H, Steinbach HL (1971). The variable manifestations of multiple enchondromatosis. *Radiology* **99**:377–388.
Schwartz HS, Zimmerman NB, Simon MA *et al.* (1987). The malignant potential of enchondromatosis. *J Bone Joint Surg A* **69**:269–274.

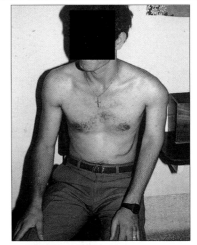

162A Note the limb shortening and deformation.

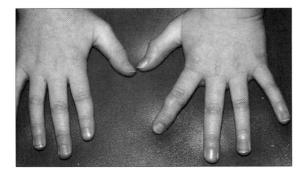

162B Note the bony lesions on the fingers.

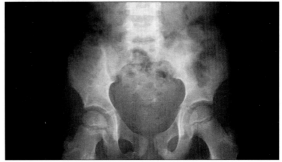

162C Note the lesions in the femoral necks.

MAFFUCCI SYNDROME   163A–163D

This is an association of enchondromatosis with skin haemangiomata. Asymmetry of the limbs can develop and the enchondromas can grow to a large size and cause a grotesque appearance. There is a risk of sarcomatous change in the enchondromata, and angiosarcomas, gliomas and adenocarcinomas also occur. The risk of malignancy is uncertain, but seems to be about 10–20%.

Genetic aspects: Uncertain, most cases are sporadic.

References
Allen BR (1978). Maffucci's syndrome. *Br J Dermatol*
Suppl.16:31–33.
Chakrabortty S, Tamaki N, Kondoh T *et al.* (1991). Maffucci's syndrome associated with intracranial enchondroma and aneurysm: case report. *Surg Neurol* **36**:216–220.
Collins PS, Han W, Williams LR *et al.* (1992). Maffucci's syndrome (hemangiomatosis osteolytica): a report of four cases. *J Vasc Surg* **16**:364–371.
Johnson TE, Nasr AM, Nalbandian RM, Cappelen-Smith J (1990). Enchondromatosis and hemangioma (Maffucci's syndrome) with

orbital involvement. *Am J Ophthalmol* **110**:153–159.
Mellon CD, Carter JE, Owen DB (1988). Ollier's disease and Maffucci syndrome: distinct entities or a continuum? Case report: enchondromatosis complicated by an intracranial glioma. *J Neurol* **235**:376–378.
Schwartz HS, Zimmerman NB, Simon MA *et al.* (1987). The malignant potential of enchondromatosis. *J Bone Joint Surg A* **69**:269–274.
Tsuchiya H, Tomita K, Yasutake H *et al.* (1991). Maffucci's syndrome combined with dedifferentiated chondrosarcoma. *Arch Orth Traum Surg* **110**:269–272.

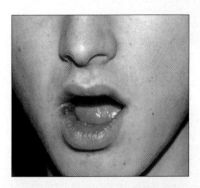

163A Note the haemangioma on the lip.

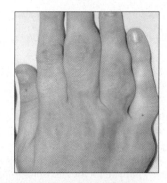

163B Note the combination of skin haemangioma and underlying enchondromata.

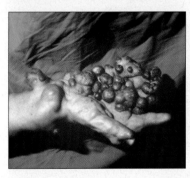

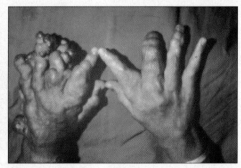

163C and 163D Note severe haemangioma and enchondromata.

MULTIPLE EXOSTOSES (DIAPHYSEAL ACLASIS)

Exostoses of the long bones occur at the periphery of the epiphyseal growth plate and the metaphysis. The exostoses can cause deformities such as bowing of the forearms, restriction of pronation and supination, tibia valga, obliquity of the distal tibial metaphysis and shortening of the fibula relative to the tibia. The pelvis and scapulae may also be involved. Sarcomatous change may occur in 5–10% of cases according to some authors, although some authors suggest that the real incidence of sarcomatous change might be nearer to 1% (Peterson). Hennekam reports that the mean age of malignant degeneration is 31 years and that this complication seldom appears before the tenth or after the fiftieth year.

Genetic aspects: Autosomal dominant. Three separate loci at 8q24, 11p11-12 and 19p11-13 have been identified by linkage analysis.

References
Baran R, Bureau H (1991). Multiple exostoses syndrome. *J Am Acad Dermatol* **25**:333–335.
Hennekam RCM (1991). Syndrome of the month. Hereditary multiple exostoses. *J Med Genet* **28**:262–266.
Menchetti G, Pompella A (1989). Hereditary multiple exostosis: pediatric aspects and differential diagnosis. *Ped Rev Commun* **3**:261–270.
Peterson HA (1989). Multiple hereditary osteochondromata. *Clin Orthop* **239**:222–230.

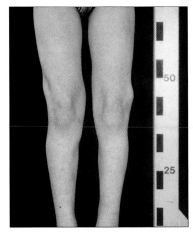
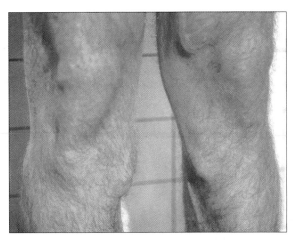

164A–164D
Note the exostoses at knees and elbows.

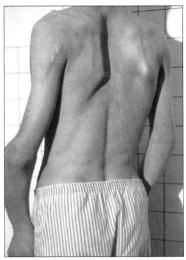
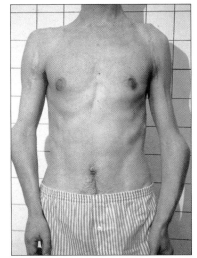
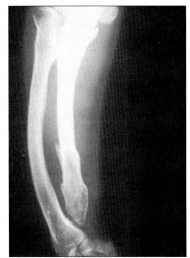

164C

164D

164E Note the exostoses at the lower end of radius and ulna.

MELNICK–NEEDLES OSTEODYSPLASTY

165A–165D

Affected females usually have short stature with prominent eyes, full cheeks, a small chin with malalignment of the teeth and a prominent forehead. Radiographs reveal delayed closure of the anterior fontanelle, sclerosis of the base of the skull, micrognathia with an increased mandibular angle, thin 'wavy' ribs, an increased height of the vertebral bodies, coxa valga and an 'S' shape to the long bones.

Genetic aspects: An X-linked dominant syndrome and male hemizygotes are more severely affected, especially where the mother carries the gene. Severely affected males can have more marked radiological features with exomphalos, an absent hallux, mild skin syndactyly and an absent cornea. Sporadic males resemble affected females, indicating a possible maternal effect in the male cases where the mother is affected.

References

Dereymaeker AM, Christens J et al. (1986). Melnick-Needles syndrome (osteodysplasty). *Helv Paediatr Acta* **41**:339–351.

Donnenfeld AE, Conrad KA, Roberts NS et al. (1987). Melnick-Needles syndrome in males: a lethal multiple congenital anomalies syndrome. *Am J Med Genet* **27**:159–173.

Eggli K, Giudici M, Ramer J et al. (1992). Melnick-Needles syndrome. Four new cases. *Pediatr Radiol* **22**:257–261.

Gardner RJM, Morrison PS, Faigan LA et al. (1990). Syndrome of a craniofacial dysostosis, limb malformation, and omphalocele. *Am J Med Genet* **36**:133–136.

Krajewska-Walasek M, Winkielman J, Gorlin RJ (1987). Melnick-Needles syndrome in males. *Am J Med Genet* **27**:153–158.

van der Lely H, Robben SGF, Meradji M, Derksen-Lubsen G (1991). Melnick-Needles syndrome (osteodysplasty) in an older male – report of a case and a review of the literature. *Br J Radiol* **64**:852–854.

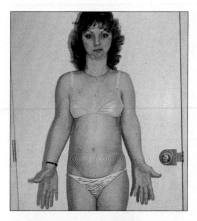

165A Note the prominent supra-orbital ridges, pointed chin and relative shortening of the upper arms.

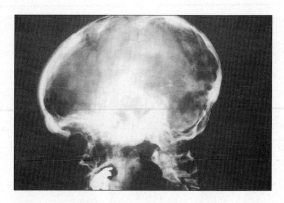

165B Note sclerosis of the base of the skull.

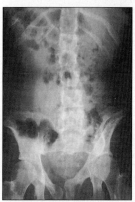

165C Note tall vertebrae, wavy ribs and flared iliac wings.

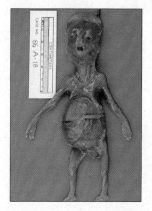

165D This severely affected male fetus has exomphalos.

LERI–WEILL DYSCHONDROSTEOSIS   165A–166B

The forearms are short and broad and Madelung deformity of the wrist is usually clinically apparent. Genu valgum is common. Stature is reduced to between 137cm and 152cm in adults. Radiographs reveal bowing of the radius and ulna, whose distal ends form a 'V' configuration between which the carpals are wedged. The ulnar styloid is usually posteriorly dislocated. In the lower limbs the tibia and fibula are short (with the latter being more severely affected).

Genetic aspects: Autosomal dominant. Homozygotes have the clinical picture of Langer mesomelic dysplasia. Expression is variable and some family members might need to be X-rayed to determine their carrier status.

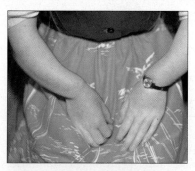

166A Note the bilateral Madelung deformity.

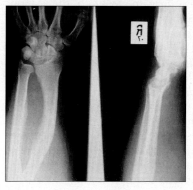

166B There is dorsal subluxation of the radius and ulna, bowing of the radius and a V-shaped configuration of the distal end of both the radius and ulna.

References

Carter AR, Currey HLF (1974). Dyschondrosteosis (mesomelic dwarfism). A family study. *Br J Radiol* **47**:634–640.

Herdman RC, Langer LO, Good RA (1966). Dyschondrosteosis. The most common cause of Madelung's deformity. *J Pediatr* **68**:432–441.

Langer LO Jr (1965). Dyschondrosteosis, a hereditable bone dysplasia with characteristic roentgenographic features. *Am J Roentgenol* **95**:178–188.

LANGER MESOMELIC DYSPLASIA

167A–167D

Langer mesomelic dysplasia is the homozygous form of dyschondrosteosis (q.v.). Affected individuals have mesomelic shortening of the limbs with severe bowing of the radii and shortening of the ulnae. The tibiae and fibulae are short and the proximal ends of the fibulae may be hypoplastic. The parents may have only mild abnormalities of the forearms.

Genetic aspects: Autosomal recessive. It may be necessary to X-ray the parents to establish whether they have Madelung deformity.

References

Espiritu C, Chen H, Woolley PV (1975). Mesomelic dwarfism as the homozygous expression of dyschondrosteosis. *Am J Dis Child* **129**:375–377.

Fryns JP, Van den Berghe H (1979). Langer type of mesomelic dwarfism as the possible homozygous expression of dyschondrosteosis. *Hum Genet* **46**:21–27.

Goldblatt J, Wallis C, Viljoen DL *et al.* (1987). Heterozygous manifestations of Langer mesomelic dysplasia. *Clin Genet* **31**:19–24.

Langer LO (1967). Mesomelic dwarfism of the hypoplastic ulna, fibula, mandible type. *Radiology* **89**:654–660.

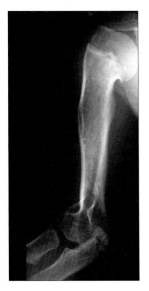 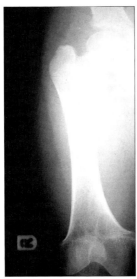 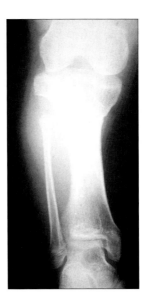 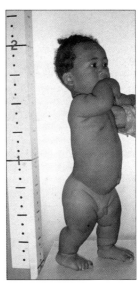

167A and 167B The other long bones are also shortened and abnormally modelled.

167C Note the severe mesomelic changes. The proximal part of the fibula is hypoplastic.

167D Note the severe mesomelic shortening of the limbs and relatively long trunk.

CLEIDOCRANIAL DYSOSTOSIS

168A–168F

The face is characterised by frontal and parietal bossing, a persistent open anterior fontanelle, often with late closure of the other sutures (including the metopic suture), small facial bones, hypertelorism and delayed eruption of the dentition. Radiological features include wormian bones, thickening of the calvarium (especially over the occiput), a narrow thorax, absent or hypoplastic clavicles, hypoplasia of the iliac wings, and failure of fusion of the symphysis pubis. Occasionally there is severe scoliosis and short distal phalanges in the hands.

Genetic aspects: Autosomal dominant. The gene maps to 6p21.

References

Chitayat D, Hodgkinson KA, Azouz EM (1992). Intrafamilial variability in cleidocranial dysplasia: a three-generation family. *Am J Med Genet* **42**:298–303.

Jarvis JL, Keats TE (1974). Cleidocranial dysostosis. A review of 40 new cases. *Am J Radiol* **121**:5–16.

Jensen BL, Kreiborg S (1990). Development of the dentition in cleidocranial dysplasia. *J Oral Pathol Med* **19**:89–93.

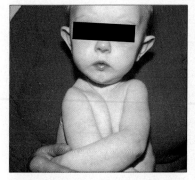
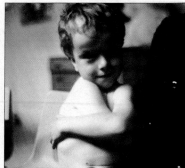

168A–168D Note short or absent clavicles allowing a proximation of the shoulders. Note broad forehead and, in **168C**, the protruding ends of the short clavicles.

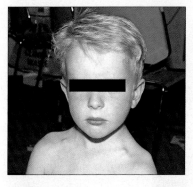
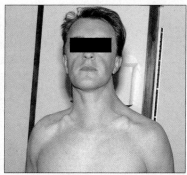

168C   168D

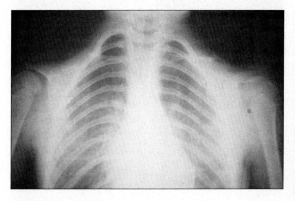
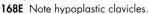

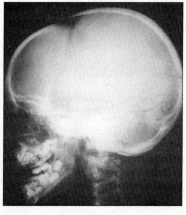

168F Note persistent anterior fontanelle and multiple wormian bones.

168E Note hypoplastic clavicles.

HAJDU–CHENEY (ACRO-OSTEOLYSIS)

The facial abnormalities may be present before skeletal abnormalities become obvious. There is micrognathia, the philtrum is long, the nares anteverted, the eyes widely spaced and down-slanting, and there is synophrys. The skull is dolichocephalic. Later optic atrophy can develop and there is early loss of teeth. Radiographs show wormian bones of the skull, an elongated pituitary fossa, persistent sutures, platybasia and absent frontal sinuses. There is a discrepancy in the length of the paired long bones, resulting in a valgus deformity of the knees or dislocation of the radial heads. The classical feature of acro-osteolysis develops only in late childhood, and it should be noted that the toes are only partially affected, leading to a triangular shape of the distal phalanges. The vertebrae are tall and the disc spaces are narrow.

Genetic aspects: Most cases are sporadic but inheritance is likely to be autosomal dominant.

References

Diren HB, Kovanlikaya I, Suller A, Dicle O (1990). The Hajdu–Cheney syndrome: a case report and review of the literature. *Pediatr Radiol* **20**:568–569.

Elias AN, Pinals RS, Anderson HC *et al.* (1978). Hereditary osteodysplasia with acro-osteolysis (the Hajdu–Cheney syndrome). *Am J Med* **65**:627–636.

Greenberg BE, Street DM (1957). Idiopathic non-familial acro-osteolysis. Report of a case observed for five years. *Radiology* **69**:259–262.

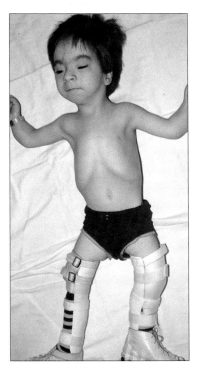

169A Note legs are in plaster because of severe osteoporosis and fractures.

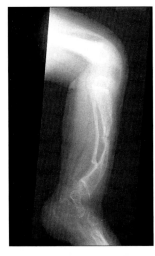

169B Note osteoporosis, bowed tibia with lytic lesion and short fibula.

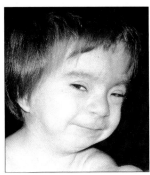

169C Note telecanthus, mild synophrys, small mouth and receding chin.

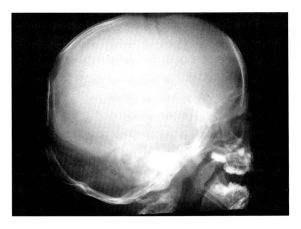

169D Note wormian bones, wide sutures, relative absence of frontal sinuses and elongated sella turcica.

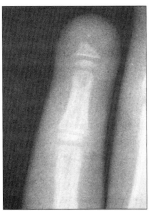

169E Note lysis of terminal phalanx.

MANDIBULO-ACRAL DYSPLASIA

This is a condition resembling pyknodysostosis and Hajdu–Cheney syndrome with features of premature ageing. There are wide fontanelles which are late closing, wormian bones, hypoplasia of the mandible and clavicles, acro-osteolysis, stiff joints and short stature. The aged appearance is caused by skin atrophy, alopecia, premature loss of teeth, and a thin face and beaked nose. Tenconi *et al.* pointed out that the mutation appears to be more frequent in Italy.

Genetic aspects: Autosomal recessive.

References

Pallotta R, Morgese G (1984). Mandibuloacral dysplasia: a rare progeroid syndrome. *Clin Genet* **26**:133–138.

Schrander-Stumpel C, Spaepen A, Fryns J-P, Dumon J (1992). A severe case of mandibuloacral dysplasia in a girl. *Am J Med Genet* **43**:877–881.

Tenconi R, Miotti F, Miotti A et al. (1986). Another Italian family with mandibuloacral dysplasia: why does it seem more frequent in Italy? *Am J Med Genet* **24**:357–364.

Welsh O (1975). Study of a family with a new progeroid syndrome. *BDOAS* **11(5)**:25–38.

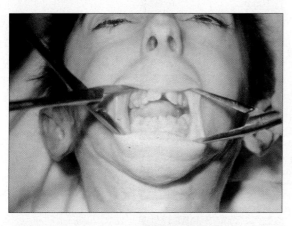

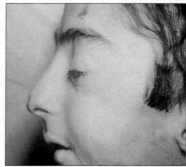

170A–170C Note the hooked thin nose, small mandible, crowded teeth, expanded tips to the fingers and atrophic skin. These are post-mortem pictures.

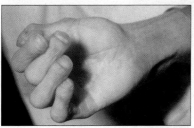

170C

PYKNODYSOSTOSIS (MAROTEAUX–LAMY SYNDROME)

The main clinical problems are short stature, dental caries, fractures of the bones and osteomyelitis. The cranium is relatively large and this is accentuated by a small face and micrognathia. The sclerae may be blue with exophthalmos. The nose is pinched with anteverted nares and the palate is high and grooved. The deciduous teeth may persist, giving a double row of teeth. The shoulders are narrow and there may be a thoracic kyphosis and lumbar lordosis. The tips of the fingers are short and bulbous, the nails thin and hypoplastic, and the skin over the dorsum of the hands wrinkled. Radiographs reveal generalised increased bone density, multiple wormian bones, osteolysis of the distal phalanges and partial aplasia of the distal ends of the clavicles. Characteristically, the mandibular angles are absent.

Genetic aspects: Autosomal recessive.

References

Edelson JG, Obad S, Geiger R et al. (1992. Pycnodysostosis. Orthopedic aspects with a description of 14 new cases. *Clin Orthop J***280**:263–276.

Elmore SM (1967). Pycnodysostosis: a review. *J Bone Joint Surg A* **49**:153.

Maroteaux P, Lamy M (1962). La pycnodystose. *Presse Med* **70**:999–1002.

Maroteaux P, Lamy M (1965). The malady of Toulouse-Lautrec. *JAMA* **191**:715–717.

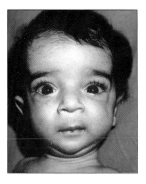
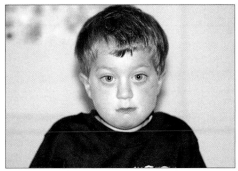
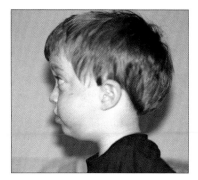

171A–171C Note prominent forehead, small chin with triangular face, prominent eyes and blue sclerae.

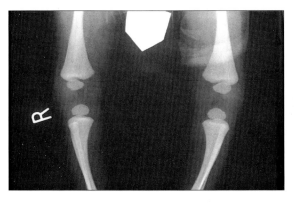
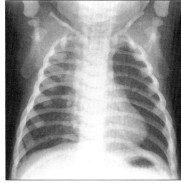

171D and 171E Note dense bones and hypoplastic clavicles.

OSTEOPETROSIS, INFANTILE (ALBERS–SCHONBERG SYNDROME)   172A–172B

From birth the bones are sclerotic with poor modelling and a 'bone within bone appearance'. Abnormal facial features become more pronounced with time and consist of macrocephaly and a square-shaped head, frontal bossing, ptosis and strabismus. Progressive pressure on cranial nerves leads to optic atrophy, deafness and facial palsy. The teeth are abnormal and decay easily. Hypochromic anaemia and pancytopenia develop and hepatosplenomegaly results. Osteomyelitis may complicate the picture. Without treatment, death is in infancy. In some cases bone marrow transplantation has produced a remission.

Genetic aspects: The severe infantile form is recessively inherited.

References
Herman TE, McAlister WH (1991). Inherited diseases of bone density in children. *Radiol Clin N Am* **29**:149–164.
Kaplan FS, August CS, Fallon MD et al. (1988). Successful treatment of infantile malignant osteopetrosis by bone-marrow transplantation. A case report. *J Bone Joint Surg A* **70**:617–623.
Loria-Cortes R, Quesada-Calvo E (1977). Osteopetrosis in children: a report of 26 cases. *J Pediatr* **91**:43–47.

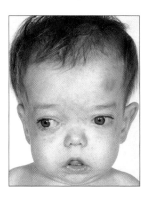

172A Note broad forehead, flat nasal bridge, prominent eyes, strabismus and bilateral facial nerve palsies.

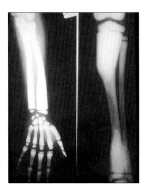

172B Note the dense and poorly modelled bones.

CAMURATI–ENGELMANN (PROGRESSIVE DIAPHYSEAL DYSPLASIA) 173A–173D

The radiological features of this condition are sclerosis and thickening of the cortex of the skull, and undermodelling and sclerosis of the diaphyses and metaphyses of the long bones. The spine is mostly spared, but occasionally there is severe scoliosis and a lumbar lordosis. This condition usually has an onset in childhood, but can occur later. The initial symptoms are mostly of muscle weakness, fatigue, poor appetite, headache and pain in the limbs. There might be a waddling gait. The tibia feels thick and prominent and there might be muscle tenderness on palpation. Pathologically, there is progressive bone formation along both the periosteal and endosteal surfaces of the long tubular bones. Symptoms can be severe early on, but there is usually spontaneous remission. Steroid therapy may help the bone pain.

Genetic aspects: Autosomal dominant.

References
Hundley JD, Wilson FC (1973). Progressive diaphyseal dysplasia. Review of the literature and report of seven cases in one family. *J Bone Joint Surg A* **55**:461–474.
Kaftori JK, Kleinhaus U, Naveh Y (1987). Progressive diaphyseal dysplasia (Camurati–Engelmann): radiographic follow-up and CT findings. *Radiology* **164**:772–782.
Minford AMB, Hardy CJ et al. (1981). Engelmann's disease and the effect of corticosteroids: a case report. *J Bone Joint Surg B* **63**:597–600.
Naveh Y, Kaftori JK, Alon U et al. (1984). Progressive diaphyseal dysplasia: genetics and clinical and radiologic manifestations. *Pediatrics* **74**:399–405.
Naveh Y, Ludatscher R, Alon U, Sharf B (1985). Muscle involvement in progressive diaphyseal dysplasia. *Pediatrics* **76**:944–949.

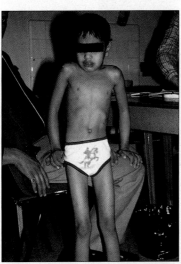
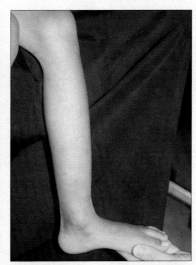

173A and 173B
Note thin slender build with poor muscle development.

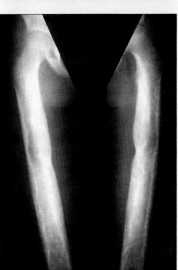
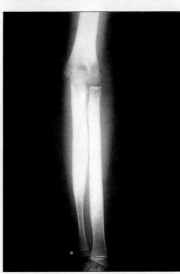

173C and 173D
Note thickening and sclerosis of the cortices of the long bones with narrowing of the medullary canals.

KENNY–CAFFEY SYNDROME (TUBULAR STENOSIS)   174A–174C

The characteristic radiological finding in this condition is excessive thickening of the cortex of the long bones, with consequent medullary stenosis. Clinical presentation is with pre- and postnatal growth retardation, hypocalcaemia leading to seizures, hypermetropia or occasionally myopia and small eyes. Intelligence is usually normal. Most data suggest that the hypocalcaemia is due to partial or complete hypoparathyroidism. Delayed closure of the anterior fontanelle and widely separated metopic sutures are common occurrences. The calvaria of the skull is often thick.

Genetic aspects: In most cases the inheritance appears to be autosomal dominant. Franceschini *et al.* reported a brother and sister, the offspring of consanguineous parents, with some features of the condition and reviewed the evidence for a rarer recessive form.

References

Abdel-Al YK, Auger LT, El-Gharbawy F (1989). Kenny–Caffey syndrome. Case report and literature review. *Clin Pediatr* **28**:175–179.

Bergada I, Schiffrin A *et al.* (1988). Kenny syndrome: description of additional abnormalities and molecular studies. *Hum Genet* **80**:39–42.

Franceschini P, Testa A, Bogetti G *et al.* (1992). Kenny–Caffey syndrome in two siblings born to consanguineous parents: evidence for an autosomal recessive variant. *Am J Med Genet* **42**:112–116.

Lee WK, Vargas A, Barnes J *et al.* (1983). The Kenny–Caffey syndrome: growth retardation and hypocalcemia in a young boy. *Am J Med Genet* **14**:773–782.

Majewski F, Rosendahl W, Ranke M *et al.* (1981). The Kenny syndrome, a rare type of growth deficiency with tubular stenosis, transient hypoparathyroidism and anomalies of refraction. *Eur J Pediatr* **136**:21–30.

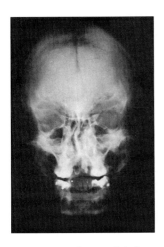
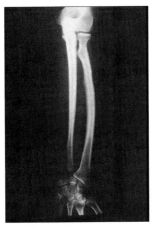
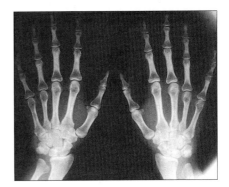

174A Note sclerosis of skull with open anterior fontanelle and metopic suture.

174B and 174C The medullary cavities of long bones are narrow.

CRANIODIAPHYSEAL DYSPLASIA   175A–175D

There is progressive overgrowth of bone affecting all areas of the skull and face, including the mandible, and of the diaphyses of the long bones. Clinically, the initial feature is often the progressive facial distortion, especially around the nose. Later, optic atrophy and deafness might develop. Radiologically, the skull is thick and the sinuses and nasal passages might be obscured. In the spine the neural arches are sometimes sclerotic and there is diaphyseal thickening of the long bones, resulting in poor bone modelling. In later stages of the disease the facial features become grotesque and mask-like.

Genetic aspects: These are still unclear. It is possible that severe cases have autosomal recessive inheritance. However, Schaefer *et al.* reported a mother and son with features of the condition.

References

Brueton LA, Winter RM (1990). Syndrome of the month. Craniodiaphyseal dysplasia. *J Med Genet* **27**:701–706.

Fosmoe RJ, Holm RS, Hildreth RC (1968). Van Buchem's disease (hyperostosis corticalis generalisata familiaris). *Radiology* **90**:771–774.

Kirkpatrick DB, Rimoin DL, Kaitila I *et al.* (1977). The craniotubular bone modelling disorders: a neurosurgical introduction to rare skeletal dysplasias with cranial nerve compression. *Surg Neurol* **7**:221–232.

McKeating JB, Kershaw CR (1987). Craniodiaphyseal dysplasia. Partial suppression of osteoblastic activity in the severe progressive form with calcitonin therapy. *J R Nav Med Serv* **73**:81–93.

Schaefer B, Stein S, Oshman D *et al.* (1986). Dominantly inherited craniodiaphyseal dysplasia: a new craniotubular dysplasia *Clin Genet* **30**:381–391.

Thurnau GR, Stein SA, Schaefer GB *et al.* (1991). Management and outcome of two pregnancies in a woman with craniodiaphyseal dysplasia. *Am J Perinatol* **8**:56–61.

Tucker AS, Klein L, Anthony GJ (1976). Craniodiaphyseal dysplasia: evolution over a five year period. *Skeletal Radiol* **1**:47–53.

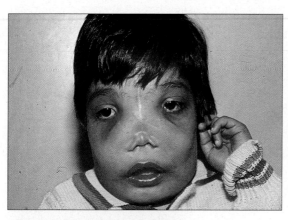

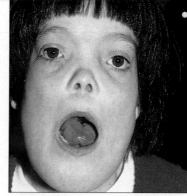

175A–175C Note enlarged mandible, marked paranasal bossing and hypertelorism.

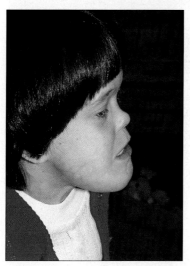

175C

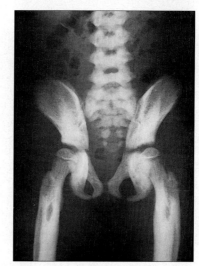

175D Note undermodelled and sclerotic femora and pelvis.

FRONTO-METAPHYSEAL DYSPLASIA

176A–176B

There is a bony overgrowth involving the supraorbital ridges, giving a visor-like appearance. The tibiae are curved backwards, with a mild valgus deformity at the knees. The fingers are long and progressive contractures develop. Extension and rotation is limited at the elbows. The muscles tend to be thin and wasted. Deafness and cranial nerve entrapment occur. Radiologically, there is patchy sclerosis of the skull, as well as the overgrowth of the supraorbital ridges. The paranasal sinuses might be obliterated. The long bones are undermodelled. The ribs are thin and irregular and the tibiae and fibulae are wavy and bowed. The carpal bones might be fused.

Genetic aspects: Inheritance is most likely X-linked, but this is not certain.

References

Abuelo DN *et al.* (1983). Picture of the month: frontometaphyseal dysplasia. *Am J Dis Child* **137**:1017–1018.

Fitzsimmons JS, Fitzsimmons EM, Barrow M (1982). Fronto-metaphyseal dysplasia. Further delineation of the clinical syndrome. *Clin Genet* **22**:195–205.

Gorlin RJ, Cohen MM Jr (1969). Frontometaphyseal dysplasia. A new syndrome. *Am J Dis Child* **118**:487–494.

Gorlin RJ, Winter RB (1980). Frontometaphyseal dysplasia – evidence for X-linked inheritance. *Am J Med Genet* **5**:81–84.

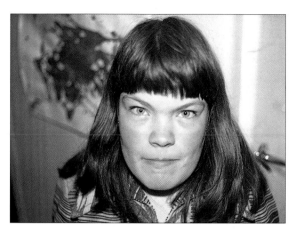 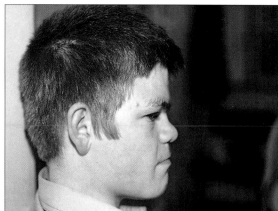

176A and 176B Note hypertelorism, prominent supraorbital ridges and prominent jaw.

CRANIOMETAPHYSEAL DYSPLASIA

The initial symptoms are often progressive nasal obstruction and mouth breathing in childhood. Later a craniotubular bone dysplasia can be shown on skeletal survey, characterised by sclerosis of the skull, including the vault and the base, and abnormal metaphyseal modelling of the long bones. Clinically, there is broadening of the nasal base with paranasal bossing, telecanthus and a prominence of the facial bones, especially the jaw. Bilateral facial weakness and progressive deafness might be other childhood signs. Intelligence is usually normal.

Genetic aspects: Most families have shown autosomal dominant inheritance although autosomal recessive inheritance has been occasionally observed, (Penchaszadeh *et al.*).

References
Beighton P, Hamersma H, Horan F (1979). Craniometaphyseal dysplasia - variability of expression within a large family. *Clin Genet* **15**:252–258.

Carlson DH, Harris GBC (1983). Craniometaphyseal dysplasia: a family with three documented cases. *Radiology* 1972;**103**:147–151.

Carnevale A, Grether P, Castillo VD. Autosomal dominant craniometaphyseal dysplasia. Clinical variability. *Clin Genet* **23**:17–22.

Key LL Jr, Volberg F, Baron R, Anast CS (1988). Treatment of craniometaphyseal dysplasia with high-dose calcitriol. *J Pediatr* **112**:583–586.

Penchaszadeh VB, Gutierrez ER *et al.* (1980). Autosomal recessive craniometaphyseal dysplasia. *Am J Med Genet* **5**:43–55.

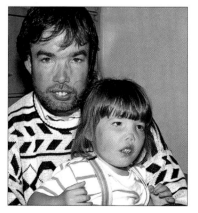

177A Note body overgrowth changes the contour of the nose. Both patients have facial nerve palsies.

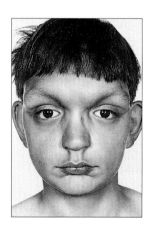

177B Note frontal bossing.

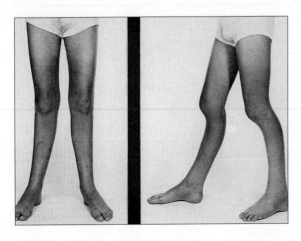

177C There is deformity of the lower limbs due to metaphyseal changes.

FIBRODYSPLASIA OSSIFICANS PROGRESSIVA (FOP)

178A–178F

The important clue to the diagnosis in the neonatal period is hypoplasia of the great toe. There may be an absent skin crease, a single phalanx and deviation of the toe laterally. The thumbs can be similarly affected. The progressive ossification which characterises this condition can occur at any time from birth to 10 years, with a mean age of onset of 3 years. Typically, there is an initial subcutaneous lump, sometimes provoked by trauma, followed 4–6 months later by radiological evidence of ossification. The main sites for these lesions are over the spine, the shoulder joints and jaw (but also elsewhere, causing restriction of movement and respiratory problems). Baldness and deafness are occasional features. Synovial osteochondromatosis may also be a feature.
Genetic aspects: Autosomal dominant (Connor *et al.*).

References

Cohen RB, Hahn GV, Tabas JA *et al.* (1993). The natural history of heterotopic ossification in patients who have fibrodysplasia ossificans progressiva. A study of forty-four cases. *J Bone Joint Surg A* **75**:215–219.

Connor JM, Evans DAP (1982). Fibrodysplasia ossificans progressiva: the clinical features and natural history of 34 patients. *J Bone Joint Surg B* **64**:76–83.

Connor JM, Skirton H, Lunt PW (1993). A three generation family with fibrodysplasia ossificans progressiva. *J Med Genet* **30**:687–689.

Kaplan FS, McCluskey W, Hahn G *et al.* (1993). Genetic transmission of fibrodysplasia ossificans progressiva. Report of a family. *J Bone Joint Surg A* **75**:1214–1220.

Rogers JG, Geho WB (1979). Fibrodysplasia ossificans progressiva: a survey of forty-two cases. *J Bone Joint Surg* **61A**:909–914.

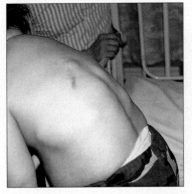

178A Note subcutaneous nodules over the back.

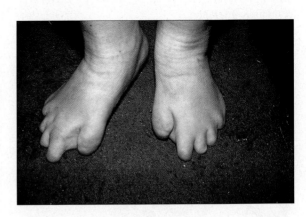

178B Note short hallux and abnormalities of the other toes.

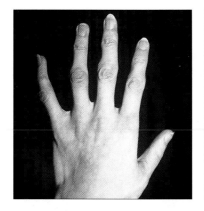

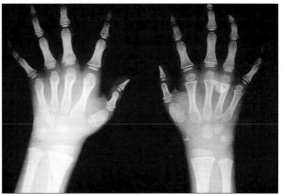

178C and 178D Note proximally placed thumbs, short first metacarpals and hypoplasia of the phalanges.

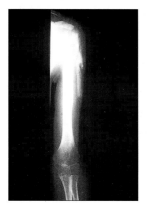

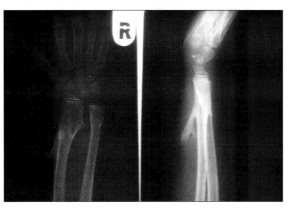

178E and 178F There are sheets of ossification in the muscles.

SYNDROMES WITH SIGNIFICANT NEUROLOGICAL ABNORMALITIES

AICARDI SYNDROME   179

This condition is characterised by infantile spasms, agenesis of the corpus callosum, hemivertebrae, block vertebrae, scoliosis, abnormal costovertebral articulations and retinal lesions. The latter are described as a 'punched-out' with a 'footprint' shape. Other ocular abnormalities include staphyloma, coloboma of the optic nerve and microphthalmia. Tsao *et al.* reported a case with a metastatic angiolipoma of the left leg and a scalp lipoma. These authors reviewed other cases from the literature with tumours. The cerebral pathology is widespread and includes cortical and sub-cortical heterotopia, and papillomas of the choroid plexus.

Genetic aspects: X-linked dominant inheritance has been postulated because most cases are isolated females. Ropers *et al.* described an affected girl with an apparently balanced X;3 translocation suggesting localisation to Xp22.

References
Bardelli AM, Hadjistilianou T, Barberi L (1985). Aicardi's syndrome. *Ophthal Paed Genet* **5**:141–144.
Donnenfeld AE, Packer RJ, Zackai E et al. (1989). Clinical, cytogenetic, and pedigree findings in 18 cases of Aicardi syndrome. *Am J Med Genet* **32**:461–467.
Molina JA, Mateos F, Merino M et al. (1989). Aicardi syndrome in two sisters. *J Pediatr* **115**:282–283.
Ropers HH, Zuffardi O, Bianchi E et al. (1982). Agenesis of the corpus callosum, ocular, and skeletal anomalies (X-linked dominant Aicardi's syndrome) in a girl with balanced X/3 translocation. *Hum Genet* **61**:364–368.
Tanaka T, Takakura H, Takashima S et al. (1985). A rare case of Aicardi syndrome with severe brain malformation and hepatoblastoma. *Brain Dev* **7**:507–512.
Tsao CY, Sommer A, Hamoudi AB (1993). Aicardi syndrome, metastatic angiosarcoma of the leg, and scalp lipoma. *Am J Med Genet* **45**:594–596.

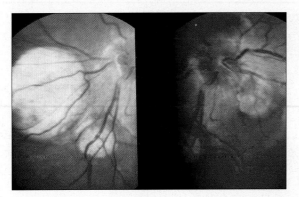

179 Note punched-out retinal lesions.

TRICHOMEGALY-CHORIORETINOPATHY (OLIVER–MACFARLANE SYNDROME) 180

The main features are sparse but abnormally long eyebrows and eyelashes which can be unusually curled, pigmentary degeneration of the retina, short stature, and mental retardation in some.

References
Corby DG, Lowe RS, Haskins RC *et al.* (1971). Trichomegaly, pigmentary degeneration of the retina, and growth retardation. *Am J Dis Child* **121**:344–345.
Delleman JW, Van Walbeek K (1975). The syndrome of trichomegaly, tapetoretinal degeneration and growth disturbances. *Ophthalmologica* **171**:313–315.
Sampson JR, Tolmie JL, Cant JS (1989). Oliver McFarlane syndrome: a 25-year follow-up. *Am J Med Genet* **34**:199–201.

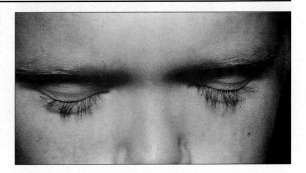

180 Note the long eyelashes.

ALOPECIA-MENTAL RETARDATION-SEIZURES 181A–181B

There are a number of case reports in which siblings have had congenital universal atrichia and mental retardation, with or without microcephaly and seizures.

Pridmore *et al.* (1992) suggest that these cases are heterogeneous and can be split into three groups. The first group contains cases with congenital total alopecia and microcephaly (Baraitser *et al.*; Mosavy; Pfeiffer and Volklein). The second group have alopecia and mental retardation, with or without seizures but without microcephaly (Richieri-Costa and Frota-Pessoa). The third group is represented by the two male infants from a consanguineous Pakistani pedigree with subtotal alopecia, microcephaly, mental retardation and seizures reported by Pridmore *et al.*
Genetic aspects: In most cases inheritance appears to be autosomal recessive, but note that the condition reported by Shokeir was inherited in a dominant manner.

References
Baraitser M, Carter CO, Brett EM (1983). A new alopecia/mental retardation syndrome. *J Med Genet* **20**:64–75.
Mosavy SH (1975). Universal alopecia and microcephaly in four siblings. *S Afr Med J* **49**:172.
Perniola T, Krajewska G *et al.* (1980). Congenital alopecia, psychomotor retardation, convulsions in two siblings of a consanguineous marriage. *J Inherit Metab Dis* **3**:49–53.
Pfeiffer RA, Volklein J (1982). Congenital universal alopecia, mental deficiency, and microcephaly in two siblings. *J Med Genet* **19**:388–389.
Pridmore C, Baraitser M, Brett EM (1992). Alopecia, mental retardation, epilepsy and microcephaly in two cousins. *Clin Dysmorphology* **1**:79–84.
Richieri-Costa A, Frota-Pessoa O (1979). Atrichia, abnormal EEG, epilepsy and mental retardation in two sisters. *Hum Hered* **29**:293–297.
Shokeir MHK (1977). Universal permanent alopecia, psychomotor epilepsy, pyorrhoea and mental subnormality. *Clin Genet* **11**:13–17.
Wessel HB, Barmada MA, Hashida Y (1987). Congenital alopecia, seizures, and psychomotor retardation in three siblings. *Pediatr Neurol* **3**:101–107.

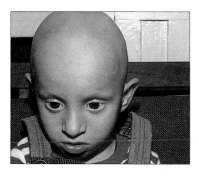

181A and 181B Note total alopecia, including sparse eyebrows.

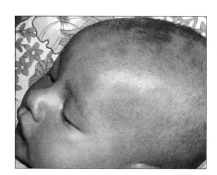

ANGELMAN SYNDROME

182A–182D

There is mental retardation associated with microcephaly, with a disproportionate emphasis on a profound speech deficit. Jerky movements affecting the trunk and upper limbs become apparent about the time that the child begins to sit. The onset of walking is significantly delayed because of ataxia and the gait is unsteady and wide-based. Most children learn to walk and the gait disturbance improves. Outbursts of laughter, often accompanied by hand flapping, are frequent and the children in general have a happy disposition. Seizures may develop but these are relatively easy to control. The EEG is characteristic (see Boyd *et al.*). The facial features may be characteristic with fair hair, a prominent chin and constant dribbling.

Genetic aspects: Deletions or rearrangements of the long arm of chromosome 15 at 15q11-q13 are seen in 60% of cases. The deletion is usually a new mutation and is always on the chromosome 15 inherited from the mother. A small proportion of cases have paternal disomy for chromosome 15 (Malcolm *et al.*). However, at least 20% of affected individuals have normal chromosomes and no evidence of disomy. Wagstaff *et al.* reported three normal sisters who had all given birth to children with Angelman syndrome. This was shown to be due to a mutation in 15q11-13

that resulted in Angelman syndrome when transmitted by females, but no phenotypic effect when transmitted by a male (i.e. the grandfather).

In cases without detectable deletions or paternal disomy there is a significant recurrence risk and evidence of maternal inheritance of an abnormal gene (Clayton-Smith *et al.*). In those with a deletion the recurrence risks are small provided that parental chromosomes are normal.

References

Boyd SG, Harden A, Patton MA (1988). The EEG in early diagnosis of the Angelman (happy puppet) syndrome. *Eur J Pediatr* **147**:508–513.

Clayton-Smith J (1992). Angelman's syndrome. *Arch Dis Child* **67**:889–890.

Clayton-Smith J, Pembrey ME (1992). Angelman syndrome. *J Med Genet* **29**:412–415.

Driscoll DJ, Waters MF, Williams CA *et al.* (1992). A DNA methylation imprint, determined by the sex of the parent, distinguishes the Angelman and Prader–Willi syndromes. *Genomics* **13**:917–924.

Malcolm S, Clayton-Smith J, Nichols M *et al.* (1991). Uniparental paternal disomy in Angelman's syndrome. *Lancet* **1**:694–697.

Wagstaff J, Knoll JHM, Glatt KA *et al.* (1992). Maternal but not paternal transmission of 15q11-13-linked nondeletion Angelman syndrome leads to phenotypic expression. *Nature Genetics* **1**:291–294.

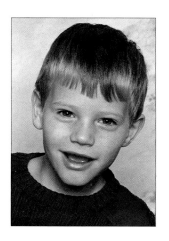

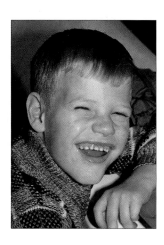

182A–182D Note wide mouth, small pointed jaw and happy disposition.

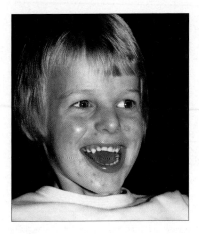

182C

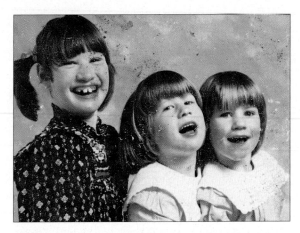

182D

RETT SYNDROME

183A–183C

This condition occurs in females with a normal pre- and perinatal history, normal development and head circumference up to 6 months of age (and often up to 12–18 months). There is subsequent regression of social and motor skills, hand-wringing or clapping with frequent mouthing, and truncal and gait ataxia. Epilepsy may be a feature and the respiratory pattern is characteristic with periods of rapid breathing and hyperventilation followed by reactive apnoea. Later on in the disease the patient becomes chair-bound with spasticity, joint contractures and a staring gaze. **Genetic aspects:** The vast majority of cases are sporadic, but familial cases have been reported. Anvret and Wahlstrom reviewed the genetics of the condition – to that date there was one report of classical Rett syndrome in a 12-year-old girl and her more mildly affected maternal aunt, three full sister pairs, two half-sister pairs, and cousins. Witt Engerstrom and Forslund reported a convincingly affected mother and daughter.

References
Anvret M, Wahlstrom J (1992). Genetics of the Rett syndrome. *Brain Dev* **14(Suppl.)**:S101–103.
Hagberg B (1992). The Rett syndrome: an introductory overview 1990. *Brain Dev* **14(Suppl.)**:S5–8.
Hagberg B, Goutieres F, Hanefeld F *et al.* (1985). Rett syndrome: criteria for inclusion and exclusion. *Brain Dev* **7**:372–373.
Opitz JM, Lewin SO (1987). Rett syndrome – a review and discussion of syndrome delineation and syndrome definition. *Brain Dev* **9**:445–450.
Witt Engerstrom I, Forslund M (1992). Mother and daughter with Rett syndrome (Letter). *Dev Med Child Neurol* **34**:1022–1023.

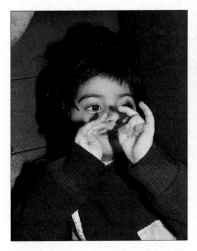

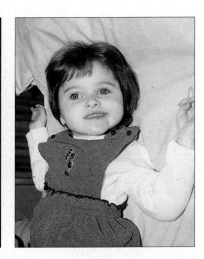

183A and 183B Note the characteristic hand posturing.

183C Note that the facial features can resemble Angelman syndrome.

CARBOHYDRATE-DEFICIENT GLYCOPROTEIN DISEASE   184A–184D

According to Jaeken *et al.* (1991) there are four stages to this condition. The stage one infantile phase is characterised by failure to thrive, hypotonia, developmental delay, liver insufficiency, pericardial and stroke-like episodes; the stage two childhood phase by ataxia, mental retardation and a pigmentary retinopathy; the stage three teenage stage by marked muscle atrophy in the legs secondary to a neuropathy; and the stage four adult phase by additional hypogonadism. All individuals previously diagnosed as having ataxic cerebral palsy should be tested for this condition.

The most characteristic clue to the diagnosis is the presence of fat pads over the outer buttocks, absent fat with unusual skin folds over the anterior aspect of the thighs, unusual fat pads on the dorsum of the fingers, areas of thick skin (like the peel of an orange), and lipoatrophic areas over the legs. Other features include inverted nipples, arachnodactyly, restricted joint movement, a high nasal bridge and a prominent jaw.

There may be a more severe sub-group where affected individuals die in the first year of life with peripheral oedema and abnormal liver function.

Diagnosis can be established by transferrin isoelectric focusing which shows evidence of reduced sialation. Prenatal diagnosis by fetal blood sampling has been attempted, but this may result in false negative diagnoses (Clayton *et al.* 1993).

Genetic aspects: Autosomal recessive.

References

Clayton PT, Winchester BG, Keir G (1992). Hypertrophic obstructive cardiomyopathy in a neonate with the carbohydrate-deficient glycoprotein syndrome. *J Inherit Metab Dis* **15**:857–860.

Clayton P, Winchester B, Di Tomaso E *et al.* (1993). Carbohydrate-deficient glycoprotein syndrome: normal glycosylation in the fetus (Letter). *Lancet* **1**:956.

Horslen SP, Clayton PT, Harding BN *et al.* (1991). Olivopontocerebellar atrophy of neonatal onset and disialotransferrin developmental deficiency syndrome. *Arch Dis Child* **66**:1027–1032.

Jaeken J, Hagberg B, Stromme P (1991). Clinical presentation and natural course of the carbohydrate-deficient glycoprotein syndrome. *Acta Paediatr Scand Suppl.* **375**:6–13.

Petersen MB, Brostrom K, Stibler H, Skovby F (1993). Early manifestations of the carbohydrate-deficient glycoprotein syndrome. *J Pediatr* **122**:66–70.

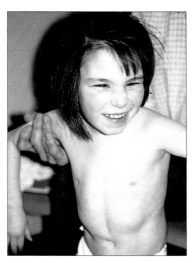

184A–184D
Note unusual fat distribution and inverted nipples.

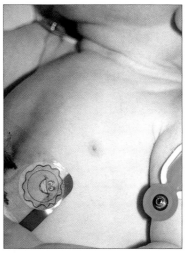

184B

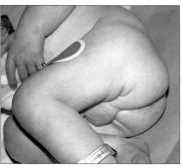

184C

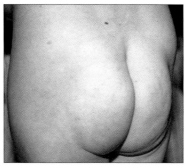

184D

MOEBIUS SYNDROME (CONGENITAL FACIAL DIPLEGIA)   185A–185D

The essential features of Moebius syndrome are unilateral or bilateral facial and abducens palsies. Other cranial nerve palsies, particularly bulbar, may be present. Associated facial features include micrognathia, epicanthic folds, structural abnormalities of the ears and defective branchial musculature. Limb defects, present in some cases, include syndactyly, polydactyly, brachydactyly, oligodactyly and absent trapezoid or pectoral muscles. There is therefore considerable overlap with Poland syndrome and the hypoglossia-hypodactyly syndrome.

Mental retardation is often absent, but Baraitser noted significant retardation in 50% of carefully diagnosed cases.

Genetic aspects: Baraitser pointed out that in the absence of limb abnormalities diagnosis can be difficult, and that cases with the limb deformity have a low recurrence risk.

References

Baraitser M (1977). Genetics of Moebius syndrome. *J Med Genet* **14**:415–417.

Bavinck JNB, Weaver DD (1986). Subclavian artery supply disruption sequence: hypothesis of a vascular etiology for Poland, Klippel-Feil, and Moebius anomalies. *Am J Med Genet* **23**:903–918.

Fujita I, Koyanagi T, Kukita J et al. (1991). Moebius syndrome with central hypoventilation and brainstem calcification: a case report. *Eur J Pediatr* **150**:582–583.

Goldblatt D, Williams D (1986). "I am smiling": Mobius syndrome inside and out. *J Child Neurol* **1**:71–78.

Kumar D (1990). Syndrome of the month. Moebius syndrome. *J Med Genet* **27**:122–126.

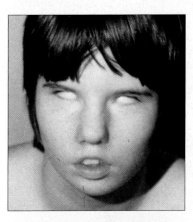
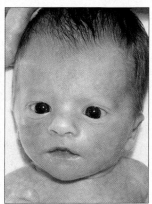

185A–185C Note the immobile face due to bilateral facial nerve palsies and the convergent squint due to bilateral sixth nerve palsies.

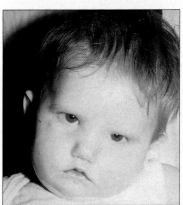

185C

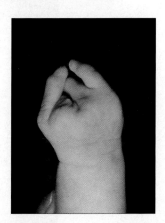

185D Symbrachydactyly.

MILLER–DIEKER LISSENCEPHALY   186A–186B

Microcephaly is common, but not invariable, and is usually not severe in the neonatal period. Characteristic facial features include a prominent forehead, bitemporal narrowing, a depressed nasal bridge, anteverted nares, mid-face hypoplasia and a thin upper lip. Vertical furrowing of the forehead is present in about only 25% of cases and is usually present only in the neonatal period. These infants have type I lissencephaly (Dobyns *et al.* 1985). CT and MRI scans show severe lissencephaly and, characteristically, a midline focus of calcification in the callosal remnant. These is post-natal growth deficiency and frequently prolonged neonatal jaundice. Other associated malformations include congenital heart defect (in cases with a large chromosome deletion) and post-axial polydactyly.

Genetic aspects: About half of the cases can be shown to have a deletion of 17p13.3 by light microscopy and a further 35–41% have a submicroscopic deletion, most easily demonstrated by fluorescent *in situ* hybridisation (FISH).

Isolated lissencephaly (i.e. without dysmorphic features) is heterogeneous. About 13% of cases have submicroscopic deletions of 17p (Ledbetter *et al.*). Intrauterine CMV infection and early placental insufficiency may be other causes. A 7% recurrence risk is suggested if a deletion is not found.

Reiner *et al.* demonstrated mutations in a gene from the beta-transducin family of G protein-like molecules (LIS1).

References
Barkovich AJ, Koch TK, Carrol CL (1991). The spectrum of lissencephaly – report of ten patients analysed by magnetic resonance imaging. *Ann Neurol* **31**:139–146.

De Rijk-van Andel JF, Arts WFM, Barth PG, Loonen MCB (1990). Diagnostic features and clinical signs of 21 patients with lissencephaly type I. *Dev Med Child Neurol* **32**:707–717.

Dobyns WB, Gilbert EF, Opitz JM (1985). Further comments on the lissencephaly syndromes. *Am J Med Genet* **22**:197–211.

Dobyns WB, Curry CJR, Hoyme HE *et al.* (1991). Clinical and molecular diagnosis of Miller–Dieker syndrome. *Am J Hum Genet* **48**:584–594.

Ledbetter SA, Kuwano A, Dobyns WB, Ledbetter DH (1992). Microdeletions of chromosome 17p13 as a cause of isolated lissencephaly. *Am J Hum Genet* **50**:182–189.

Reiner O, Carrozzo R, Shen Y *et al.* (1993). Isolation of a Miller–Dieker lissencephaly gene containing G protein beta-subunit-like repeats. *Nature* **364**:717–721.

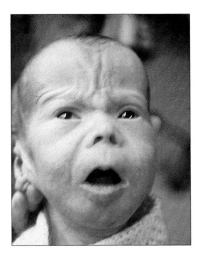

186A Note the vertical furrows on the forehead.

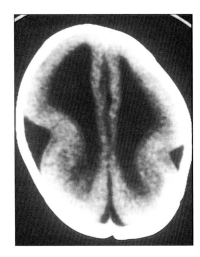

186B Note the figure of '8' configuration and the lack of gyral indentations because of the smooth cortex.

PROGRESSIVE ENCEPHALOPATHY-OEDEMA-HYPSARRHYTHMIA-OPTIC ATROPHY (PEHO)   187A–C

Starting from 2 weeks to 3 months of age there is severe hypotonia, hyperreflexia, infantile spasms and marked oedema, especially of the extremities. The facies are characterised by a narrow forehead, puffy cheeks, a receding chin, protruding earlobes, epicanthic folds, mid-face hypoplasia, a high-arched palate and an open mouth. The patients become almost inactive after 3–4 years of age and die in childhood. Neuropathological studies reveal a small cerebellum, wide ventricles or internal hydrocephalus, spongy vacuolation in the cerebral cortex, loss of Purkinje cells and granule cells with proliferation of Bergmann's glia in the cerebellum and small cystic or haemorrhagic changes in the basal ganglia.

Genetic aspects: Autosomal recessive.

References
Salonen R, Somer M, Haltia M *et al.* (1991). Progressive encephalopathy with edema, hypsarrhythmia, and optic atrophy (PEHO syndrome). *Clin Genet* **39**:287–293.

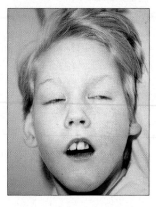

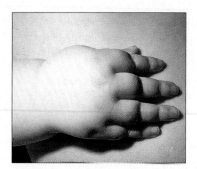

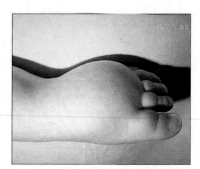

187B and 187C Note puffiness of hands and feet.

187A Note the bitemporal narrowing and round face.

MENTAL RETARDATION-APHASIA-SHUFFLING GAIT-ADDUCTED THUMBS (MASA) SYNDROME 188

The main clinical features are mental retardation, delayed speech development, adducted or contracted thumbs, clinodactyly of the index and little fingers, a shuffling gait and increased reflexes in the lower limbs. CT scans can show hydrocephalus and partial agenesis of the corpus callosum.

Genetic aspects: X-linked recessive. The gene maps to Xq28 and has been identified as the X-linked cell adhesion molecule L1 (L1CAM), mutations of which also cause X-linked aqueduct stenosis.

References
Fryns JP, Schrander-Stumpel C, de Die-Smulders C *et al.* (1992). MASA syndrome: delineation of the clinical spectrum at prepubertal age. *Am J Med Genet* **43**:402–407.
Kenwrick S, Ionasescu V, Ionasescu G *et al.* (1986). Linkage studies of X-linked recessive spastic paraplegia using DNA probes. *Hum Genet* **73**:264–266.
Macias VR, Day DW, King TE, Wilson GN (1992). Clasped-thumb mental retardation (MASA) syndrome: confirmation of linkage to Xq28. *Am J Med Genet* **43**:408–414.
Straussberg R, Blatt I, Brand N *et al.* (1991). X-linked mental retardation with bilateral clasped thumbs: report of another affected family. *Clin Genet* **40**:337–341.
Winter RM, Davies KE, Bell MV *et al.* (1989). MASA syndrome: further clinical delineation and chromosomal localisation. *Hum Genet* **82**:367–370.

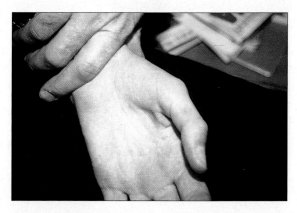

188 Note atrophy of the thenar eminence in this patient with spastic paraparesis of the lower limbs.

KEARNS–SAYRE SYNDROME 189

The age of onset might be in early childhood, especially if short stature is one of the features. Ptosis, abnormalities of eye movement and a retinal dystrophy may become evident before the age of 20 years. Cardiac conduction defects are common. Proximal muscle weakness, deafness, ataxia and a cardiomyopathy may develop. All cases will have ragged red fibres on muscle biopsy. The list of abnormalities in this condition has been extended to include basal ganglia calcification and a lipid myopathy. There have been reports of cytochrome-c-oxidase deficiency, and some cases have been shown to have mitochondrial DNA deletions. There is evidence that some cases with Pearson syndrome may go on to develop symptoms of this disorder.

Genetic aspects: Although many cases have a mitochondrial DNA mutation, most are single within a family. At present, recurrence risks are in the vicinity of 5%.

References

Clarke LA (1992). Mitochondrial disorders in pediatrics. Clinical, biochemical, and genetic implications. *Pediatr Clin N Am* **39**:319–334.

Inui K, Fukushima H, Tsukamoto H *et al.* (1992). Mitochondrial encephalomyopathies with the mutation of the mitochondrial tRNA Leu (UUR) gene. *J Pediatr* **120**:62–66.

Moraes CT *et al.* (1989). Mitochondrial DNA deletions in progressive external ophthalmoplegia and Kearns–Sayre syndrome. *New Engl J Med* **320**:1293–1299.

Reichmann H, Degoul F, Gold R *et al.* (1991). Histological, enzymatic and mitochondrial DNA studies in patients with Kearns–Sayre syndrome and chronic progressive external ophthalmoplegia. *Eur Neurol* **31**:108–113.

Tulinius MH, Holme E, Kristiansson B *et al.* (1991). Mitochondrial encephalomyopathies in childhood. II. Clinical manifestations and syndromes. *J Pediatr* **119**:251–259.

Zeviani M, Moraes CT, Dimauro S *et al.* (1988). Deletions of mitochondrial DNA in Kearns–Sayre syndrome. *Neurology* **38**:1339–1346.

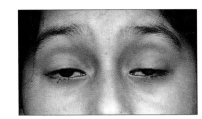

189 Note the bilateral ptosis. The patient also has an external ophthalmoplegia.

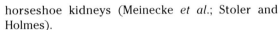

AGNATHIA-HOLOPROSENCEPHALY

In this condition the mandible and tongue are extremely small or absent and the ears are low-set, in the most extreme cases meeting in the midline under the chin. The facial features may reflect underlying holoprosencephaly of the brain. Pauli *et al.* (1983) reported two stillborn sisters with this condition. The mandible was extremely small in both, but whereas one had the facial features of cebocephaly the other had down-slanting, normally placed palpebral fissures. One case had alobar holoprosencephaly and the other had agenesis of both olfactory bulbs. One infant had tetralogy of Fallot, malrotation of the gut and a hypoplastic kidney on one side. Subsequent chromosome analysis on one sibling showed a 46,XX,der18,t(6;18)(pter→p24::p11.21→qter) karyotype with a balanced translocation in the father. Some cases have had situs inversus, anal atresia and horseshoe kidneys (Meinecke *et al.*; Stoler and Holmes).

Genetic aspects: Most cases of agnathia (about 80 cases in the literature) are sporadic. The genetics of agnathia with additional anomalies, as described above, is uncertain.

References

Ades LC, Sillence DO (1992). Agnathia-holoprosencephaly with tetramelia (case report). *Clin Dysmorphol* **1**:182–184.

Meinecke P, Padberg B, Laas R (1990). Agnathia, holoprosencephaly, and situs inversus: a third report. *Am J Med Genet* **37**:286–287.

Pauli RM, Graham J Jr, Barr M Jr (1981). Agnathia, situs inversus, and associated malformations. *Teratology* **23**:85–93.

Pauli RM, Pettersen JC, Arya S (1983). Familial agnathia-holoprosencephaly. *Am J Med Genet* **14**:677–698.

Stoler JM, Holmes LB (1992). A case of agnathia, situs inversus, and a normal central nervous system. *Teratology* **46**:213–216.

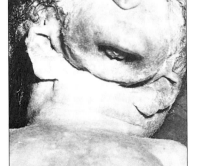

190A Note absent jaw, low-set ears and cebocephaly nostril.

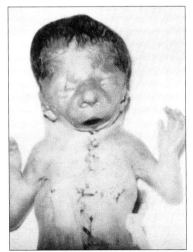

190B Note the absent jaw and low-set ears.

HOLOPROSENCEPHALY

The incidence of holoprosencephaly with normal chromosomes is 1 in 16 000–53 000. Facial abnormalities include a range of severity including hypotelorism, midline clefting of the upper lip with premaxillary agenesis, a single nostril, cyclopia and a midline proboscis. CT or MRI scans show fusion of the cerebral hemispheres in the lobar form, or absence of the olfactory tracts in the semilobar form. **Genetic aspects:** Autosomal dominant inheritance is rare, but certainly exists. In an autosomal dominant family there can be incomplete penetrance and variable expression. Some gene carriers may have a single central maxillary incisor and mild hypotelorism and anosmia. The brain scan in these presumptive carriers is usually normal. The risk of an obligate carrier having a severely affected infant is 16–21%; the risk of milder manifestations is 13–14%. Cohen *et al.* (1989) review autosomal recessive families. Recurrence risks after an isolated case of holoprosencephaly with normal chromosomes are 5–6%.

Several chromosomal aberrations are consistently associated with holoprosencephaly including del(18p), del(2p21), del(7q36), dup(3p24-pter) and del(21q22.3).

References

Balci S, Onol B, Ercal MD *et al* (1993). Autosomal recessive alobar holoprosencephaly with cyclops in three female siblings: prenatal ultrasonographic diagnosis at 18th week. *Clin Dysmorphol* **2**:165–168.

Cohen MM Jr (1989). Perspectives on holoprosencephaly: part I. Epidemiology, genetics, and syndromology. *Teratology* **40**:211–235.

Collins AL, Lunt PW, Garrett C, Dennis NR (1990). Holoprosencephaly: a family showing dominant inheritance and variable expression. *J Med Genet* **30**:36–40.

Corsello G, Buttitta P, Cammarata M et al. (1993). Holoprosencephaly: examples of clinical variability and etiologic heterogeneity. *Am J Med Genet* **37**:244–249.

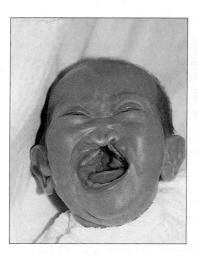 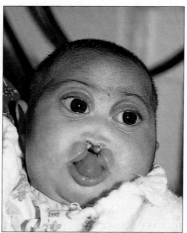

191A and 191B Note premaxillary agenesis.

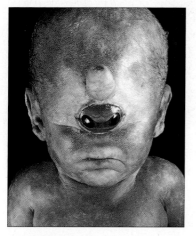

191C Note hypotelorism with single nostril (cebocephaly).

191D Cyclopian fetus.

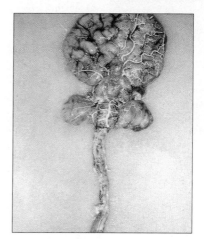

191E Note undivided cerebral hemispheres.

NEURAL TUBE DEFECTS

The diagnosis is usually straightforward. The recurrence risk is 4% and preconceptional folic acid is recommended to reduce recurrence risks.

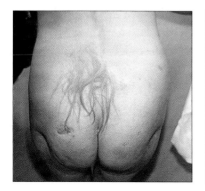

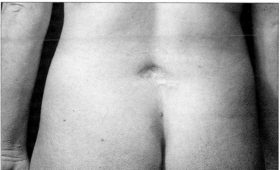

192A and 192B
Closed spina bifida.

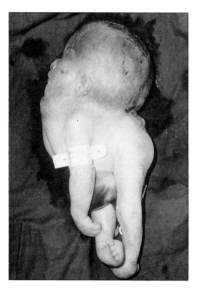

192C
Iniencephaly.

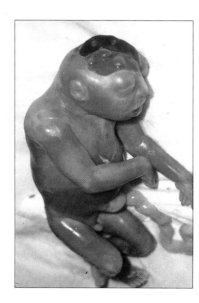

192D
Anencephaly.

SIRENOMELIA/CAUDAL REGRESSION

The lower limbs are fused together, sometimes with a single femur, with two tibiae and fibulae being rotated by 180 degrees. Associated malformations include absent external genitalia, imperforate anus, lumbosacral vertebral and pelvic abnormalities and renal agenesis. The condition has been thought to be part of the caudal regression spectrum. Sirenomelia occurs in about 1 in 65 000 livebirths and may be more common in one of monozygotic twins.

References

Di Lorenzo M, Brandt ML, Veilleux A (1991). Sirenomelia in an identical twin: a case report. *J Pediatr Surg* **26**:1334–1336.

Kallen B, Castilla EE, Lancaster PAL et al. (1992). The cyclops and the mermaid: an epidemiological study of two types of rare malformation. *J Med Genet* **29**:30–35.

Kapur RP, Mahony BS, Nyberg DA et al. (1991). Sirenomelia associated with a "vanishing twin". *Teratology* **43**:103–108.

Martinez-Frias ML, Cucalon F, Urioste M (1992). New case of limb body-wall complex associated with sirenomelia sequence. *Am J Med Genet* **44**:583–585.

Tang TT, Oechler HW, Hinke DH et al. (1991). Limb body-wall complex in association with sirenomelia sequence. *Am J Med Genet* **41**:21–25.

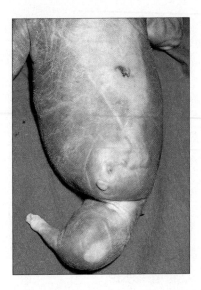

193 Note the fusion of the lower limbs.

SYNDROMES WITH ENDOCRINE AND GROWTH ABNORMALITIES

ALBRIGHT – PSEUDO, AND PSEUDO-PSEUDOHYPOPARATHYROIDISM   194A–194F

Most authors now accept that Albright's hereditary osteodystrophy and pseudo-pseudohypoparathyroidism are variants of the same condition. The main features are hypocalcemia, hyperphosphatemia, obesity, a short stocky build, a round face, short bones in the fingers, especially the fourth and fifth metacarpals, and subcutaneous calcification. Cataracts can occur, osteoporosis and an advanced bone age are probably common manifestations, and less well known is the frequent shortening of the distal phalanx of the thumb. Mental retardation occurs in about 70% of cases. Ectopic calcification frequently occurs in the kidneys, brain and other tissues. In the skin the histological appearance can be that of osteoma cutis.

In type I the urinary cAMP response to administered parathyroid hormone (PTH) is absent. In type II a cAMP response occurs but there is no phosphate diuresis.

Genetic aspects: The sex ratio is F:M, 2:1, although autosomal dominant inheritance seems most likely. The condition is caused by a defective G protein (Spiegel *et al.*) (the G proteins are a family of guanine-binding proteins that mediate signal transduction across cell membranes – Patten *et al.*). Type I cases are now divided into type Ia (with G protein defect) and type Ib (without G protein defect).

References

Faull CM, Welbury RR, Paul B, Kendall-Taylor P (1991). Pseudohypoparathyroidism: its phenotypic variability and associated disorders in a large family. *Q J Med* **78**:251–264.

Fitch N (1982). Albright's hereditary osteodystrophy: a review. *Am J Med Genet* **11**:11–29.

Patten JL, Johns DR, Valle D *et al.* (1990). Mutation in the gene encoding the stimulatory G protein of adenylate cyclase in Albright's hereditary osteodystrophy. *New Engl J Med* **322**:1412–1419.

Smit L, van Wijk RM, Rico RE, Sitalsing AD (1988). Intracerebral bilateral symmetrical calcifications, demonstrated in a patient with pseudohypoparathyroidism. *Clin Neurol Neurosurg* **90**:145–150.

Spiegel AM (1990). Albright's hereditary osteodystrophy and defective G proteins (Editorial). *New Engl J Med* **322**:1461–1462.

Stirling HF, Darling JAB, Barr DGD (1991). Plasma cyclic AMP response to intravenous parathyroid hormone in pseudohypoparathyroidism. *Acta Paediatr Scand* **80**:333–338.

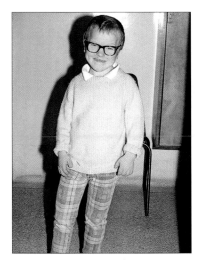
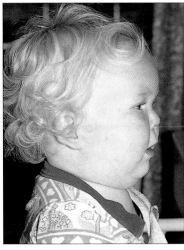

194A and 194B Note flat nasal bridge and short stature.

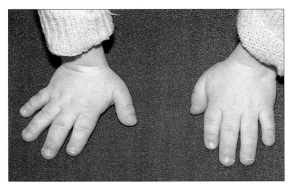
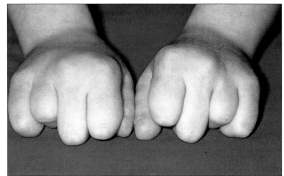

194C and 194D Note short stubby fingers and especially short fourth and fifth metacarpals.

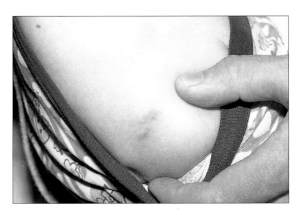
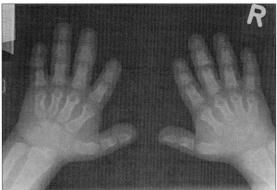

194E Note subcutaneous calcification.

194F Note short metacarpals and cone-shaped epiphyses.

McCUNE–ALBRIGHT SYNDROME – POLYOSTOTIC FIBROUS DYSPLASIA 195

This is the association between polyostotic fibrous dysplasia, cutaneous pigmentation and precocious puberty. The fibrous dysplasia may involve any bone, although some sites are preferentially affected, such as the upper end of the femur. Involvement of long bones results in bowing, pain and sometimes fractures. Involvement of the bones of the skull results in facial asymmetry, prognathism and proptosis. Radiographs of the skull may reveal hyperostosis. Cafe au lait spots of the skin are characteristic; they are usually large and are distributed asymmetrically with an irregular border. Oral pigmentation can occur. Precocious puberty occurs in 50% of affected females and in some males. Hyperthyroidism and Cushing's syndrome are complications. When this occurs in the neonatal period the bone lesions may not be typical and there may be diffuse osteoporosis without obvious fibrous dysplasia or widening of metaphyses with scattered irregular lucencies in the vertebrae, pelvis and long bones.

Genetic aspects: Almost all cases are sporadic. The condition has been shown to be caused by somatic mutation of the GNAS1 gene, coding for the alpha-subunit of G-protein, leading to overactivity of adenylyl cyclase (Schwingdinger *et al.*). Loss of function of the same gene leads to Albright hereditary osteodystrophy (q.v.).

References

Feuillan PP, Shawker T, Rose SR *et al.* (1990). Thyroid abnormalities in the McCune–Albright syndrome: ultrasonography and hormonal studies. *J Clin Endocr Metab* **71**:1596–1601.

Lee PA, Van Dop C, Migeon CJ (1986). McCune–Albright syndrome. Long-term follow-up. *JAMA* **256**:2980–2984.

Roth JG, Esterly NB (1991). McCune–Albright syndrome with multiple bilateral cafe au lait spots. *Pediatr Dermatol* **8**:35–39.

Schwindinger WF, Francomano CA, Levine MA (1992). Identification of a mutation in the gene encoding the alpha subunit of the stimulatory G protein of adenylyl cyclase in McCune–Albright syndrome. *Proc Nat Acad Sci* **89**:5152–5156.

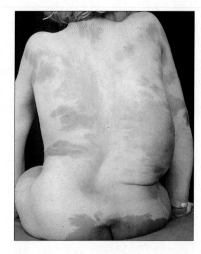

195 Note large patches of pigmentation with irregular borders ('coast of Maine appearance'), and scoliosis.

MULTIPLE ENDOCRINE ADENOMATOSIS TYPE 2B 196A–196B

There is a marfanoid habitus with thickened lips and sometimes ectropion. Mucosal ganglioneuromas, presenting as nodules on the tongue or lips, become evident. Medullated nerve fibres may be seen in the cornea. Medullary carcinoma of the thyroid, phaeochromocytoma and parathyroid tumours can occur. Some cases have Hirschsprung disease. Gene carriers can now be identified by DNA techniques and presymptomatic screening should be carried out on at-risk individuals.

Genetic aspects: Autosomal dominant. Point mutations in the RET proto-oncogene have been demonstrated in this condition, as well as in MEN 2A (Hofstra *et al.*; Eng *et al.*). These appear to be 'gain of function' mutations, rather than 'loss of function' mutations (van Heyningen).

References

Eng C, Smith DP, Mulligan LM *et al.* (1994). Point mutation within the tyrosine kinase domain of the RET proto-oncogene in multiple endocrine neoplasia type 2B and related sporadic tumours. *Hum Molec Genet* **3**:237–241.

Hofstra RMW, Landsvater RM, Ceccherini I *et al.* (1994). A mutation in the RET proto-oncogene associated with multiple endocrine neoplasia type 2B and sporadic medullary thyroid carcinoma. *Nature* **367**:375–376.

Van Heyningen V (1994). One gene – four syndromes. *Nature* **367**:319–320.

Vasen HFA, van der Feltz M, Raue F *et al.* (1992). The natural course of multiple endocrine neoplasia type IIb: a study of 18 cases. *Arch Intern Med* **152**:1250–1252.

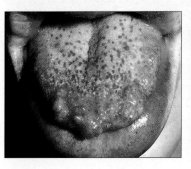
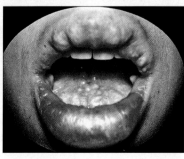

196A and 196B Note the multiple neuromas of the tongue and lips. The lips appear prominent.

DIGEORGE SYNDROME

DiGeorge syndrome is characterised by thymic aplasia or hypoplasia, hypoparathyroidism and cardiac malformations. The dysmorphic features are 'soft' and consist of hypertelorism, low-set ears and micrognathia. The cardiac defects are variable but the two most common are an interrupted aortic arch, often with a VSD, and a persistent truncus arteriosus – so-called 'cono-truncal' anomalies.

The condition is thought to be compatible with a developmental field defect involving the third and fourth pharyngeal arches. Infants might present with hypocalcaemia, absent T-cells and failure to thrive. CNS abnormalities occur in one-third and arhinencephaly, lissencephaly, a simple gyral pattern, and microcephaly have all been described. There is phenotypic overlap with the velocardiofacial syndrome. **Genetic aspects:** On cytogenetic investigation about a third of cases have partial monosomy of the proximal long arm of chromosome 22 (Wilson *et al.*). In patients without visible cytogenetic deletions of 22q, molecular techniques show a deletion in a high proportion of cases (Scambler *et al.*). In one study 21 out of 22 cases had molecular deletions whereas only six out of the 16 cases tested had cytogenetic deletions (Carey *et al.*). Routine FISH analysis is now available.

References

Carey AH, Kelly D, Hulford S *et al.* (1992). Molecular genetic study of the frequency of monosomy 22q11 in DiGeorge syndrome. *Am J Hum Genet* **51**:964–970.

Desmaze C, Scambler P, Prieur M *et al.* (1993). Routine diagnosis of DiGeorge syndrome by fluorescent in situ hybridisation. *Hum Genet* **90**:663–665.

Driscoll DA, Budarf ML, Emanuel BS (1992). A genetic etiology for DiGeorge syndrome: consistent deletions and microdeletions of 22q11. *Am J Hum Genet* **50**:924–933.

Rein AJJT, Dollberg S, Gale R (1990). Genetics of conotruncal malformations: review of the literature and report of a consanguineous kindred with various conotruncal malformations. *Am J Med Genet* **36**:353–355.

Scambler PJ, Kelly D, Lindsay E *et al.* (1992). Velo-cardio-facial syndrome associated with chromosome 22 deletions encompassing the DiGeorge locus. *Lancet* **1**:1138–1139.

Wilson DI, Cross IE, Goodship JA *et al.* (1992). A prospective cytogenetic study of 36 cases of DiGeorge syndrome. *Am J Hum Genet* **51**:957–963.

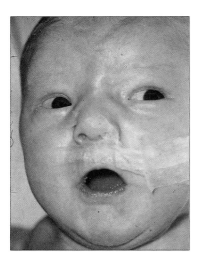

197A Note the hypertelorism and small jaw.

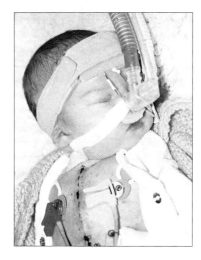

197B Note abnormal ear helix. This child has an interrupted aortic arch.

MOORE–FEDERMAN SYNDROME

The main clinical features of the condition in the original family were short stature, a hoarse voice, hypermetropia, mild hepatosplenomegaly, tight skin, decrease in joint mobility and a tendency to asthma. The proband had retinal detachment and glaucoma. There is marked similarity to acromicric dysplasia, which may be the same condition (Winter *et al.*). Fell and Stanhope reported two further cases, including a follow-up of one of the cases of Winter *et al.*. **Genetic aspects:** Autosomal dominant.

References

Fell JME, Stanhope R (1993). Reviving the Moore–Federman syndrome. *J Royal Soc Med* **86**:52–53.

Moore WT, Federman DD (1965). Familial dwarfism and "stiff joints": report of a kindred. *Arch Intern Med* **115**:398–404.

Winter RM, Patton MA, Challener J *et al.* (1989). Moore–Federman syndrome and acromicric dysplasia: are they the same entity? *J Med Genet* **26**:320–325.

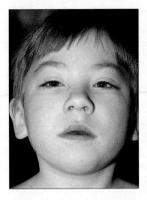
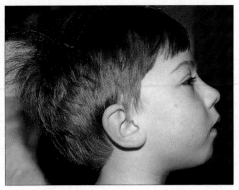
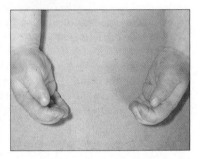

198C There is short stature with a lumbar lordosis.

198A and 198B Note round cheeks and narrow palpebral fissures.

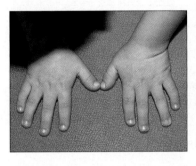
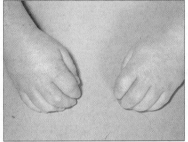
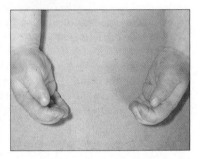

198D and 198F The fingers are short and there is inability to make a fist.

RUSSELL–SILVER SYNDROME

199A–199D

Prenatal growth retardation with a normal head circumference and asymmetry of the limbs are the main features of this condition. The face is small and triangular with frontal bossing, blue sclerae, thin lips with downturned corners, and micrognathia. The normal head circumference gives the impression of 'pseudohydrocephalus'. Minor abnormalities include increased sweating, clinodactyly of the fifth fingers and cafe au lait patches. Intelligence is usually normal. Occasional cases have a very severe form of the condition with developmental delay (Donnai *et al.*).

Genetic aspects: Most cases are sporadic - although there is a possibility that this syndrome is autosomal dominant in some families (Duncan *et al.*).

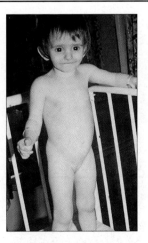

199A and 199B Note the triangular face, proportionally large head (pseudohydrocephalus) and short stature.

References
Davies PSW, Valley R, Preece MA (1988). Adolescent growth and pubertal progression in the Silver–Russell syndrome. *Arch Dis Child* **63**:130–136.

Donnai D, Thompson E *et al.* (1989). Severe Silver-Russell syndrome. *J Med Genet* **26**:447–451.

Duncan PA, Hall JG, Shapiro LR, Vibert BK (1990). Three-generation dominant transmission of the Silver-Russell syndrome. *Am J Med Genet* **35**:245–250.

Patton MA (1988). Syndrome of the month: Russell–Silver syndrome. *J Med Genet* **25**:557–560.

Stanhope R, Preece MA, Hamill G (1991). Does growth hormone treatment improve final height attainment of children with intrauterine growth retardation? *Arch Dis Child* **66**:1180–1183.

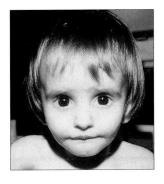

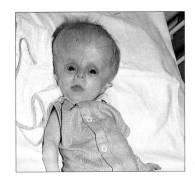

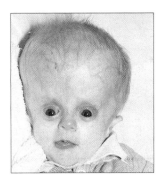

199B

199C and 199D This child has a more severe form of the condition.

THREE M SLENDER BONED DWARFISM

200A–200F

This is a form of low birth-weight dwarfism. The face is said to be 'hatchet-shaped' when viewed from the side and there can be relative macrocephaly. The heels are prominent. Radiographs reveal slender ribs and long bones, and tall vertebrae. These features are rather subjective so that there is a distinct risk of over-diagnosis. The name derives from the initials of the first authors to describe the condition.

Genetic aspects: Autosomal recessive.

References

Cantu JM, Garcia-Cruz D, Sanchez JC et al. (1981). 3-M slender boned nanism. A distinct autosomal recessive intrauterine growth retardation syndrome. *Am J Dis Child* **135**:905–908.

Hennekam RCM, Bijlsma JB, Spranger J (1987). Further delineation of the 3-M syndrome with review of the literature. *Am J Med Genet* **28**:195–209.

Spranger J, Opitz JM, Nourmand A (1976). A new familial intrauterine growth retardation syndrome – the '3-M syndrome'. *Eur J Pediatr* **123**:115–124.

Winter RM, Baraitser M, Grant DB et al. (1984). The 3-M syndrome. *J Med Genet* **21**:124–128.

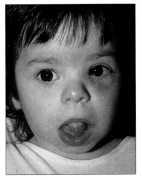

200A Note the triangular face with squared off chin.

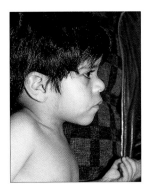

200B The profile is said to be 'hatchet'-faced.

200C and 200D Note the short stature and prominent heels.

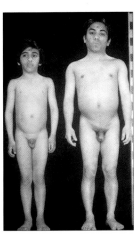

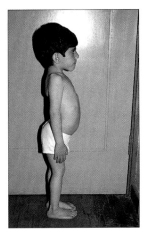

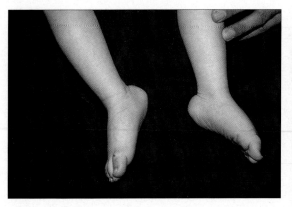

200E Note prominent heels.

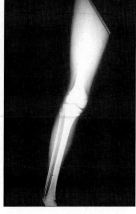

200F Note the slender bones.

MULIBREY NANISM

The main features of the condition are short stature, a large and unusually shaped cranium, muscle wasting, an enlarged liver and yellow spots in the retina. The enlarged liver is most likely due to cardiovascular abnormalities (constrictive pericarditis). In the original report of Perheentupa *et al.*, one patient died at 16 months of a myocardial infarction and another had subendocardial fibrosis. The craniofacies resemble those of Russell–Silver syndrome, but body asymmetry is not present. The name 'Mulibrey' is derived from the words muscle, liver, brain and eye.
Genetic aspects: Autosomal recessive.

References

Cummings GR, Kerr D, Ferguson CC (1976). Constrictive pericarditis with dwarfism in two siblings (mulibrey nanism). *J Pediatr* **88**:569–572.

Perheentupa J, Autio S, Leisti S et al. (1973). Mulibrey nanism, an autosomal recessive syndrome with pericardial constriction. *Lancet* **2**:351–355.

Raitta C, Perheentupa J (1974). Mulibrey nanism: an inherited dysmorphic syndrome with characteristic ocular findings. *Acta Ophthalmol* **52**:162–171.

Tarkkanen A, Raitta C, Perheentupa J (1982). Mulibrey nanism, an autosomal recessive syndrome with ocular involvement. *Acta Ophthalmol* **60**:628–633.

Thoren L (1973). The so-called mulibrey nanism with pericardial constriction. *Lancet* **2**:731.

Voorhees ML, Husson GS, Blackman MS (1976). Growth failure with pericardial constriction: the syndrome of mulibrey nanism. *Am J Dis Child* **130**:1146–1148.

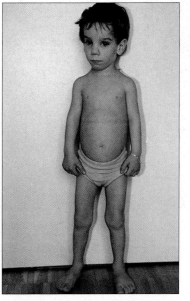

201A There is short stature with a relatively large head.

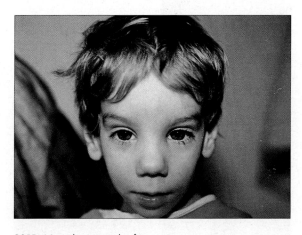

201B Note the triangular face.

FLOATING-HARBOR SYNDROME 202A–202E

This is a distinct, but difficult to diagnose, short stature syndrome. The first two patients were seen at the Boston Floating and Harbor General Hospitals, hence the name. The birth-weight is reduced and subsequent height remains below the third centile. The neck is short but with a low/normal posterior hairline. The eyes are deep-set, but normally placed. The nose is broad with flared nostrils, the mouth is large and the ears are low-set and posteriorly rotated. Affected children have had mild developmental delay, especially of language. Radiographic clues to the diagnosis include a delayed bone-age and pseudarthroses of the clavicles. Coeliac disease is an occasional association.

Genetic aspects: Sporadic, but there have been too few cases to be certain about aetiology.

References

Leisti J *et al.* (1975). The Floating-Harbor syndrome. *BDOAS* **11(5)**:305.

Patton MA, Hurst J, Donnai D *et al.* (1991). Syndrome of the month: Floating-Harbor syndrome. *J Med Genet* **28**:201–204.

Robinson PL, Shohat M, Winter RM *et al.* (1988). A unique association of short stature, dysmorphic features, and speech impairment (Floating-Harbor syndrome). *J Pediatr* **113**:703–705.

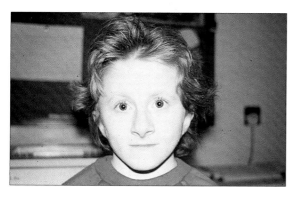
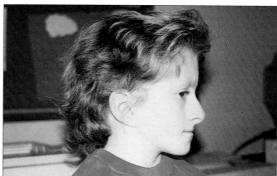

202A–202E Note relatively large nose with prominent columella and flared nostrils. The philtrum is short, the eyes deep-set and the ears posteriorly rotated.

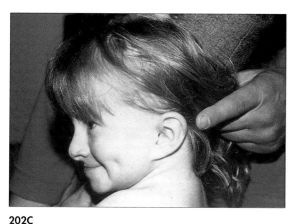
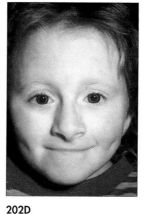
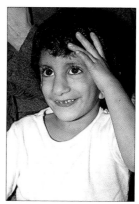

202C **202D** **202E**

SOTOS SYNDROME (CEREBRAL GIGANTISM) 203A–203C

There is early overgrowth associated with a characteristic facial appearance and sometimes mental retardation. The birth-weight may be increased with an enlarged head circumference. The face is characterised by macrocephaly, a high prominent forehead, down-slanting palpebral fissures, a long pointed chin, and a high-arched palate. In childhood height is excessive, with an advanced bone-age and large hands and feet, although final adult height may not be increased. The cerebral ventricles may appear mildly dilated on CT scan.

Genetic aspects: Most cases are sporadic, but occasional convincing autosomal dominant families have been reported.

References

Cole TRP, Hughes HE (1990). Syndrome of the month. Sotos syndrome. *J Med Genet* **27**:571–576.

Karlberg J, Wit JM (1991). Linear growth in Sotos syndrome. *Acta Paediatr Scand* **80**:956–957.

Rutter SC, Cole TRP (1991). Psychological characteristics of Sotos syndrome. *Dev Med Child Neurol* **33**:898–902.

Winship IM (1985). Sotos syndrome – autosomal dominant inheritance substantiated. *Clin Genet* **28**:243–246.

Wit JM, Beemer FA, Barth PG et al. (1985). Cerebral gigantism (Sotos syndrome). Compiled data of 22 cases. Analysis of clinical features, growth and plasma somatomedin. *Eur J Pediatr* **144**:131–140.

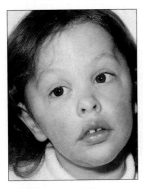 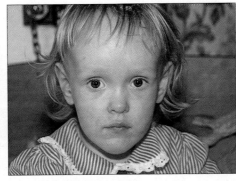 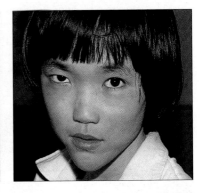

203A–203C Note the broad and high forehead, mild hypertelorism, down-slanting palpebral fissures and small pointed chin.

WEAVER SYNDROME   204A–204C

Most infants are large at birth, but overgrowth may not be apparent until a few months of age. The bone age is significantly advanced. Deceleration of growth may occur in childhood. The face is distinctive with a broad forehead, large ears, hypertelorism, micrognathia (but with a prominent, dimpled fleshy part of the chin) and a long philtrum. There might be a positional deformity of the elbows and knees with limitation of extension, as well as camptodactyly. The thumbs may be broad and prominent fingertip pads are seen. A general connective tissue abnormality is suggested by loose skin and hernias. Radiographs may show flaring of the metaphyses. Development is usually mildly delayed but can be normal.

Genetic aspects: Most cases have been sporadic.

References

Cole TRP, Dennis NR, Hughes HE (1992). Syndrome of the month: Weaver syndrome. *J Med Genet* **29**:332–337.

Fitch N (1980). The syndromes of Marshall and Weaver. *J Med Genet* **17**:174–178.

Ramos-Arroyo MA, Weaver DD, Banks ER (1991). Weaver syndrome: a case without early overgrowth and review of the literature. *Pediatrics* **88**:1106–1111.

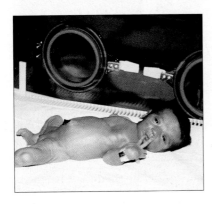 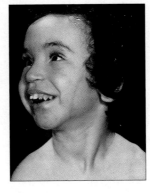 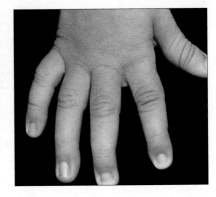

204A Note the broad forehead, flat nasal bridge, hypertelorism, loose skin and small jaw.

204B Note how the phenotype changes with age but the jaw is still small and the cheeks are prominent.

204C Note the narrow nails, broadening of the middle phalanges and camptodactyly.

MARSHALL–SMITH SYNDROME 205A–205B

Infants with this disorder have increased length and bone-age at birth, but tend to be underweight and fail to thrive. There is dolichocephaly with a prominent forehead, prominent eyes, micrognathia and anteverted nostrils. The proximal and middle phalanges are broad and occasional abnormalities have included choanal atresia, exomphalos, a hypoplastic epiglottis and an absent corpus callosum. Mental retardation is the rule. The differential diagnosis is with Weaver and Sotos syndromes.
Genetic aspects: Uncertain.

References
Charon A, Gillerot Y, Van Maldergem L *et al.* (1990). The Marshall–Smith syndrome. *Eur J Pediatr* **150**:54–55.

Cohen MM Jr (1989). A comprehensive and critical assessment of overgrowth and overgrowth syndromes. Marshall–Smith syndrome. *Adv Hum Genet* **18**:254–261.

Eich GF, Silver MM, Weksberg R *et al.* (1991). Marshall–Smith syndrome: new radiographic, clinical, and pathologic observations. *Radiology* **181**:183–188.

Fitch N (1980). The syndromes of Marshall and Weaver. *J Med Genet* **17**:174–178.

Roodhooft AM, Van Acker KJ *et al.* (1988). Marshall–Smith syndrome: new aspects. *Neuropediatrics* **19**:179–182.

Tipton RE, Wilroy R Jr, Summitt RL (1973). Accelerated skeletal maturation in infancy syndrome. Report of a third case. *J Pediatr* **83**:829–832.

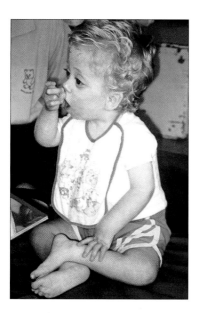
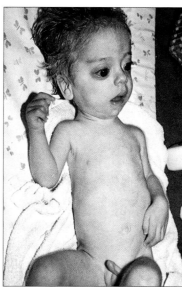

205A and 205B Note the combination of overgrowth with failure to thrive. The length and head circumferences are above the 95th centile and the head is often dolichocephalic.
Note also the prominent forehead, prominent eyes and small jaw.

SIMPSON–GOLABI–BEHMEL SYNDROME 206A–206B

This overgrowth syndrome presents in the neonatal period with a high birth-weight, coarse features, thickened lips, a wide mouth, a large tongue, a high-arched or cleft palate, a short neck and hepatosplenomegaly. Later a husky voice, malposition of the teeth, and a prominent jaw may become evident. Post-axial polydactyly of the hands or feet may be present. There is a possible association with embryonal tumours, particularly Wilms', neuroblastoma and perhaps hepatoblastoma (Hughes-Benzie *et al.*).
Genetic aspects: X-linked recessive. Some heterozygous females may also have overgrowth. Hughes-Benzie *et al.* mapped the gene to Xq13-q21.

References
Behmel A, Plochl E, Rosenkranz W (1988). A new X-linked dysplasia gigantism syndrome: follow up in the first family and report on a second Austrian family. *Am J Med Genet* **30**:275–285.

Golabi M, Rosen L (1984). A new X-linked mental retardation- overgrowth syndrome. *Am J Med Genet* **17**:345–358.

Gurrieri F, Cappa M, Neri G (1992). Further delineation of the Simpson–Golabi–Behmel (SGB) syndrome. *Am J Med Genet* **44**:136–137.

Hughes-Benzie RM, Hunter AGW, Allanson JE, MacKenzie AE (1992). Simpson–Golabi–Behmel syndrome associated with renal dysplasia and embryonal tumor: localization of the gene to Xqcen- q21. *Am J Med Genet* **43**:428–435.

Neri G, Marini R, Cappa M *et al.* (1988). Simpson–Golabi–Behmel syndrome: an X-linked encephalo-tropho-schisis syndrome. *Am J Med Genet* **30**:287–299.

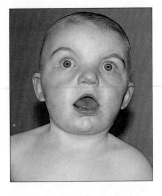

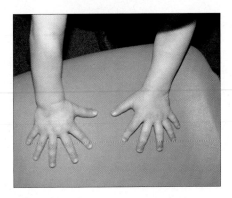

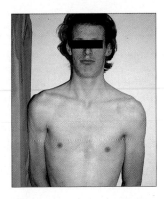

206A This child had a high birth-weight. The face is slightly coarse and the tongue large.

206B Note the post-axial polydactyly.

206C The uncle of the child in **206A**. He is a large man with supernumerary nipples.

PRADER–WILLI SYNDROME

Severe hypotonia is usually present at birth, and feeding difficulties and failure to thrive may predominate in the first year of life. In the second year over-eating may begin, with subsequent obesity. Short stature, mental retardation, hypogonadism and small hands and feet complete the clinical picture. Average adult height in males is 155cm and in females 147cm. Mental retardation is mild to moderate, although up to 10% of adults are said to have an IQ within the normal range. Excessive skin 'picking' and thick saliva have been noted as unusual signs. Fair hair and skin have been noted in many patients, especially those with a deletion of chromosome 15 (see below). Holm *et al.* present a good review of the consensus diagnostic criteria.

Genetic aspects: 55–70% patients can be shown to have a small, paternally derived deletion of the proximal part of the long arm of chromosome 15 by cytogenetic analysis. Of cases without a cytogenetic deletion 40% have deletions detectable at the DNA level and 60% have maternal disomy for part or all of chromosome 15.

References

Cassidy SB, Lai L-W, Erickson RP *et al.* (1992) Trisomy 15 with loss of the paternal 15 as a cause of Prader–Willi syndrome due to maternal disomy. *Am J Hum Genet* **51**:701–708.

Holm VA, Cassidy SB, Butler MG, *et al.* (1993). Prader–Willi syndrome: consensus diagnostic criteria. *Pediatrics* **91**:398–402.

Robinson WP, Bottani A, Yagang X *et al.* (1991). Molecular, cytogenetic, and clinical investigations of Prader–Willi syndrome patients. *Am J Hum Genet* **49**:1219–1234.

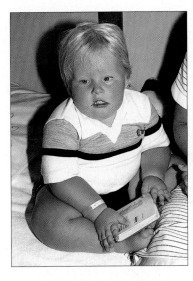

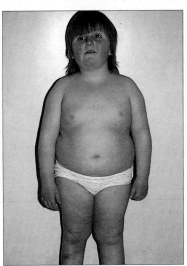

207A Note the obesity and blond hair.

207B and 207C Note that the obesity involves trunk, limbs and face.

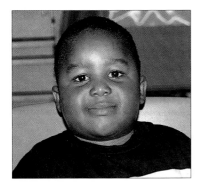

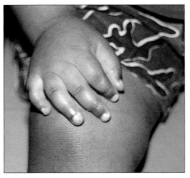

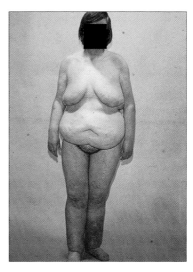

207D Note that the facial dysmorphic features are not distinctive.

207E The hands are small.

207F An older patient with this condition.

COHEN SYNDROME

Affected individuals have microcephaly (in about half of the cases), prominent central incisors, a prominent nasal bridge, a short philtrum with maxillary and mandibular hypoplasia (not severe and not constant), and an open mouth appearance. The children have mild to moderate mental retardation, are short and have a truncal obesity, with concentration of fat around the lower abdomen. The face may not look obese. Hypotonia is common and puberty might be delayed. The fingers are characteristically long and tapered and a third of patients have a choreoretinopathy. Colobomata of the iris or retina have been described.

Genetic aspects: Autosomal recessive. Tahvanainen *et al.* mapped the gene to 8q22-q23 in Finnish families.

References

Cohen MM Jr, Hall BD, Smith DW *et al.* (1973). A new syndrome with hypotonia, obesity, mental deficiency, and facial, oral, ocular and limb anomalies. *J Pediatr* **83**:280–284.

Kondo I, Nagataki S, Miyagi N (1990). The Cohen syndrome: does mottled retina separate a Finnish and Jewish type? *Am J Med Genet* **37**:109–113.

Norio R, Raitta C, Lindahl E (1984). Further delineation of the Cohen syndrome: report on chorioretinal dystrophy, leukopenia and consanguinity. *Clin Genet* **25**:1–14.

Steinlein O, Tariverdian G, Boll HU, Vogel F (1991). Tapetoretinal degeneration in brothers with apparent Cohen syndrome: nosology with Mirhosseini–Holmes–Watson syndrome. *Am J Med Genet* **41**:196–200.

Tahvanainen E, Norio R, Karila E *et al.* (1994). Cohen syndrome gene assigned to the long arm of chromosome 8 by linkage analysis. *Nature Genetics* **7**:201–204.

Young ID, Moore JR (1987). Intrafamilial variation in Cohen syndrome. *J Med Genet* **24**:488–492.

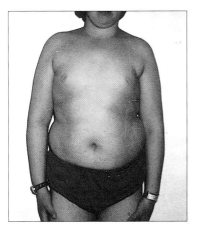

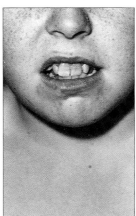

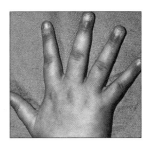

208A–208C Note truncal obesity, prominent incisors and long, tapering fingers.

BARDET–BIEDL (LAURENCE–MOON–BARDET–BIEDL) SYNDROME 209A–209F

Bardet–Biedl syndrome presents with polydactyly, retinal dystrophy, mental handicap, obesity and hypogenitalism. 70% of cases have post-axial polydactyly. Syndactyly and brachydactyly are also common. Renal problems are present in 90% of cases when looked for (Harnett *et al.*). Abnormalities include calyceal clubbing, cysts or diverticulae, fetal lobulations, renal cortical loss and a reduced ability to concentrate urine – renal failure can occur. The picture can be that of juvenile nephronophthisis.

Visual abnormalities characteristically consist of an atypical pigmentary retinopathy with early macular involvement. Electrophysiological studies reveal a cone-rod dystrophy. Onset of visual impairment is in the second or third decade and in one study 63.6% of patients were legally blind by the age of 20 years (Fulton *et al.*).

Mental retardation might not always be present. Green *et al.* found this in 41% of cases. The frequency of other abnormalities is obesity (90%), diabetes mellitus (50%), hypogonadism in males (88%) and menstrual problems in females (100%) (Green *et al.*).

In general four of the five major manifestations are necessary for a positive diagnosis.

Genetic aspects: Autosomal recessive. Kwitek-Black *et al.* found linkage to markers at 16q13-q22 in a large inbred Bedouin family. However, in a second family linkage was excluded, suggesting genetic heterogeneity. Leppert *et al.* showed linkage to markers at 11q13 in some families.

References

Fulton AB, Hansen RM, Glynn RJ (1993). Natural course of visual functions in the Bardet–Biedl syndrome. *Arch Ophthalmol* **111**:1500–1506.

Green JS, Parfrey PS, Harnett JD et al. (1989). The cardinal manifestations of Bardet–Biedl syndrome, a form of Laurence–Moon–Biedl syndrome. *New Engl J Med* **321**:1002–1009.

Harnett JD, Green JS, Cramer BC et al. (1988). The spectrum of renal disease in Laurence–Moon–Biedl syndrome. *New Engl J Med* **319**:615–618.

Kwitek-Black AE, Carmi R, Duyk GM et al. (1993). Linkage of Bardet–Biedl syndrome to chromosome 16q and evidence for non-allelic genetic heterogeneity. *Nature Genetics* **5**:392–396.

Leppert M, Baird L, Anderson KL et al. (1994). Bardet–Biedl syndrome is linked to DNA markers on chromosome 11q and is genetically heterogeneous. *Nature Genetics* **7**:108–112.

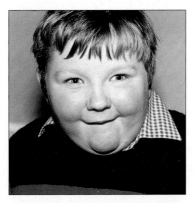

209A–209D Note varying degrees of obesity.

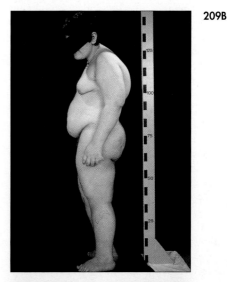

209B

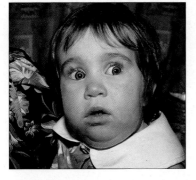

209C

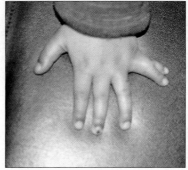

209D

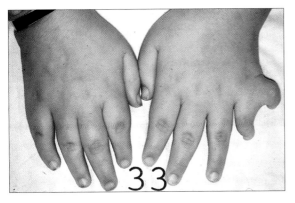
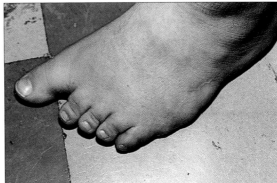

209E and 209F Note postaxial polydactyly.

SYNDROMES ASSOCIATED WITH PREDISPOSITION TO MALIGNANCY

ANIRIDIA-WILMS' TUMOUR / WAGR SYNDROME 210

It has been suggested that about 1 in 70–90 children with Wilms' tumour will be found to have aniridia, and 20% of children with aniridia will develop a Wilms' tumour (data from Friedman). The WAGR syndrome includes ambiguous genitalia and mental retardation in addition to aniridia and Wilms' tumour.

Screening for Wilms' tumour in these cases is controversial, but many authors recommend ultrasound examination every three months until the age of 5 years and then yearly until growth is complete (25% of children with Wilms' tumour are older than 5 years) (Clericuzio).

Genetic aspects: In most cases the association is due to an interstitial chromosomal deletion involving the WT-1 gene at 11p13. This deletion is not always evident by conventional chromosome analysis and FISH may be necessary to demonstrate it (Fantes *et al.*). Pax-6 gene deletions are responsible for the aniridia

and mutations of this gene have also been demonstrated in non-syndromic forms of human aniridia (Davis and Cowell).

References

Clericuzio CL (1993). Clinical phenotypes and Wilms tumor. *Med Pediatr Oncol* **21**:182–187.

Davis A, Cowell JK (1993). Mutations in the PAX6 gene in patients with hereditary aniridia. *Hum Molec Genet* **2**:2093–2098.

Fantes JA, Bickmore WA, Fletcher JM *et al.* (1992). Submicroscopic deletions at the WAGR locus, revealed by nonradioactive in situ hybridisation. *Am J Hum Genet* **51**:1286–1294.

Friedman AL (1986). Wilms' tumor detection in patients with sporadic aniridia. *Am J Dis Child* **140**:173–174.

Ton CCT, Huff V, Call KM *et al.* (1991). Smallest region of overlap in Wilms tumor deletions uniquely implicates an 11p13 zinc finger gene as the disease locus. *Genomics* **10**:293–297.

Ton CCT, Hirvonen H, Miwa H *et al.* (1991). Positional cloning and characterization of a paired box- and homeobox-containing gene from the aniridia region. *Cell* **67**:1059–1074.

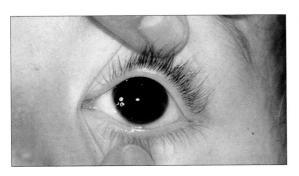

210 Note the absent iris.

BECKWITH–WIEDEMANN (EMG) SYNDROME

Characteristic features include macroglossia, abdominal wall defects, hypoglycaemia, visceromegaly (liver, spleen, kidneys, adrenals) and gigantism, often but not always present at birth. Ear creases or pits on either the front or the back of the pinna should be looked for. A facial nevus flammeus and mid-facial hypoplasia may be present. Hemihypertrophy should be sought. There is a known association with certain malignancies, especially Wilms' tumour, and hemihypertrophy is found in 40% of cases who develop this tumour. The overall risk of malignancy is 7.5%, and if hemihypertrophy is absent, closer to 1%.

Genetic aspects: Chromosome analysis is usually normal but 11p duplications and translocations have been found in some cases. The syndrome can be caused by disomy for the segment of 11p15.5 containing the Igf2 gene. In cases with a duplication of 11p15.5 the parental origin is usually paternal. On the other hand cases with a balanced 11p15.5 translocation or insertion are maternal in origin. In Wilms' tumours in these patients there is usually evidence of disomy for paternal 11p15 markers.

References

Henry I, Puech A, Riesewijk A *et al* (1993). Somatic mosaicism for partial paternal isodisomy in Wiedemann–Beckwith syndrome: a post-fertilization event. *Eur J Hum Genet* **1**:19–29.

Mannens M, Hoovers JMN, Redeker E *et al.* (1994). Parental imprinting of human chromosome region 11p15.3-pter involved in the Beckwith–Wiedemann syndrome and various human neoplasia. *Eur J Hum Genet* **2**:3–23.

Martinez y Martinez R, Martinez-Carboney R, Ocampo-Campos R *et al.* (1992). Wiedemann–Beckwith syndrome: clinical, cytogenetical and radiological observations in 39 new cases. *Genetic Counseling* **3**:67–76.

Norman AM, Read AP, Clayton-Smith J *et al.* (1992). Recurrent Wiedemann–Beckwith syndrome with inversion of chromosome (11)(p11.2p15.5). *Am J Med Genet* **42**:638–641.

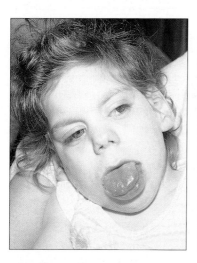
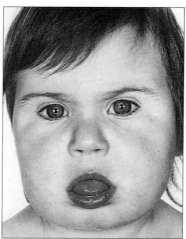
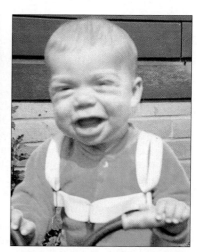

211A–211C Note large tongue and heavy face.   **211C**

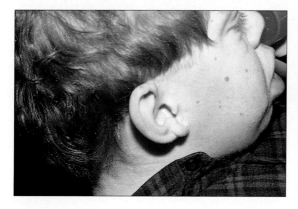
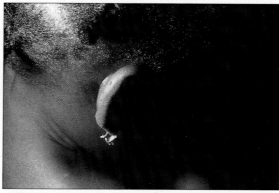

211D Note ear creases.   **211E** Note pit behind helix of ear.

PERLMAN SYNDROME

There is overgrowth at birth and bilateral renal hamartomas with a tendency to nephroblastomatosis. The face is said to be characteristic with deep-set eyes, a small nose, a depressed nasal bridge, serrated alveolar margins, low-set ears and an everted lower lip. Polyhydramnios in pregnancy, cryptorchidism, fetal ascites, hepatomegaly, diaphragmatic hernia, and congenital heart defects are also part of the condition. One patient has had pancreatic islet cell hyperplasia with hypoglycaemia. The case of Greenberg *et al.* had an interrupted aortic arch, polysplenia, and hypospadias.

Genetic aspects: There are similarities to Beckwith syndrome, but the inheritance pattern appears to be autosomal recessive.

References

Greenberg F, Copeland K, Gresik MV (1988). Expanding the spectrum of the Perlman syndrome. *Am J Med Genet* **29**:773–776.

Grundy RG, Pritchard J, Baraitser M et al. (1992). Perlman and Wiedemann–Beckwith syndromes: two distinct conditions associated with Wilms' tumour. *Eur J Pediatr* **151**:895–898.

Perlman M (1986). Perlman syndrome: familial renal dysplasia with Wilms tumor, fetal gigantism, and multiple congenital anomalies (Letter). *Am J Med Genet* **25**:793–795.

Perlman M, Goldberg GM, Bar-Ziv J et al. (1973). Renal hamartomas and nephroblastomas with fetal gigantism: a familial syndrome. *J Pediatr* **83**:414–418.

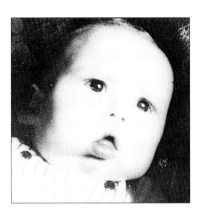 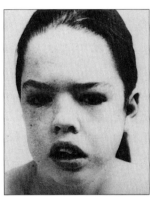

212A and 212B   Note the deep-set eyes and everted lower lip.

ATAXIA-TELANGIECTASIA (LOUIS–BAR SYNDROME)

This is a progressive form of ataxia associated with telangiectasia of the conjunctiva ears and face, developmental delay, immunodeficiency and tendency to malignancies. Early development is usually normal but walking might be delayed and when it occurs a truncal ataxia is noted. This worsens and dysarthria develops. Extra-pyramidal signs such as athetosis and dystonia are often features. Signs of a peripheral neuropathy may be evident from the second decade. The mean age of loss of walking is 10 years (Woods and Taylor). Eye movements are jerky and oculomotor apraxia is common. Investigations reveal a raised serum alpha-fetoprotein and reduced synthesis of IgA, IgG and IgM. Cultured cells are sensitive to X-radiation and there is an increased risk of lymphomas and leukaemias.

Genetic aspects: Autosomal recessive. Several genetic complementation groups have been demonstrated (see Jaspers *et al.* for review). The loci map to 11q22-q23 in families with type A, C and D, although there is evidence that AT-C lies outside the linkage group for AT-A and AT-D.

Swift *et al.* have suggested an increased incidence of cancer in heterozygotes (particularly breast cancer in women).

References

Chessa L, Petrinelli P, Antonelli A et al. (1992). Heterogeneity in ataxia-telangiectasia: classical phenotype associated with intermediate cellular radiosensitivity. *Am J Med Genet* **42**:741–746.

Foroud T, Wei S, Ziv Y et al. (1991). Localization of an ataxia-telangiectasia locus to a 3-cM interval on chromosome 11q23: linkage analysis of 111 families by an international consortium. *Am J Hum Genet* **49**:1263–1279.

Jaspers NGJ, Gatti RA, Baan C et al. (1988). Genetic complementation analysis of ataxia telangiectasia and Nijmegen breakage syndrome: a survey of 50 patients. *Cytogenet Cell Genet* **49**:259–263.

Llerena J Jr, Murer-Orlando M et al. (1989). Spontaneous and induced chromosome breakage in chorionic villus samples: a cytogenetic approach to first trimester prenatal diagnosis of ataxia telangiectasia syndrome. *J Med Genet* **26**:174–178.

Swift M, Reitnauer PJ et al. (1987). Breast and other cancers in families with ataxia-telangiectasia. *New Engl J Med* **316**:1289–1294.

Woods CG, Taylor AMR (1992). Ataxia telangiectasia in the British Isles: the clinical and laboratory features of 70 affected individuals. *Q J Med* **82**:169–179.

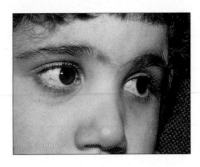

213 Note the conjunctival telangiectasia.

BLOOM SYNDROME

214A–214C

Characteristic skin abnormalities, consisting of photosensitive telangiectatic erythematous lesions, appear on the face in infancy, especially over the butterfly area, and occasionally over the dorsa of the hands and feet. Later, the skin lesions become scarred, atrophic and depigmented, and the eyelashes may fall out. The other cardinal features are marked short stature and microcephaly, of prenatal onset but persisting into childhood and adulthood. The lateral incisors can be absent and mild retardation has been reported. Whereas most patients are Jewish in origin this is not exclusively the case, and a number of affected Japanese children have been reported. Specialised cytogenetic analysis reveals that increased sister chromatid exchange and malignancy, especially lymphomas or leukaemia, may develop. The average age of mani-festation of leukaemias is 22 years and of solid tumours 35 years (German).

Genetic aspects: Autosomal recessive. Prenatal diagnosis has been performed, looking at sister chromatid exchange.

References

Bloom D (1954). Congenital telangiectatic erythema resembling lupus erythematosus in dwarfs: probably a syndrome entity. *Am J Dis Child* **88**:754–758.

Bloom D (1966). The syndrome of congenital telangiectatic erythema and stunted growth. *J Pediatr* **68**:103–113.

German J (1969). Bloom's syndrome. I. Genetical and clinical observations in the first 27 patients. *Am J Hum Genet* **21**:196–227.

Nicotera TM (1991). Molecular and biochemical aspects of Bloom's syndrome. *Cancer Genet Cytogen* **53**:1–13.

Sullivan NF, Willis AE (1992). Cancer predisposition in Bloom's syndrome. *BioEssays* **14**:333–336.

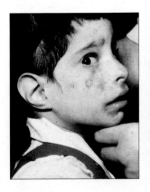 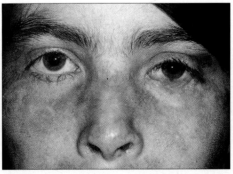 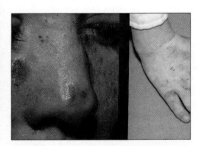

214A–214C Malar hypoplasia and talangiectatic erythema on face and hands.   **214C**

VON HIPPEL–LINDAU SYNDROME

215A–215B

This is the association between retinal, cerebellar and spinal angiomatous lesions, cysts of the pancreas, liver and kidneys, hypernephromas and phaeochromocytomas. 60% of individuals have ocular lesions, 60% cerebellar lesions, 13% spinal lesions, 28% renal tumours and 7% phaeochromocytomas. The characteristic intracranial lesion is a cerebellar haemangioblastoma, but supratentorial lesions have also been reported. The average age at diagnosis is 26 years and 97% of gene carriers have some manifestations by 60 years (Maher *et al.*). Those at risk need yearly ophthalmological examination from the age of five years, a yearly urinary VMA and metadrenaline estimation from the age of 10 years, a CT brain scan every 2 years from the age of 15, and a CT kidney scan every 2 years from the age of 20 (Huson *et al.*; Jennings *et al.*). The prevalence is around 1 in 36 000.

Genetic aspects: Autosomal dominant. The gene has been identified as tumour suppressor gene mapping to 3p25-26.

References

Huson SM, Harper PS, Hourihan MD *et al.* (1986). Cerebellar hae-mangioblastoma and von Hippel–Lindau disease. *Brain* **109**:1297–1300.

Jennings AM, Smith C, Cole DR *et al.* (1988). Von Hippel–Lindau disease in a large British family: clinicopathological features and recommendations for screening and follow-up. *Q J Med* **66**:233–250.

Latif F, Tory K, Gnarra J *et al.* (1993). Identification of the von Hippel–Lindau disease tumor suppressor gene. *Science* **260**:1317–1320.

Maher ER, Yates JRW, Harries R *et al.* (1990). Clinical features and natural history of von Hippel–Lindau disease. *Q J Med* **77**:1151–1163.

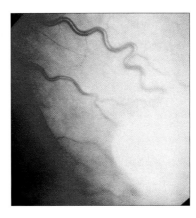

215A and 215B Note the retinal angioma with tortuous and dilated feeding vessels.

NEVOID BASAL CELL CARCINOMA SYNDROME (GORLIN)

216A–216D

The multiple nevoid basal cell carcinomas appear after puberty, especially on the face and neck, but also on the trunk and elsewhere. Ulceration is common. Other skin lesions include pits (punctate lesions) on the palmar and plantar areas, cysts and comedones. The facial features can be characteristic with macrocephaly, frontal and temporoparietal bossing, and prominent supraorbital ridges. The jaw is prognathic, the nasal root is broad and there might be telecanthus or even true hypertelorism. Bifurcation of the ribs, jaw cysts, kyphoscoliosis, short metacarpals, and a Sprengel deformity are fre-

quent. Other features include dural calcification, mild mental retardation, agenesis of the corpus callosum, medulloblastomas, ovarian fibromas, lymphomesenteric cysts and hypogonadism.

Genetic aspects: Autosomal dominant. The gene maps to 9q22-31 (Farndon *et al.*).

References

Farndon PA, Evans DGR, Del Mastro RG, Kilpatrick MW (1992). Location of gene for Gorlin syndrome. *Lancet* **1**:581–582.

Gorlin RJ (1987). Nevoid basal-cell carcinoma syndrome. *Medicine* **66**:98–113.

216A and 216B Note the basal cell nevi and carcinomata on the face.

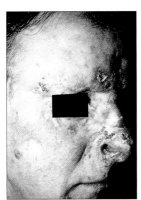
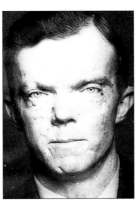

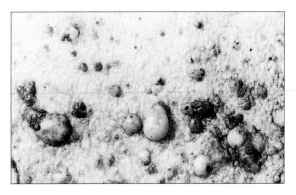

216C A close-up of the skin lesions.

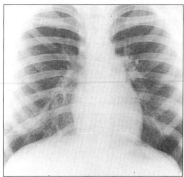

216D The bifid ribs on the chest X-ray are commonly seen.

SYNDROMES WITH METABOLIC DEFECTS

HURLER SYNDROME (MUCOPOLYSACCHARIDOSIS TYPE IH)   217A–217E

The features of Hurler syndrome are well known. There are coarse facies, macrocephaly, corneal clouding, hepatosplenomegaly, joint contractures, umbilical and inguinal herniae and radiological features of dysostosis multiplex. Onset is insidious but features should be obvious in the second year of life. After this mental deterioration becomes apparent and death occurs around 10 years in severe cases. Bone marrow transplantation has had some effect on ameliorating the condition.

Genetic aspects: Autosomal recessive. There are cases with typical features except for the mildness of the mental defect and prolonged survival. Some of these cases may be homozygous for a milder mutation, but some may be so-called Hurler–Scheie compound heterozygotes with a mild and a severe allele for the alpha-L-iduronidase gene.

References

Beighton P (1993). *McKusick's Heritable Disorders of Connective Tissue*. Johns Hopkins, Baltimore. 378–391.

Collins MLZ, Traboulsi EI, Maumenee IH (1990). Optic nerve head swelling and optic atrophy in the systemic mucopolysaccharidoses. *Ophthalmology* **97**:1445–1449.

Roubicek M, Gehler J, Spranger J (1985). The clinical spectrum of alpha-L-iduronidase deficiency. *Am J Med Genet* **20**:471–481.

Scott HS, Ashton LJ, Eyre HJ et al. (1990). Chromosomal location of the human alpha-L-iduronidase gene (IDUA) to 4p16.3. *Am J Hum Genet* **47**:802–807.

Semenza GL, Pyeritz RE (1988). Respiratory complications of mucopolysaccharide storage disorders. *Medicine* **67**:209–219.

Whitley CB, Belani KG, Chang P-N et al. (1993). Long-term outcome of Hurler syndrome following bone marrow transplantation. *Am J Med Genet* **46**:209–218.

Young EP (1992). Prenatal diagnosis of Hurler disease by analysis of alpha-iduronidase in chorionic villi. *J Inherit Metab Dis* **15**:224–230.

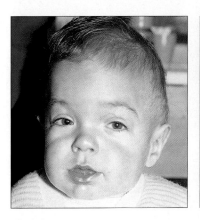

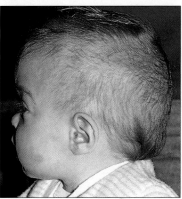

217A and 217B Note coarse facial features.

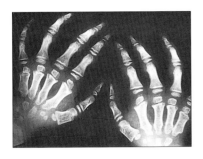

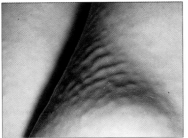

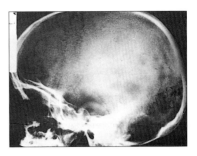

217C Note the proximal tapering of the metacarpals, coarse trabeculation and irregular epiphyses.

217D Note deposits of aminoglycans underneath the skin.

217E Note the J-shaped sella turcica.

HUNTER SYNDROME (MUCOPOLYSACCHARIDOSIS TYPE II)   218

This X-linked form of mucopolysaccharidosis presents with coarse facies, a large head, frontal bossing and an enlarged tongue. Hydrocephaly may develop. Corneal clouding is not usually present. Conductive or sensorineural hearing loss is common. There may be progressive joint stiffness and claw hands. Hepatosplenomegaly, inguinal and umbilical herniae, thickened heart valves, carpal tunnel syndrome and upper airway obstruction are all seen. Radiographs show features of dysostosis multiplex.

Affected cases fall into two main groups. In the severe form the diagnosis is made by about three years and mental impairment is obvious by about four years. Death occurs around 15 years. Onset in the milder form is later, survival is into adulthood and mental deterioration may not be a major feature. Treatment with bone marrow transplantation has been attempted.

Genetic aspects: X-linked recessive. Female carriers may have intermediate levels of the enzyme iduronate-2-sulphatase in serum, and carrier detection looking at levels in individual hair bulbs has been tried. However, neither of these methods is completely reliable. Direction mutation analysis of the gene is likely to replace these methods.

References

Flomen RH, Green PM, Bentley DR *et al.* (1992). Detection of point mutations and a gross deletion in six Hunter syndrome patients. *Genomics* **13**:543–550.

Schroder W, Petruschka L, Wehnert M *et al.* (1993). Carrier detection of Hunter syndrome (MPS II) by biochemical and DNA techniques in families at risk. *J Med Genet* **30**:210–213.

Stone S, Adinolfi M (1992). Carrier detection of deletions of the Hunter gene by in situ hybridisation. *Ann Hum Genet* **56**:93–97.

Winchester B, Young E, Geddes S *et al.* (1992). Female twin with Hunter disease due to nonrandom inactivation of the X-chromosome: a consequence of twinning. *Am J Med Genet* **44**:834–838.

Young ID, Harper PS (1983). The natural history of the severe form of Hunter's syndrome: a study based on 52 cases. *Dev Med Child Neurol* **25**:481–489.

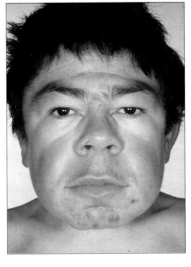

218 Note the coarse facial features, prominent supraorbital ridges, thick eyebrows, broad bulbous nose, and thick lips.

SANFILIPPO SYNDROME (MUCOPOLYSACCHARIDOSIS TYPE III)   219A–219B

Intellectual deterioration may be the presenting feature, although mild coarsening of the facial features, hirsutism, or minimal signs of dysostosis multiplex, may be noted. Corneal clouding and hepatosplenomegaly are usually absent. Increased growth with advanced bone-age can occur early on but later growth may be retarded. Thickening of the mitral valve can be severe. Biochemically, the defect is in the breakdown of heparan sulphate. This can be the most difficult form of mucopolysaccharidosis to diagnose because of the relatively mild dysmorphic features and the absence of mucopolysaccharides in the urine by some screening tests.

Genetic aspects: Autosomal recessive. Four separate enzyme defects have been recognised, giving types A, B, C and D.

References

Sewell AC, Pontz BF, Benischek G (1988). Mucopolysaccharidosis type IIIC (Sanfilippo): early clinical presentation in a large Turkish pedigree. *Clin Genet* **34**:116–121.

Siciliano L, Fiumara A, Pavone L *et al.* (1991). Sanfilippo syndrome type D in two adolescent sisters. *J Med Genet* **28**:402–405.

Turki I, Kresse H, Scotto J, Tardieu M (1989). Sanfilippo disease, type C: three cases in the same family. *Neuropediatrics* **20**:90–92.

van Schrojenstein-de Valk HMJ *et al.* (1987). Follow-up on seven adult patients with mild Sanfilippo B-disease. *Am J Med Genet* **28**:125–130.

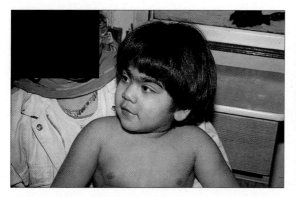
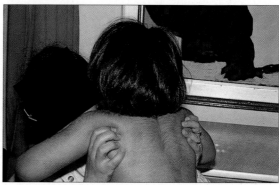

219A and 219B Note the mildly coarse facial features and hirsutism over the back.

MORQUIO SYNDROME (MUCOPOLYSACCHARIDOSIS TYPE IV) 220A–220B

Clinically, the condition is characterised by severe skeletal abnormalities with cloudy corneae and aortic regurgitation. Onset may be in the first 2 years of life with genu valgum, a short trunk and neck, pectus carinatum and coarse facies. Clouding of the cornea is mild but deafness may be a problem. The joints may be loose without the claw hand seen in other mucopolysaccharidoses. Odontoid hypoplasia leads to atlantoaxial instability. Radiographs reveal severe dysostosis multiplex. Patients with the severe form may not survive beyond their twenties. Intelligence is often normal.

Genetic aspects: Autosomal recessive. This form of mucopolysaccharidosis is subdivided according to the particular enzyme defect responsible (see Beck *et al.*).

References

Beck M, Glossl J, Grubisic A, Spranger J (1986). Heterogeneity of Morquio disease. *Clin Genet* **29**:325–331.

Giugliani R, Jackson M, Skinner SJ *et al.* (1987). Progressive mental regression in siblings with Morquio disease Type B (mucopolysaccharidosis IVB). *Clin Genet* **32**:313–325.

Nelson J, Broadhead D, Mossman J (1988). Clinical findings in 12 patients with MPS IV A (Morquio's disease). Further evidence for heterogeneity. Part I: Clinical and biochemical findings. *Clin Genet* **33**:111–121.

Nelson J, Kinirons M (1988). Clinical findings in 12 patients with MPS IV A (Morquio's disease). Further evidence for heterogeneity. Part II: Dental findings. *Clin Genet* **33**:121–126.

Oshima A, Yoshida K, Shimmoto M *et al.* (1991). Human beta-galactosidase gene mutations in Morquio B disease. *Am J Hum Genet* **49**:1091–1093.

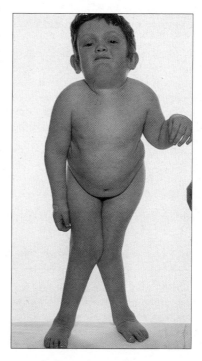

220A Note the short neck, short trunk, prominent joints and restricted movement.

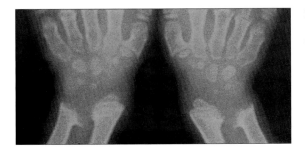

220B Note the epiphyseal changes at the wrist with metaphyseal flaring and irregularity. The metacarpals are pointed at their proximal ends.

SIALIDOSIS TYPE 2

This disorder of oligosaccharide metabolism manifests with a cherry-red spot in the macula, myoclonus, coarse facies, deafness, short stature, changes of dysostosis multiplex on radiography, ataxia and spasticity. Onset can be variable, there is an infantile form manifesting at birth with the additional features of ascites, hepatosplenomegaly, pericardial effusion and nephrotic syndrome (nephrosialidosis), and a juvenile form with later onset. There is increased urinary excretion of abnormal sialyloligosaccharides and a deficiency of the enzyme N-acetyl-neuraminic acid hydrolase (sialidase, neuraminidase). Sialidosis type 1 presents with a cherry-red spot and myoclonus but no dysmorphic features.

Genetic aspects: Autosomal recessive.

References
Aylsworth AS, Thomas GH, Hood J (1980). A severe infantile sialidosis: clinical, biochemical, and microscopic features. *J Pediatr* **96**:662–668.
Lowden JA, O'Brien JS (1979). Sialidosis: a review of human neuraminidase deficiency. *Am J Hum Genet* **31**:1–18.
Winter RM, Swallow DM, Baraitser M *et al.* (1980). Sialidosis type 2 [acid neuraminidase deficiency]: clinical and biochemical features of a further case. *Clin Genet* **18**:203–210.
Young ID, Young EP, Mossman J *et al.* (1987). Neuraminidase deficiency: case report and review of the phenotype. *J Med Genet* **24**:283.

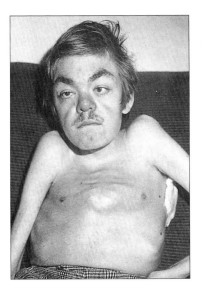

221A Note the coarse facial features and chest deformity.

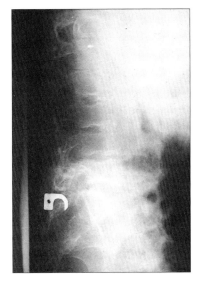

221B There is an anterosuperior deficiency of the vertebral bodies in lateral projection.

I-CELL DISEASE (MUCOLIPIDOSIS TYPE II)

Most cases present in the first year with poor weight gain and coarse facial features with prominent gums. The skin is often thick, tight and hirsute. Joint movement might be limited and fractures or periosteal cloaking are seen on X-ray. Later there is psychomotor retardation, short stature, Hurler-like features and signs of dysostosis multiplex on X-ray. The name 'I-cell' (inclusion-cell) comes from the marked cytoplasmic inclusions seen in culture fibroblasts. Prognosis is poor. There is a deficiency of GlcNAc-P-transferase in fibroblasts and leukocytes. An 'I-cell screen' reveals increased levels of a number of lysosomal enzymes in the medium surrounding the cultured fibroblasts.

Genetic aspects: Autosomal recessive. Prenatal diagnosis by analysis of amniotic fluid cell cultures is possible.

References

Leroy JG, Spranger JW, Feingold M *et al.* (1971). I-cell disease: a clinical picture. *J Pediatr* **79**:360–365.

Okada S, Owada M, Sakiyama T *et al.* (1985). I-cell disease: clinical studies of 21 Japanese cases. *Clin Genet* **28**:207–215.

Poenaru L, Mezard C, Akli S *et al.* (1990). Prenatal diagnosis of mucolipidosis type II on first-trimester amniotic fluid. *Prenatal Diagn* **10**:231–235.

Whelan DT, Chang PL, Cockshott PW (1983). Mucolipidosis II. The clinical, radiological and biochemical features in three cases. *Clin Genet* **24**:90–96.

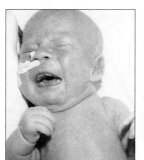 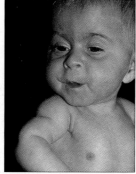 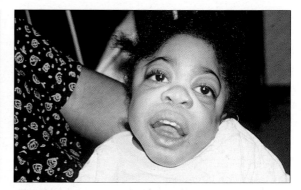

222A–222C Note coarse facial features. The patient in **222C** has a craniosynostosis which can be a consequence of the disease.

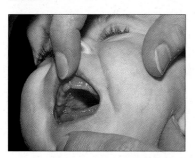

222D Note gum hypertrophy.

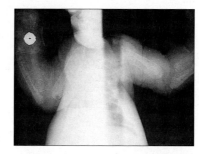

222E Note the periosteal cloaking of the bones.

ASPARTYLGLUCOSAMINURIA 223

This condition should be considered in the differential diagnosis of the mucopolysaccharidoses and the mucolipidoses. The majority of cases have been described in Finland, but a handful of patients have no Finnish ancestry. Recurrent respiratory infections are characteristic, as are umbilical and inguinal hernias, delayed speech, attention deficits, clumsiness and aggressive behaviour. The early facial features are described as 'a sagging face with a low bridge of the nose and a big mouth'. Liver and cardiac involvement do occur but are uncommon) angiokeratoma corporis diffusum has been described. The diagnosis is first suspected by finding vacuolated lymphocytes and oligosaccharides in the urine, and can be confirmed by thin layer chromotography of urine and enzymology.

Genetic aspects: Autosomal recessive inheritance. The gene has been mapped to 4q.

References

Aula P, Mattila K, Piiroinen O *et al.* (1989). First-trimester prenatal diagnosis of aspartylglucosaminuria. *Prenatal Diagn* **9**:617–620.

Borud O, Stromme JH, Lie SO, Torp KH (1978). Aspartylglucosaminuria in Northern Norway in eight patients: clinical heterogeneity and variations with the diet. *J Inherit Metab Dis* **1**:95–97.

Chitayat D, Nakagawa S *et al.* (1988). Aspartylglucosaminuria in a Puerto Rican family: additional features of a panethnic disorder. *Am J Med Genet* **31**:527–532.

Mononen T, Mononen I, Matilainen R, Airaksinen E (1991). High prevalence of aspartylglycosaminuria among school-age children in eastern Finland. *Hum Genet* **87**:266–268.

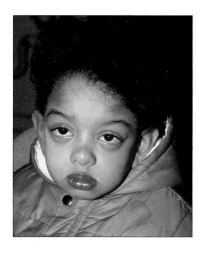

223 Note heavy face with prominent lips. The hair tends to be coarse.

MANNOSIDOSIS 224

This autosomal recessive storage disorder results from accumulation of mannose-containing residues due to a deficiency of alpha-mannosidase. The phenotype resembles a mucopolysaccharidosis but is generally milder with moderate coarsening of the face becoming apparent after 2–3 years, a lumbar gibbus, sensorineural deafness, hepatomegaly and dysostosis multiplex on X-ray. All cases have mild to moderate mental retardation. Diagnosis is made by finding vacuolated lymphocytes in the peripheral blood, abnormal oligosaccharides in the urine and reduced enzyme levels. There is a severe infantile form (type I) with rapid mental deterioration and a milder juvenile form (type II), although there is considerable overlap between the two.
Genetic aspects: Autosomal recessive.

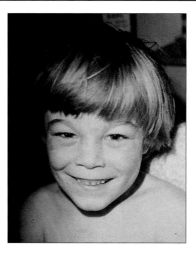

224 Note coarse facial features (prominent supraorbital ridges, full eyebrows and broad bridge to nose) and wide-spaced teeth.

References

Autio S, Louhimo T, Helenius M (1982). The clinical course of mannosidosis. *Ann Clin Res* **14**:93–97.

Dietemann JL, Filippi De La Palavesa MM, Tranchant C, Kastler B (1990). MR findings in mannosidosis. *Neuroradiology* **32**:485–487.

Jansen PHP, Schoonderwaldt HC *et al.* (1987). Mannosidosis: a study of two patients, presenting clinical heterogeneity. *Clin Neurol* **89**:185–192.

Noll RB, Netzloff ML, Kulkarni R (1989). Long-term follow-up of biochemical and cognitive functioning in patients with mannosidosis. *Arch Neurol* **46**:507–509.

Yunis JJ, Lewandowski R Jr *et al.* (1976). Clinical manifestations of mannosidosis – a longitudinal study. *Am J Med* **61**:841–848.

FABRY SYNDROME (ANGIOKERATOMA CORPORIS DIFFUSUM) 225

In this lysosomal storage disorder, unusual skin manifestations are associated with neurological abnormalities and renal impairment. Initial symptoms in childhood are usually episodes of pain, lasting from minutes to weeks, of an intense burning nature, felt deep to the skin. This often occurs in the fingers and toes but also in the abdomen and genitalia, and is influenced by temperature. Patients seek cool environments. At the same time skin lesions appear, consisting of clusters of dark red papules of about 1mm in diameter. These develop on the lower trunk and become more profuse during the third and fourth decades, spreading to the genitalia and other areas. Ocular signs include opacification of the cornea, said to be whirl-like in configuration. Oedema of the eyelids and retinal vessel thrombosis have also been described. Death usually occurs as a result of renal failure in middle life. Cardiac defects occur in 30% of patients and include mitral valve prolapse and cardiomyopathy. **Genetic aspects:** X-linked recessive. The deficient enzyme is acid hydrolase alpha-galactosidase A. The gene has been cloned and mutations have been identified. Heterozygote can be achieved by direct mutation analysis in many cases, or by linkage where the pedigree structure is appropriate.

References

Anonymous (1990). Anderson–Fabry disease (Editorial). *Lancet* **2**:24–25.

Ishii S, Sakuraba H, Shimmoto M *et al.* (1991). Fabry disease: detection of 13-bp deletion in alpha-galactosidase A gene and its application to gene diagnosis of heterozygotes. *Ann Neurol* **29**:560–564.

Morgan SH, Rudge P, Smith SJM *et al.* (1990). The neurological complications of Anderson–Fabry disease (alpha-galactosidase A deficiency) – investigation of symptomatic and presymptomatic patients. *Q J Med* **75**:491–507.

Sakuraba H, Oshima A, Fukuhara Y *et al.* (1990). Identification of point mutations in the alpha-galactosidase A gene in classical and atypical hemizygotes with Fabry disease. *Am J Hum Genet* **47**:784–789.

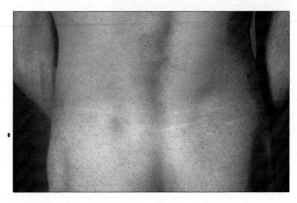

225 Punctate angiomatous lesions of the skin.

MENKES SYNDROME

This X-linked recessive condition is caused by a defect of copper transport and metabolism. Onset is in infancy with lethargy, abnormal temperature regulation, abnormal tone and seizures. Frequently, there is prematurity. The face is said to be characteristic with pallor, full cheeks, tangled eyebrows and a pronounced cupid's bow to the upper lip. The hair may be normal at birth but becomes depigmented, thin and brittle. Microscopic analysis reveals pili torti. It has been described as 'kinky' or 'steely'. Neurological deterioration is progressive and death occurs before the age of 3. Pathological examination of the brain reveals neuronal degeneration, gliosis, optic degeneration and tortuous arteries with an abnormal intima and occlusion. Therapy with subcutaneous administration of copper-histidine has been attempted. Sarkar *et al.* reviewed the long-term results in seven patients, two of whom were thought to have done well neurologically as a result of the treatment. If delivery is induced at 35 weeks and treatment commenced then, neurological features may be much milder. **Genetic aspects:** X-linked recessive. The gene maps to Xq13. Chelly *et al.* and Mercer *et al.* reported the isolation of a candidate gene. There was homology with bacterial heavy metal binding protein genes. This was most similar to a copper-transporting ATPase.

References

Chelly J, Tumer Z, Tonnesen T *et al.* (1993). Isolation of a candidate gene for Menkes disease that encodes a potential heavy metal binding protein. *Nature Genetics* **3**:14–19.

Johnsen DE, Coleman L, Poe L (1991). MR of progressive neurodegenerative change in treated Menkes' kinky hair disease. *Neuroradiology* **33**:181–182.

Mercer JFB, Livingston J, Hall B *et al.* (1993). Isolation of a partial candidate gene for Menkes disease by positional cloning. *Nature Genetics* **3**:20–25.

Sarkar B, Lingertat-Walsh K, Clarke JTR (1993). Copper-histidine therapy of Menkes disease. *J Pediatr* **123**:828–830.

Tonnesen T, Kleijer WJ, Horn N (1991). Incidence of Menkes disease. *Hum Genet* **86**:408–410.

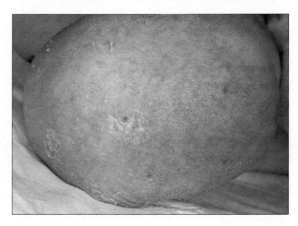

226 Note the sparse stubby (kinky) hair.

LOWE (OCULO-CEREBRO-RENAL) SYNDROME

227A–227B

Males with this X-linked recessive condition have cataracts, hypotonia, mental retardation, a generalised aminoaciduria and renal tubular acidosis with hypophosphataemia. There is a characteristic facial appearance after infancy because the eyes are sunken. Diagnosis is made in a retarded male with cataracts and a generalised aminoaciduria. Attree *et al.* showed that in an affected female with an X–autosome translocation, a gene with homology to inositol polyphosphate-5-phosphatase was interrupted.

Genetic aspects: X-linked recessive. Heterozygous females may have fine lenticular opacities – a sign that can be used for carrier detection.

References
Attree O, Olivos IM, Okabe I *et al.* (1992). The Lowe's oculocerebrorenal syndrome gene encodes a protein highly homologous to inositol polyphosphate-5-phosphatase. *Nature* **358**:239–242.

Charnas LR, Gahl WA (1991). The oculocerebrorenal syndrome of Lowe. *Adv Pediatr* **38**:75–102.

Fagerholm P, Anneren G, Wadelius C (1991). Lowe's oculocerebrorenal syndrome - variation in lens changes in the carrier state. *Acta Ophthalmol* **69**:102–104.

Pueschel SM, Brem AS, Nittoli P (1992). Central nervous system and renal investigations in patients with Lowe syndrome. *Child's Nerv Syst* **8**:45–48.

Redfield VA, Mimouni F, Strife FC, Tsang RC (1991). Severe rickets in Lowe syndrome: treatment with continuous nasogastric infusion. *Pediatr Nephrol* **5**:696–699.

227A and 227B The eyes are deep-set and the face hypotonic.

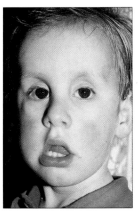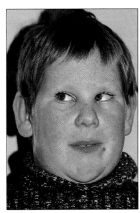

LESCH–NYHAN SYNDROME

228A–228C

This syndrome presents with choreoathetosis, self mutilation, spasticity and developmental delay. Onset is within the first few months with developmental retardation, and the full clinical picture develops before 2 years. The self mutilation is distressing to the patient and consists of biting the lips and limbs. A few cases have had congenital abnormalities such as anal atresia, Hirschsprung's disease and cryptorchidism. There is an acceleration of *de novo* purine synthesis, leading to hyperuricemia with gouty symptoms and renal uric acid stones. A deficiency of the enzyme hypoxanthine-guanine phosphoribosyltransferase can be demonstrated.

Genetic aspects: X-linked recessive.

References
Mizuno T (1986). Long-term follow-up of ten patients with Lesch–Nyhan syndrome. *Neuropediatrics* **17**:158–161.

Sculley DG, Dawson PA, Emmerson BT, Gordon RB (1992). A review of the molecular basis of hypoxanthine-guanine phosphoribosyltransferase (HPRT) deficiency. *Hum Genet* **90**:195–207.

Stout JT, Caskey CT (1988). The Lesch–Nyhan syndrome: clinical, molecular and genetic aspects. *Trend Genet* **4**:175–178.

Tarle SA, Davidson BL, Wu VC *et al.* (1991). Determination of the mutations responsible for the Lesch–Nyhan syndrome in 17 subjects. *Genomics* **10**:499–501.

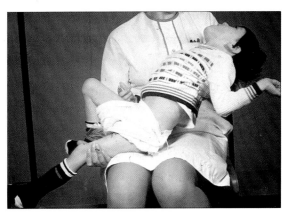

228A and 228B Note the abnormal posture due to extrapyramidal movements.

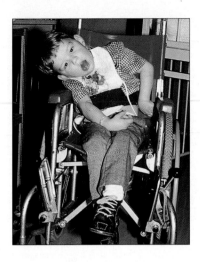

228B

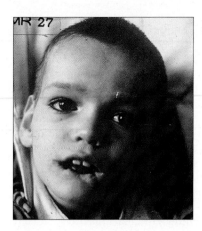

228C There is self-mutilation around the mouth.

ZELLWEGER (CEREBRO-HEPATO-RENAL) SYNDROME   229A–229D

These infants are severely hypotonic at birth and may have nystagmus and seizures. The face is characteristic with a tall forehead, hypoplastic supraorbital ridges and lack of expression. The presence of epicanthic folds and Brushfield spots has sometimes led to the misdiagnosis of Down syndrome. Other findings include cataracts, camptodactyly, club feet, a large liver, stippled epiphyses and stippling of the patellae. Peroxisomes are missing in the liver and kidneys and the activities of multiple peroxisomal enzymes are reduced, leading to deficiency of ether-glycolipids, and accumulation of very long chain fatty acids, pipecolic acid and bile acid intermediates.

Genetic aspects: Autosomal recessive. At the molecular level the disease is likely to be heterogeneous. Shimozawa *et al.* demonstrated a point mutation in both alleles of the peroxisome assembly factor-1 gene (PAF-1; PMP35) in a single patient. Gartner *et al.* found a mutation in the 70K peroxisomal membrane protein gene (PMP70) in two patients. This gene maps to chromosome 1.

References

Clayton PT, Thompson E (1988). Dysmorphic syndromes with demonstrable biochemical abnormalities. *J Med Genet* **25**:463–472.

Gartner J, Moser H, Valle D (1992). Mutations in the 70K peroxisomal membrane protein gene in Zellweger syndrome. *Nature Genetics* **1**:16–23.

Moser HW (1986). Peroxisomal disorders . *J Pediatr* **108**:89–91.

Shimozawa N, Suzuki Y, Orii T *et al.* (1993). Prenatal diagnosis of Zellweger syndrome using DNA analysis (Letter). *Prenatal Diagn* **13**:149.

Wanders RJA, Heymans HSA, Schutgens RBH *et al.* (1988). Peroxisomal disorders in neurology. *J Neurol Sci* **88**:1–39.

Wilson GN, Holmes RD, Hajra AK (1988). Peroxisomal disorders: clinical commentary and future prospects. *Am J Med Genet* **30**:771–792.

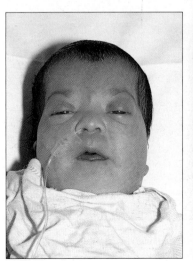

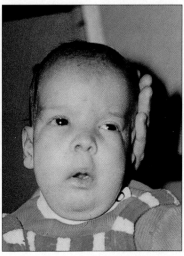

229A–229C Note the high forehead, expressionless face, and shallow supraorbital ridges.

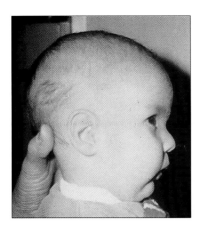

229C

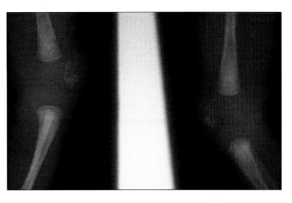

229D Note the stippling of the patella.

SYNDROMES WITH THE APPEARANCE OF PREMATURE AGEING

PROGERIA

230A–230B

After the first year progressive signs of apparent ageing appear; there is loss of scalp hair, eyebrows and eyelashes, prominent scalp veins and a small triangular face with a relatively large cranial vault. Birthweight may be low, less than 2 500g, but major problems with growth do not occur until after the first year, when growth may almost cease. The mandible is small with crowded teeth that erupt late. The nose is thin and beaked. The skin becomes dry and thin and the nails are brittle and short (reflecting shortening of the underlying distal phalanges). There is generalised wasting with a cachectic appearance and prominent joints. Hypertension, cardiomegaly and early atheroma can occur. Death is in the second decade in most cases.

Genetic aspects: Most cases are sporadic, although there have been a few reports of affected siblings.

References

Khalifa MM (1989). Hutchinson–Gilford progeria syndrome: report of a Libyan family and evidence of autosomal recessive inheritance. *Clin Genet* **35**:125–132.

Mallory SB, Krafchik BR (1990). Hutchinson–Gilford syndrome. *Pediatr Dermatol* **7**:317–319.

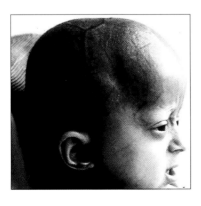

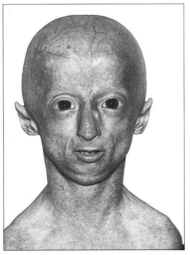

230A and 230B Note total alopecia, pinched nose and aged appearance.

WIEDEMANN–RAUTENSTRAUCH SYNDROME (NEONATAL PROGERIA)   231

This syndrome is recognisable at birth with an aged face, wrinkled skin, reduced subcutaneous fat and neonatal teeth. Birth-weight is low, subsequent growth is very poor and development delayed. The scalp hair is sparse and the children have the appearance of pseudo-hydrocephaly with a persistent anterior fontanelle. Fat distribution is abnormal, especially over the buttocks.

Genetic aspects: Autosomal recessive.

References

Rautenstrauch T, Snigula F, Krieg T *et al.* (1977). Progeria: a cell culture study and clinical report of familial incidence. *Eur J Pediatr* **124**:101–111.

Toriello HV (1990). Syndrome of the month: Wiedemann–Rautenstrauch syndrome. *J Med Genet* **27**:256–257.

Wiedemann H-R (1979). An unidentified neonatal progeroid syndrome: follow-up report. *Eur J Pediatr* **130**:65–70.

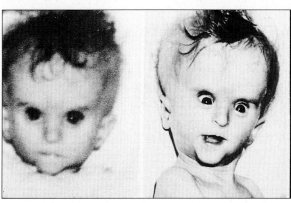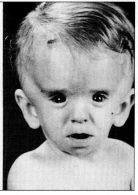

231 Three affected children at 8 months of age showing triangular face with pseudo-hydrocephalic appearance, and paucity of subcutaneous tissue giving premature aged appearance.

ACROGERIA   232

This condition has been classified Ehlers Danlos Syndrome Type IV, as in some cases a type III collagen defect can be demonstrated (Pope *et al.*). The facial features consist of premature ageing because of thin skin, a pinched nose, prominent eyes and a thin, drawn appearance. The skin of the hands and feet is atrophic with prominent tortuous veins. Death can occur in the second or third decade of life due to aortic or other vascular rupture.

Genetic aspects: There are severe recessive and milder recessive and autosomal dominant forms.

References

De Groot WP, Tafelkruyer J, Woerdeman MJ (1980). Familial acrogeria (Gottron). *Br J Dermatol* **103**:213–223.

Gilkes JJH, Sharvill DE, Wells RE (1974). The premature ageing syndromes. Report of eight cases and description of a new entity named metageria. *Br J Dermatol* **91**:243–262.

Greally JM, Boone LY, Lenkey SG *et al.* (1992). Acrometageria: a spectrum of "premature ageing" syndromes. *Am J Med Genet* **44**:334–339.

Ho A, White SJ, Rasmussen JE (1987). Skeletal abnormalities of acrogeria, a progeroid syndrome. *Skeletal Radiol* **16**:463–468.

Pope FM, Nicholls AC, Jones PM *et al.* (1980). EDS IV (acrogeria): new autosomal dominant and recessive types. *J Royal Soc Med* **73**:180–186.

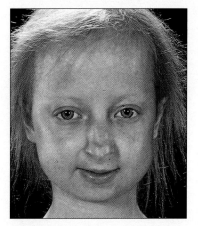

232 Note thin pinched nose, sparse hair and overall impression of premature ageing.

HALLERMANN–STREIFF SYNDROME – OCULO-MANDIBULO-DYSCEPHALY; HYPOTRICHOSIS   233A–233B

The nose is thin and pointed and the overlying skin is atrophic. The mandible is very small and the combined appearance with microphthalmia, cataracts and prominent cheeks results in a very characteristic facial appearance. Neonatal teeth may be present but there is later hypodontia. Feeding and respiratory problems can be severe early on. The scalp hair is thin and wispy. Mental retardation may occur in about 15% of cases. Radiological features include poor ossification of the skull with wormian bones and large fontanelles, thin ribs and long bones, metaphyseal widening, mild bowing of the radius and ulna in the neonatal period and platyspondyly.

Genetic aspects: Most cases are sporadic, but the possibility of autosomal dominant inheritance has not been completely ruled out.

References

Christian CL, Lachman RS, Aylsworth AS *et al.* (1991). Radiological findings in Hallermann–Streiff syndrome: report of five cases and a review of the literature. *Am J Med Genet* **41**:508–514.

Cohen MM Jr (1991). Hallermann–Streiff syndrome: a review. *Am J Med Genet* **41**:488–499.

Harrod MJ, Friedman JM (1991). Congenital cataracts in mother, sister, and son of a patient with Hallermann–Streiff syndrome: coincidence or clue? *Am J Med Genet* **41**:500–502.

Salbert BA, Stevens CA, Spence JE (1991). Tracheomalacia in Hallermann–Streiff syndrome. *Am J Med Genet* **41**:521–523.

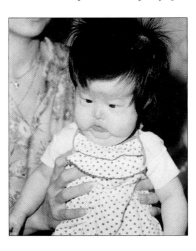 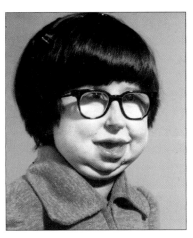

233A and 233B Note frontal bossing, small eyes, jaw and mouth, sagging cheeks and thin pointed nose.

COCKAYNE SYNDROME   234A–234F

This is a progressive neurological disorder that has a characteristic facial appearance. Obvious signs of the disorder develop between the second and fourth years but might not be present at birth. There is a loss of facial tissue, giving the appearance of premature ageing, deep-set eyes and a prominent nasal bridge. A photosensitive skin rash is almost always present. After the onset of clinical features of the disorder the head circumference becomes small and there is growth retardation. A sensorineural hearing loss is common. Both central and peripheral demyelination results in loss of skills, and features of a neuropathy. A retinopathy occurs late and may be accompanied by optic atrophy. Calcification in the cortex and in the basal ganglia is a common feature. Some cases have early onset in the neonatal period and the features overlap with COFS syndrome. Nance and Berry provide an excellent review. Chromosome breakage is seen on exposure of cells to UV light, and there is a slow recovery of DNA and RNA synthesis.

Genetic aspects: Autosomal recessive. Prenatal diagnosis looking at chromosomal breakage has been successful.

References

Jaeken J, Klocker H, Schwaiger H *et al.* (1989). Clinical and biochemical studies in three patients with severe early infantile Cockayne syndrome. *Hum Genet* **83**:339–346.

Lehmann AR, Francis AJ, Giannelli FB (1985). Prenatal diagnosis of Cockayne's syndrome. *Lancet* **1**:486–488.

Lowry RB (1982). Invited editorial comment: early onset Cockayne syndrome. *Am J Med Genet* **13**:209–210.

Nance MA, Berry SA (1992). Cockayne syndrome: review of 140 cases. *Am J Med Genet* **42**:68–84.

Patton MA, Giannelli F, Francis AJ *et al.* (1989). Early onset Cockayne's syndrome: case reports with neuropathological and fibroblast studies. *J Med Genet* **26**:154–159.

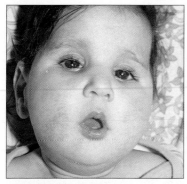
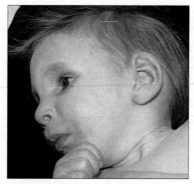
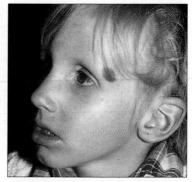

234A–234F Note the sunken eyes and beaked nose. The patient in **234A** is at an early stage of the condition, and the patient in **234F** is in his late 20s.

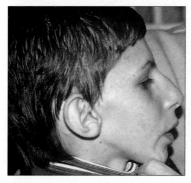
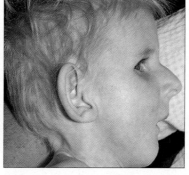
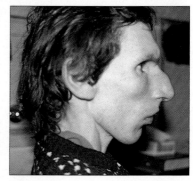

234D   **234E**   **234F**

BERARDINELLI LIPODYSTROPHY (LAWRENCE–SEIP SYNDROME)   235A–235B

Paediatricians need to consider this condition when faced with a child who appears thin but muscular. This is due, at least in part, to a lack of subcutaneous adipose tissue. Acanthosis nigricans may become apparent. Most children develop an insulin resistant non-ketotic diabetes in late childhood and they may succumb to the complications of liver cirrhosis. Neutral fats are increased in concentration in the plasma. Moller and Flier provide an excellent review of syndromes characterised by insulin resistance.

Genetic aspects: Autosomal recessive.

References

Moller DE, Flier JS (1991). Insulin resistance – mechanisms, syndromes, and implications. *New Engl J Med* **325**:938–948.

Reed WB, Dexter R, Corley C *et al.* (1965). Congenital lipodystrophic diabetes in acanthosis nigricans. *Arch Dermatol* **91**:326–334.

Seip M (1975). The syndrome of generalized lipodystrophy. *BDOAS* **11(2)**:325–327.

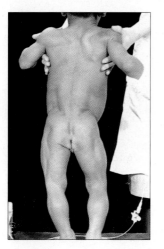

235A and 235B Note lack of subcutaneous fat causing muscles to look prominent.

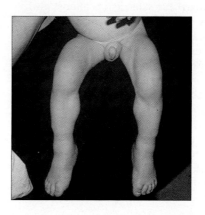

WERNER SYNDROME 236

This syndrome is characterised by features of premature ageing and endocrinological abnormalities appearing in early adulthood. The main features are short stature, a slender body habitus, a beaked nose, a high-pitched, weak or hoarse voice, juvenile cataracts, and hyperreflexia in the legs. Scleroderma-like changes are seen with tight atrophic skin, telangiectasia, soft tissue calcifications and circumscribed hyperkeratosis. Diabetes or abnormal glucose tolerance is common as is hypogonadism . Premature atherosclerosis is a feature.

Genetic aspects: Autosomal recessive. Goto *et al.*, (1992) demonstrated linkage to markers on 8p12.

References

Cerimele D, Cottoni F *et al.* (1982). High prevalence of Werner's syndrome in Sardinia: description of six patients and estimate of the gene frequency. *Hum Genet* **62**:25–30.

Epstein CJ, Martin GM, Schultz AL *et al.* (1966). Werner's syndrome. *Medicine* **45**:177–221.

Fleischmajer R, Nedwich A (1973). Werner's syndrome. *Am J Med* **54**:111–118.

Goto M, Hariuchi Y, Tanimoto K *et al.* (1978). Werner's syndrome: analysis of 15 cases with a review of the Japanese literature. *J Am Geriatr Soc* **26**:341–347.

Goto M, Rubenstein M, Weber J *et al.* (1992). Genetic linkage of Werner's syndrome to five markers on chromosome 8. *Nature* **355**:735–738.

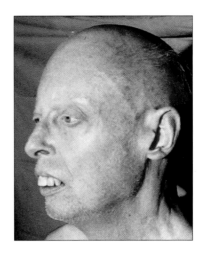

236 Note the relative alopecia and premature ageing of this young adult.

MULVIHILL–SMITH SYNDROME 237A–237B

This presents with intrauterine growth retardation, thin pinched facies, multiple pigmented nevi resembling lentigines, and developmental delay. Other manifestations are photosensitivity, thin taut dry skin, telangiectases, sparse thin hair, absent axillary hair, oligodontia, diminished muscle mass, hypospadias and diabetes. The face becomes progressively aged in appearance with hypoplasia of the facial bones.

Genetic aspects: Uncertain; all cases have been sporadic.

References

Baraitser M, Insley J, Winter RM (1988). A recognisable short stature syndrome with premature ageing and pigmented naevi. *J Med Genet* **25**:53–56.

Bartsch O, Tympner K-D, Schwinger E, Gorlin RJ (1994). Mulvihill–Smith syndrome: case report and review. *J Med Genet* **31**:707–711.

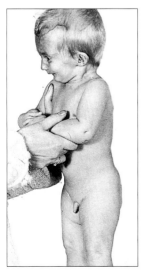

237A Note the premature ageing with decreased fat over the face and neck.

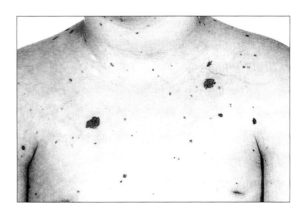

237B Note the hyperpigmented nevi.

LEPRECHAUNISM

There is intrauterine growth retardation, hirsutism, an aged face with thickened lips and prominent ears, failure to thrive and enlargement of the breasts and genitalia. The hands and feet are relatively large and acanthosis nigricans and lipodystrophy may be features. Hyperplasia of the pancreatic islet cells is seen at autopsy as well as cystic changes of the gonads. Hyperinsulinaemia can be demonstrated. Several cases have been reported with insulin receptor mutations. The extreme failure to thrive does raise the differential diagnosis of the diencephalic syndrome and it might be worthwhile to include a CT brain scan in the investigations to exclude this possibility.

Genetic aspects: Autosomal recessive.

References

Der Kaloustian VM, Kronfol NM et al. (1971). Leprechaunism: a report of two new cases. *Am J Dis Child* **122**:442–445.

Donohue WL, Uchida I (1954). Leprechaunism: a euphemism for a rare familial disorder. *J Pediatr* **45**:505–519.

Elsas LJ, Endo F, Strumlauf E, et al. (1985). Leprechaunism: an inherited defect in a high-affinity insulin receptor. *Am J Hum Genet* **37**:73–88.

Flier JS (1992). Lilly Lecture; syndromes of insulin resistance. From patient to gene and back again. *Diabetes* **41**:1207–1219.

Gross-Kieselstein E, Ben-Galim E et al. (1973)Leprechaunism (Donohue syndrome). *Am J Dis Child* **126**:500–503.

Moller DE, Flier JS (1991). Insulin resistance – mechanisms, syndromes, and implications. *New Engl J Med* **325**:938–948.

Taylor SI (1992). Lilly lecture: molecular mechanisms of insulin resistance. Lessons from patients with mutations in the insulin-receptor gene. *Diabetes* **41**:1473–1490.

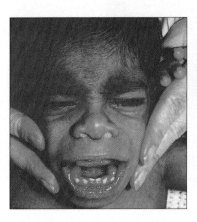 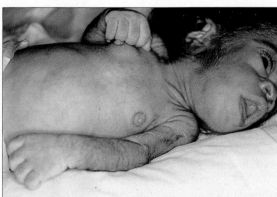

238A and 238B
Note hirsutism, thick lips, wide mouth and gum hypertrophy. There is profound failure to thrive.

SYNDROMES WITH DERMATOLOGICAL ABNORMALITIES

KLIPPEL–TRENAUNAY–WEBER SYNDROME

The features consist of a cutaneous vascular nevus over the trunk or limbs in an asymmetrical distribution, varicosities and asymmetrical hypertrophy of all or part of a limb. Some patients have lymphoedema. The hypertrophy of the limbs is due to hyperplasia of both bone and soft tissue. It does not seem to be secondary to arteriovenous anastamosis in most cases. The central nervous system is rarely affected, although macrocrania and an intracranial vascular malformation have been described. The condition must be differentiated from the Proteus syndrome, in which the limb hypertrophy can be much more severe and progressive. There is also an overlap with Sturge–Weber syndrome, in that vascular nevi involving a limb or the trunk (even with hypertrophy) are not uncommonly found in that condition.

Genetic aspects: Mostly sporadic. In a questionnaire survey of affected individuals, Aelvoet *et al.* found that two out of 86 cases had another affected family member and one relative had hemihypertrophy. Seven out of 400 relatives had naevi flammei.

References

Aelvoet GE, Jorens PG, Roelen LM (1992). Genetic aspects of the Klippel–Trenaunay syndrome. *Br J Dermatol* **126**:603–607.

Servelle M (1985). Klippel and Trenaunay's syndrome. 768 operated cases. *Ann Surg* **201**:365–373.

Sooriakumaran S, Lal Landham T (1991). The Klippel–Trenaunay syndrome. *J Bone Joint Surg B* **73**:169–170.

Viljoen DL (1988). Klippel–Trenaunay–Weber syndrome (angio-osteohypertrophy syndrome). *J Med Genet* **25**:250–252.

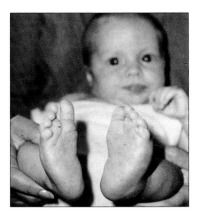

239A–239D Note the vascular nevi and asymmetrical limb hypertrophy.

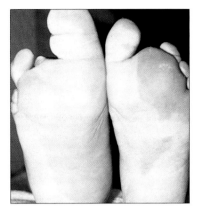

239B

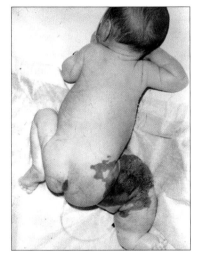

239C

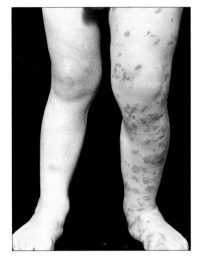

239D

STURGE–WEBER SYNDROME

240A–240D

This is the association of facial capillary haemangiomas with angiomas of the meninges. The involvement of the ophthalmic division of the trigeminal nerve is necessary for the diagnosis. Plain skull radiographs show 'tram-line' calcification. Seizures and mental retardation may be complications. The risk of glaucoma where a haemangioma is in the ophthalmic division is between 7% and 24%.

Genetic aspects: Most cases are sporadic.

References

Aicardi J, Arzimanoglou A (1991). Sturge–Weber syndrome. *Int Pediatr* **6**:129–134.

Marti-Bonmati L, Menor F, Poyatos C, Cortina H (1992). Diagnosis of Sturge–Weber syndrome: comparison of the efficacy of CT and MR imaging in 14 cases. *Am J Roentgenol* **158**:867–871.

Marti-Bonmati L, Menor F, Mulas F (1993). The Sturge–Weber syndrome: correlation between the clinical status and radiological CT and MRI findings. *Child's Nerv Syst* **9**:107–109.

Sullivan TJ, Clarke MP, Morin JD (1992). The ocular manifestations of the Sturge–Weber syndrome. *J Ped Ophthal Strab* **29**:349–356.

Tallman B, Tan OT, Morelli JG *et al.* (1991). Location of port-wine stains and the likelihood of ophthalmic and/or central nervous system complications. *Pediatrics* **87**:323–327.

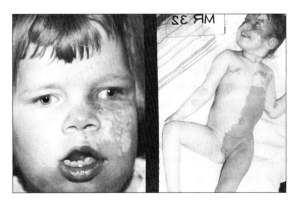

240A and 240B Note the port-wine stain over the face (and trunk) including the first division of the Vth cranial nerve.

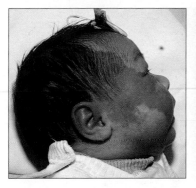

240B

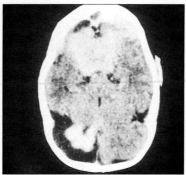

240C Note the gyral calcification and atrophy.

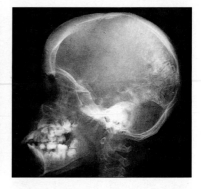

240D Note the intracranial tramline calcification.

RENDU–OSLER–WEBER HEREDITARY TELANGIECTASIA 241A–241B

Individuals with this autosomal dominant condition have small angiomas of the skin, mucous membranes and internal organs. Recurrent epistaxis is the presenting feature in 90% of cases. The cutaneous telangiectases appear between the ages of 5 and 20 years and occur on the palms and nailbeds, the lips and tongue and the face. More serious complications are caused by cerebrovascular, gastrointestinal and pulmonary arteriovascular malformations. There is some evidence that the lesions increase in size and number during puberty and pregnancy.

Genetic aspects: Autosomal dominant. The gene has been mapped to 9q32-33 in some families. However, there is evidence for genetic heterogeneity.

References
Aesch B, Lioret E, De Toffol B, Jan M (1991). Multiple cerebral angiomas and Rendu-Osler-Weber disease. *Neurosurgery* **29**:599–602.
Porteous MEM, Burn J, Proctor SJ (1992). Hereditary haemorrhagic telangiectasia: a clinical analysis. *J Med Genet* **29**:527–530.

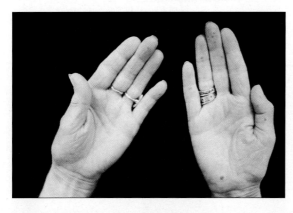

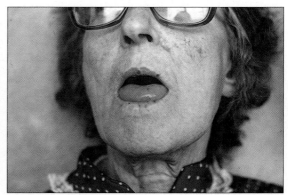

241A and 241B Note the punctate telangiectasia of the skin and mucous membranes.

CUTIS MARMORATA TELANGIECTASIA CONGENITA 242

The skin in this condition is characterised by a reticular vascular pattern which is present from birth and often improves with age. Sometimes the skin lesion persists, and there are associated features such as hemihypertrophy or hemiatrophy, aplasia cutis congenita or mild developmental delay. Rare patients have seizures and macrocephaly. Glaucoma (Miranda *et al.*; Mayatepek *et al.*) and terminal transverse defects of the limbs (Bjornsdottir *et al.*) have also been reported.
Genetic aspects: Mostly sporadic.

References

Bjornsdottir US *et al.* (1988). Cutis marmorata telangiectatica congenita with terminal transverse limb defects. *Acta Paediatr Scand* **77**:780–782.

Del Giudice SM, Nydorf ED (1986). Cutis marmorata telangiectatica congenita with multiple congenital anomalies. *Arch Dermatol* **122**:1060–1061.

Mayatepek E, Krastel H, Volcker HE *et al.* (1991). Congenital glaucoma in cutis marmorata telangiectatica congonita. *Ophthalmologica* **202**:191–193.

Miranda I, Alonso MJ, Jimenez M *et al.* (1990). Cutis marmorata telangiectatica congenita and glaucoma. *Ophthal Paed Genet* **11**:129–132.

Picascia DD, Esterly NB (1989). Cutis marmorata telangiectatica congenita: report of 22 cases. *J Am Acad Dermatol* **20**:1098–1104.

Powell ST, Su WPD (1984). Cutis marmorata telangectatica congenita: report of nine cases and review of the literature. *Cutis* **34**:305–312.

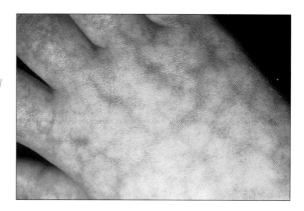

242 Note the reticulate vascular patterning.

BLUE RUBBER BLEB NEVUS SYNDROME 243

This condition is characterised by cutaneous cavernous haemangiomata, often associated with haemangiomas of the gastrointestinal tract. The skin lesions are soft, have a rubbery texture and can occasionally be either pedunculated or resemble phlebectasias. They are blue in colour and may be tender on palpation. Lesions have been described in the liver, GI-tract and the brain. Intra-oral lesions are not unusual. Histologically, there are large, irregular blood-filled spaces in the lower dermis and in subcutaneous tissue. A chronic iron deficiency anaemia from gastrointestinal bleeding may be the presenting sign, and some patients develop a chronic consumptive coagulopathy.

Genetic aspects: Nearly all cases to date have been single.

References

Hofhuis WJD, Oranje AP, Bouquet J, Sinaasappel M (1990). Blue rubber-bleb naevus syndrome: report of a case with consumption coagulopathy complicated by manifest thrombosis. *Eur J Pediatr* **149**:526–528.

Morris SJ, Kaplan SR *et al.* (1978). Blue rubber-bleb nevus syndrome. *JAMA* **239**:1887.

Munkvad M (1983). Blue rubber bleb nevus syndrome. *Dermatologica* **167**:307–309.

Satya-Murti S, Navada S, Eames F (1986). Central nervous system involvement in blue-rubber-bleb-nevus syndrome. *Arch Neurol* **43**:1184–1186.

Talbot S, Wyatt EH (1970). Blue rubber bleb naevi (report of a family in which only males were affected). *Br J Dermatol* **82**:37–39.

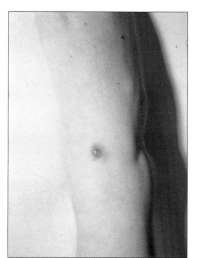

243 Note raised blue nevus on arm.

PROTEUS SYNDROME

This condition is characterised by massive overgrowth and asymmetry. Different types of skin lesion are seen, including linear verrucous epidermal nevi, intradermal nevi, shagreen patches, haemangiomas, lipomas and varicosities. There may be a characteristic warty, hyperplastic plantar overgrowth that has been termed a 'moccasin lesion'. Craniofacial anomalies include hydrocephalus, macrocephaly, hemimegalencephaly, facial and ocular asymmetry, retinal detachment, scleral tumours, prognathism, malocclusion and hyperostoses. Mental retardation may be present but is rare.

Genetic aspects: Almost all cases are sporadic, but see the paper by Goodship *et al.*

References

Clark RD, Donnai D, Rogers J et al. (1987). Proteus syndrome: an expanded phenotype. *Am J Med Genet* **27**:99–118.

Goodship J, Redfearn A, Milligan D et al. (1991). Transmission of Proteus syndrome from father to son? *J Med Genet* **28**:781–785.

Malamitsi-Puchner A, Dimitriadis D, Bartsocas C, Wiedemann H-R (1990). Proteus syndrome: course of a severe case. *Am J Med Genet* **35**:283–285.

Mayatepek E, Kurczynski TW et al. (1989). Expanding the phenotype of the proteus syndrome: a severely affected patient with new findings. *Am J Med Genet* **32**:402–406.

McCall S, Ramzy MI, Cure JK, Pai GS (1992). Encephalocraniocutaneous lipomatosis and the Proteus syndrome: distinct entities with overlapping manifestations. *Am J Med Genet* **43**:662–668.

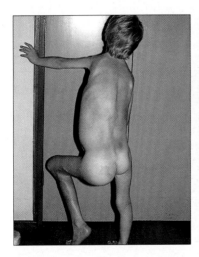

244A Note the severe hypertrophy on the left.

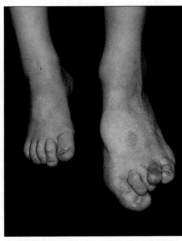

244B The foot is involved.

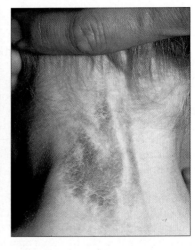

244C Note the linear sebaceous nevus at the back of the neck.

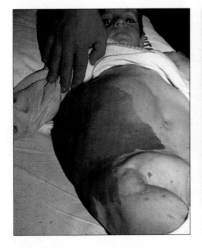

244D Note the vascular nevus which might not be present at birth.

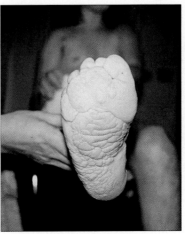

244E Note the characteristic rugate striate lesions underneath the foot (a moccasin lesion).

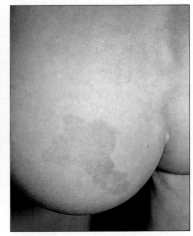

244F Note hypertrophy of the buttock with a vascular nevus overlying it.

ENCEPHALOCRANIOCUTANEOUS LIPOMATOSIS 245A–245B

There is macrocephaly, lipodermoids involving the conjunctiva, sclera or eyelids, and lipomatous swellings over the cranium or face. Mental retardation is often a feature and a CT brain scan might show cerebral atrophy, sometimes unilateral, or porencephalic cysts. Intracranial calcifications have also been described. At autopsy the lipomatous lesions might be more widespread intracranially and the cranial bones might be infiltrated. The differentiation from Proteus syndrome and the linear sebaceous nevus syndrome can be difficult and it is possible that encephalocutateous lipomatosis is a localised form of one of these conditions.

Genetic aspects: Sporadic.

References

Dean JCS, Cole GF, Appleton RE *et al.* (1990). Cranial hemihypertrophy and neurodevelopmental prognosis. *J Med Genet* **27**:160–164.

Fishman MA (1987). Encephalocraniocutaneous lipomatosis. *J Child Neurol* 1987|**2**:186–193.

Fryer AE (1992). Scalp lipomas and cerebral malformations – report of a case and review of the literature. *Clin Dysmorphol* **1**:99–102.

Haberland C, Perou MB (1970). Encephalocraniocutaneous lipomatosis: a new example of ectomesodermal dysgenesis. *Arch Neurol* **22**:144–155.

Loggers HE, Oosterwijk JC, Overweg-Plandsoen WCG *et al.* (1992). Encephalocraniocutaneous lipomatosis and oculocerebrocutaneous syndrome. A differential diagnostic problem? *Ophthal Paed Genet* **13**:171–177.

McCall S, Ramzy MI, Cure JK, Pai GS (1992). Encephalocraniocutaneous lipomatosis and the Proteus syndrome: distinct entities with overlapping manifestations. *Am J Med Genet* **43**:662–668.

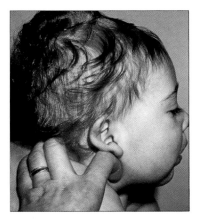

245A Note scalp lipoma.

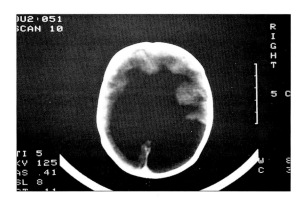

245B Note gross porencephaly.

LINEAR SEBACEOUS NEVUS SYNDROME 246A–246C

The cutaneous manifestations of this condition are linear, verrucous, pigmented lesions, ichthyosis hystrix, acanthosis nigricans, haemangiomas and café au lait spots. Associated complications include mental retardation (Feuerstein–Mims syndrome), seizures, cranial nerve palsies, hydrocephalus, renal tumours, vitamin D-resistant rickets, bone cysts and deformity, and kyphosis/scoliosis. There have been cases with diffuse pulmonary haemangiomatosis, vitamin D dependent rickets and bone cysts. Epibulbar dermoids (choristomas) appear to be associated – some of these cases may have encephalocraniocutaneous lipomatosis (q.v.).

Genetic aspects: Most case are sporadic.

References

Carey DE, Drezner MK, Hamdan JA *et al.* (1986). Hypophosphatemic rickets/osteomalacia in linear sebaceous nevus syndrome: a variant of tumor-induced osteomalacia. *J Pediatr* **109**:994–1000.

El-Shanti H, Bell WE, Waziri MH (1992). Epidermal nevus syndrome: subgroup with neuronal migration defects. *J Child Neurol* **7**:29–34.

Pavone L, Curatolo P, Rizzo R *et al.* (1991). Epidermal nevus syndrome: a neurologic variant with hemimegalencephaly, mental retardation, seizures, and facial hemihypertrophy. *Neurology* **41**:266–271.

Rogers M (1992). Epidermal nevi and the epidermal nevus syndromes: a review of 233 cases. *Pediatr Dermatol* **9**:342–344.

Sakuta R, Aikawa H, Takashima S, Ryo S (1991). Epidermal nevus syndrome with hemimegalencephaly: neuropathological study. *Brain Dev* **13**:260–265.

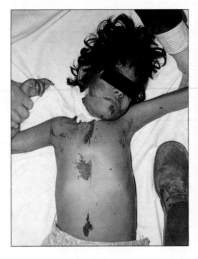 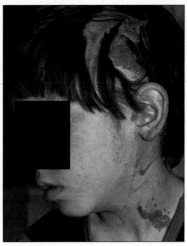 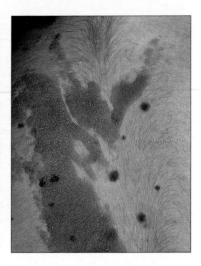

246A–246C Note the hyperpigmented raised lesions with dermatomal distribution. The alopecia in **246B** is part of the clinical picture.

OCULOCEREBROCUTANEOUS (DELLEMAN) SYNDROME

247A–247C

Aplasia, hypoplasia, and punched-out areas of skin over the ears, behind the ears, on the scalp, trunk and lips occur. There are orbital cysts and frequently microphthalmia, and a persistent hyaloid artery. Numerous skin tags involving the eyelids, especially at their lateral margins, but also on the cheeks, may be seen. Mental retardation, hydrocephalus, porencephaly, agenesis of the corpus callosum and meningo-encephaloceles have been reported. There may be overlap with encephalocraniocutaneous lipomatosis (Loggers *et al.*).

Genetic aspects: Most cases have been single but the numbers are small.

References

Al-Gazali LI, Donnai D, Berry SA *et al.* (1988). The oculocerebrocutaneous (Delleman) syndrome. *J Med Genet* **25**:773–778.

De Cock R, Merizian A (1992). Delleman syndrome: a case report and review. *Br J Ophthalmol* **76**:115–116.

Delleman JW, Oorthuys JWE *et al.* (1984). Orbital cyst in addition to congenital cerebral and focal dermal malformations: a new entity. *Clin Genet* **25**:470–472.

Loggers HE, Oosterwijk JC, Overweg-Plandsoen WCG *et al.* (1992) Encephalocraniocutaneous lipomatosis and oculocerebrocutaneous syndrome. A differential diagnostic problem? *Ophthal Paed Genet* **13**:171–177.

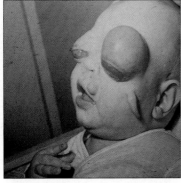 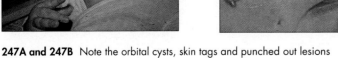 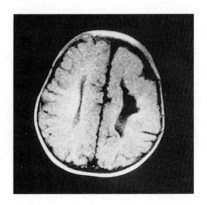

247A and 247B Note the orbital cysts, skin tags and punched out lesions above the ear.

247C Note the frontal lobe atrophy.

NEUROFIBROMATOSIS TYPE 1

This common autosomal dominant condition occurs in about one in 3 000 individuals. The manifestations are protean and well known. The most common presenting features are café au lait patches (more than six greater than 1.5cm in diameter) and peripheral neurofibromata. Complications can include optic nerve gliomas, macrocephaly, short stature, scoliosis, pseudarthrosis of the tibia, hypertension due to renal artery stenosis, phaeochromocytoma, plexiform neurofibromas, neurofibrosarcomas, and meningiomas. Acoustic neuromas may be confined to the so-called central form of the disease. Subtle signs of the disorder include Lisch nodules of the iris. About 5% of gene carriers may have mild mental retardation, and a third have serious complications at some stage during their life.

Genetic aspects: Autosomal dominant. The gene maps to 17q11 and mutations have been found in the gene in about 20% of cases.

References

Ainsworth PJ, Rodenhiser DI, Costa MT (1993). Identification and characterization of sporadic and inherited mutations in exon 31 of the neurofibromatosis (NF1) gene. *Hum Genet* **91**:151–156.

Dunn DW, Purvin V (1990). Optic pathway gliomas in neurofibromatosis. *Dev Med Child Neurol* **32**:820–824.

Gutmann DH, Collins FS (1992). Recent progress toward understanding the molecular biology of von Recklinghausen neurofibromatosis. *Ann Neurol* **31**:555–561.

Huson SM (1987). The different forms of neurofibromatosis. *Br Med J* **294**:1113–1114.

Huson SM (1989). Recent developments in the diagnosis and management of neurofibromatosis. *Arch Dis Child* **64**:745–749.

Riccardi VM (1991). Neurofibromatosis: past, present, and future (Editorial). *New Engl J Med* **324**:1283–1285.

Upadhyaya M, Fryer A, MacMillan J et al. (1992). Prenatal diagnosis and presymptomatic detection of neurofibromatosis type 1. *J Med Genet* **29**:180–183.

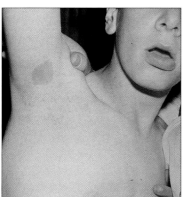

248A Note the axillary freckling and café au lait patch.

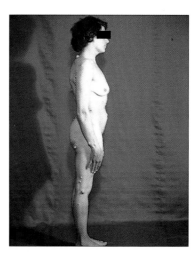

248B and 248C Note the multiple cutaneous neurofibromata.

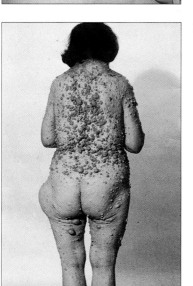

248C

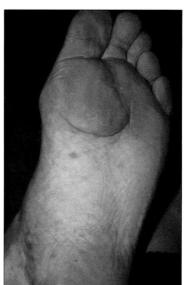

248D Note the plexiform neuroma of the sole.

PEUTZ–JEGHERS SYNDROME

Mucocutaneous pigmentation appears in childhood as brown-black or blue-black freckles around the mouth, on the buccal mucosa, and on the hands. Intestinal polyps characteristically develop in the jejunum, but also in other parts of the gastrointestinal tract. Malignant change is rare, but extra-intestinal tumours have been reported in the ovaries, breasts, urinary tract, bronchus and nose.

Genetic aspects: Autosomal dominant.

References

Burdick D, Prior JT (1982). Peutz–Jeghers syndrome: clinicopathologic study of a large family with a 27-year follow-up. *Cancer* **50**:2139–2146.

Chen KTK (1986). Female genital tract tumors in Peutz–Jeghers syndrome. *Hum Pathol* **17**:858–861.

Dorfman S, Talbot IC, Cardozo J et al. (1991). The Peutz-Jeghers syndrome: case reports. *Invest Clinica* **32**:59–65.

Foley TR, Mcgarrity TJ, Abt AB (1988). Peutz–Jeghers syndrome: a clinicopathologic survey of the "Harrisburg family" with a 49-year follow-up. *Gastroenterology* **95**:1535–1540.

Giardiello FM, Welsh SB, Hamilton SR et al. (1987). Increased risk of cancer in the Peutz–Jeghers syndrome. *New Engl J Med* **316**:1151–1154.

Laughlin EH (1991). Benign and malignant neoplasms in a family with Peutz–Jeghers syndrome: study of three generations. *South Med J* **84**:1205–1209.

Spigelman AD, Murday V, Phillips RKS (1989). Cancer and the Peutz–Jeghers syndrome. *Gut* **30**:1588–1590.

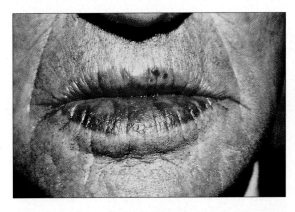

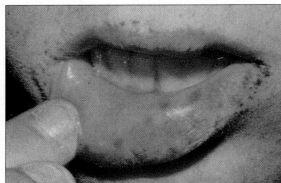

249A and 249B Note the macular pigmentation around the lips.

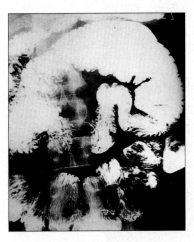

249C There are multiple small bowel polyps.

TUBEROUS SCLEROSIS

The first abnormal skin lesion might be a depigmented macule or a tuft of white hair. The characteristic warty macules ('adenoma sebaceum') appear in childhood. These are angiofibromas. They occur around the nasolabial folds and butterfly region around the nose, but are said to spare the upper lip. Shagreen patches may be seen, especially in the lumbosacral region. These are raised plaques of thickened slightly pigmented skin. Skin tags around the neck and café au lait spots may also be present. A search should be made for gingival fibromas, pits in the enamel of the teeth, periungual fibromas and ocular phakomata. Hypopigmented macules and facial angiomas occur in up to 90% of cases, shagreen patches in 20–40%, ungual fibromas in up to 50%, subependymal nodules on CT scan in 90% with cortical lesions in 50%, renal angiolipomas in 60%, renal cysts in 20%, radiological abnormalities of the bones (sclerotic patches, pseudocysts, periosteal new bone formation) in 60%, poliosis in 20%, gum fibromas in 10%, and dental pits in 70%. Cardiac rhabdomyomata are said to be characteristic of the condition. It has been suggested that at least 50% of infants with a cardiac rhabdomyoma have TS, but this is likely to be a considerable underestimate. Renal cysts can occur and can manifest before the other features of the condition, and mimic autosomal dominant polycystic kidney disease. Seizures occur in 60% of cases and mental retardation in about 40%. The condition has a prevalence of about 1 in 30 000–50 000, but may account for about 0.5% of cases of significant mental retardation.

Genetic aspects: Recurrence risks to normal parents of an isolated case are less than 5%, but not negligible.

There is evidence that mutations at more than one locus can give rise to the condition. In 30–50% of families the gene maps to 9q34 and the remainder of families may map to 16p.

References

Fryer AE, Chalmers AH, Osborne JP (1990). The value of investigation for genetic counselling in tuberous sclerosis. *J Med Genet* **27**:217–223.

Harris RM, Carter NP, Griffiths B *et al.* (1993). Physical mapping within the tuberous sclerosis linkage group in region 9q32-q34. *Genomics* **15**:265–274.

Kandt RS, Haines JL, Smith M *et al.* (1992). Linkage of an important gene locus for tuberous sclerosis to a chromosome 16 marker for polycystic kidney disease. *Nature Genetics* **2**:37–41.

Webb DW, Thomas RD, Osborne JP (1992). Echocardiography and genetic counselling in tuberous sclerosis. *J Med Genet* **29**:487–489.

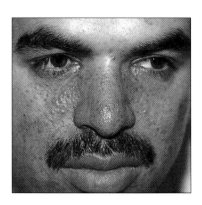
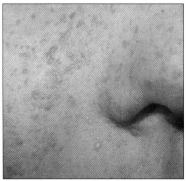
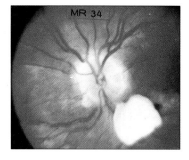

250A and 250B Note the adenoma sebaceum in a butterfly distribution around the nose.

250C Note the retinal phakoma inferior to the disc.

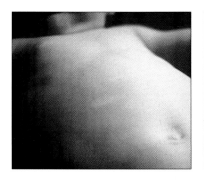
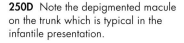
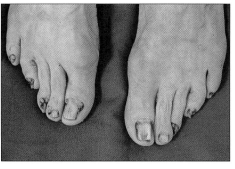
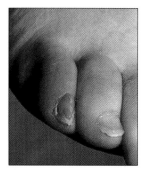

250D Note the depigmented macule on the trunk which is typical in the infantile presentation.

250E and 250F Note the periungual fibromas.

250F

GIANT PIGMENTED HAIRY NEVUS SYNDROME

A giant pigmented hairy nevus is usually situated on the trunk. The lesions are slightly raised, darkly pigmented and hairy. Some cases have concomitant leptomeningeal melanosis and an occipital nevus is said to be a pointer to this complication. In 2–13% of cases the skin nevi become malignant, 50% before the age of five years (Kaplan).

Genetic aspects: Most cases are sporadic.

References

Kaplan EN (1974). The risk of malignancy in large congenital nevi. *Plast Reconstr Surg* **53**:421–428.

Ruiz-Maldonado R, Tamayo L, Laterza AM, Duran C (1992). Giant pigmented nevi: clinical, histopathologic, and therapeutic considerations. *J Pediatr* **120**:906–911.

Salisbury JR, Rose PE (1989). Primary central nervous malignant melanoma in the bathing trunk naevus syndrome. *Postgrad Med J* **65**:387–389.

Voigtlander V, Jung EG (1974). Giant pigmented hairy nevus in two siblings. *Humangenetik* **24**:79–84.

Zack LD, Stegmeier O, Solomon LM (1988). Pigmentary regression in a giant nevocellular nevus: a case report and a review of the subject. *Pediatr Dermatol* **5**:178–183.

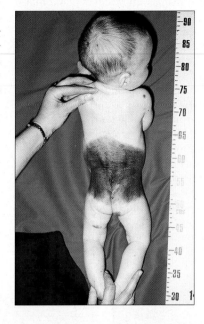

251 Note the giant pigmented hairy nevus.

NEUROCUTANEOUS MELANOSIS

252A–252B

Neurocutaneous melanosis is a form of phakomatosis in which there is a proliferation of melanocytes in skin and meninges. The most common skin lesion is a giant pigmented hairy naevus, but diffuse pigmentation can also occur. Infiltration of the pia and arachnoid by melanocytes can usually be seen macroscopically. It has been estimated that there is a 2–13% risk of malignant change in skin and a 50% risk of malignant change in the meninges. Neurological abnormalities include hydrocephalus (thought to be secondary to obstruction at the fourth ventricle foramina or the basal cisterns), epilepsy, intracranial haemorrhage, cranial nerve palsies and psychiatric disturbance.

Genetic aspects: Most cases are sporadic.

References

Findler G, Hoffman HJ, Thomson HG *et al.* (1981). Giant nevus of the scalp associated with intracranial pigmentation. *J Neurosurg* **54**:108–112.

Kadonaga JN, Barkovich AJ, Edwards MSB, Frieden IJ (1992). Neurocutaneous melanosis in association with the Dandy–Walker complex. *Pediatr Dermatol* **9**:37–43.

Leaney BJ, Rowe PW, Klug GL (1985). Neurocutaneous melanosis with hydrocephalus and syringomyelia. Case report. *J Neurosurg* 148–152.

Reed WB, Becker SW *et al.* (1965). Giant pigmented nevi, melanoma and leptomeningeal melanocytosis. *Arch Dermatol* **91**:100–119.

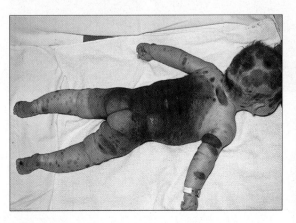

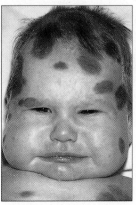

252A and 252B Note the large bathing-trunk naevus with small lesions elsewhere, especially over the scalp.

HYPERTRICHOSIS-GINGIVAL FIBROMATOSIS 253A–253C

This might well be a heterogeneous group of conditions. Those with seizures could be different from cases without neurological abnormalities. Hirsutism begins at or soon after birth. The gum hypertrophy occurs later and intelligence is usually normal. Occasionally, mental retardation is a feature. There is a suggestion that the hypertrichosis in those situations in which epilepsy and oligophrenia are present is not as severe as in cases with no neurological abnormalities (Witkop). The differential diagnosis includes forms of mucopolysaccharidosis and mucolipidosis (in the early stages) and Zimmermann–Laband syndrome in which there is nail dysplasia.

Genetic aspects: Both recessive and dominant families have been reported. Gingival fibromatosis can also occur on its own, segregating as an autosomal dominant or recessive condition – see Takagi *et al.* for a good review.

References

Anderson J, Cunliffe WJ *et al.* (1969). Hereditary gingival fibromatosis. *Br Med J* **3**:218–219.

Horning GM, Fisher JG, Barker BF *et al.* (1985). Gingival fibromatosis with hypertrichosis: a case report. *J Periodontol* **56**:344–347.

Jorgenson RJ (1971). Gingival fibromatosis. *BDOAS* **7(7)**:278–280.

Takagi M, Yamamoto H, Mega H *et al.* (1991). Heterogeneity in the gingival fibromatoses. *Cancer* **68**:2202–2212.

Vontobel F (1973). Idiopathic gingival hyperplasia and hypertrichosis associated with acromegaloid features. *Helv Paediatr Acta* **28**:401–411.

Witkop CJ (1971). Heterogeneity in gingival fibromatosis. *BDOAS* **7(7)**:210.

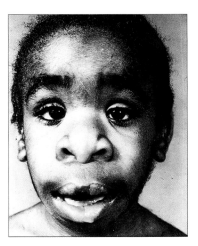
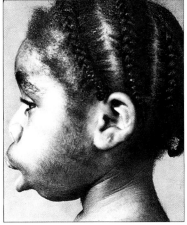
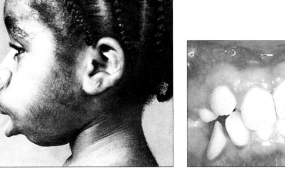

253A and 253B Note the hairiness and the distortion of lower face due to the gum hypertrophy.

253C Note gum hypertrophy.

HYPERTRICHOSIS UNIVERSALIS CONGENITA 254A–254B

In this condition the hair gradually lengthens and covers the whole body, except for the palms and soles, labia minora, the prepuce and the glans of the penis. Intelligence is normal. The condition is also called hypertrichosis lanuginosa universalis and edentate hypertrichosis.

Genetic aspects: Autosomal dominant pedigrees have been described.

References

Beighton P (1970). Congenital hypertrichosis lanuginosa. *Arch Dermatol* **101**:669–672.

Felgenhauer WR (1969). Hypertrichosis lanuginosa universalis. *J Genet Hum* **17**:1–44.

Freire-Maia N, Felizali J *et al.* (1976). Hypertrichosis lanuginosa in a mother and son. *Clin Genet* **10**:303–306.

Partridge JW (1987). Congenital hypertrichosis lanuginosa: neonatal shaving. *Arch Dis Child* **62**:623–625.

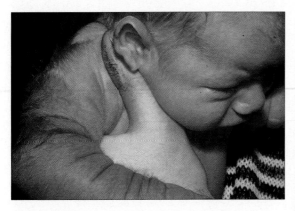

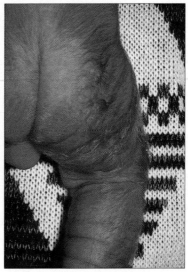

254A and 254B Note the excessive hair over the whole body, especially the arms and legs.

HYPOMELANOSIS OF ITO   255A–255C

The cutaneous lesions consist of linear areas of depigmentation or hyperpigmentation over the trunk and limbs following the lines of Blaschko. The lesions also appear as whorls. The most serious consequence of this condition is mental retardation and/or seizures. Eye abnormalities are not infrequent and include microphthalmia and other structural abnormalities. A CT brain scan might show cerebral atrophy, sometimes involving the whole side of one hemisphere. Many other abnormalities have been reported, and this reflects the probability that the condition is heterogeneous (see below).

Genetic aspects: Most cases are sporadic and it is now apparent that many of these cases are in fact mosaic for different types of chromosome aberration. A large variety of different abnormalities have been recorded. Skin biopsy might be needed to demonstrate mosaicism.

References
Donnai D, Read AP, McKeown C, Andrews T (1988). Hypomelanosis of Ito: a manifestation of mosaicism or chimerism. *J Med Genet* **25**:809–818.

Flannery DB (1990). Invited editorial comment: pigmentary dysplasias, hypomelanosis of Ito, and genetic mosaicism. *Am J Med Genet* **35**:18–21.

Glover MT, Brett EM, Atherton DJ (1989). Hypomelanosis of Ito: spectrum of the disease. *J Pediatr* **115**:75–80.

Pascual-Castroviejo I *et al.* (1988). Hypomelanosis of Ito. Neurological complications in 34 cases. *Can J Neurol Sci* **15**:124–129.

Ruiz-Maldonado R, Toussaint S, Tamayo L *et al.* (1992). Hypomelanosis of Ito: diagnostic criteria and report of 41 cases. *Pediatr Dermatol* **9**:1–10.

Sybert VP (1990). Hypomelanosis of Ito (Commentary). *Pediatr Dermatol* **7**:74–76.

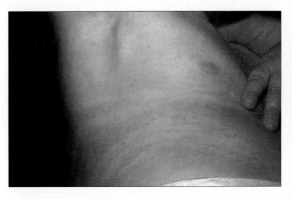

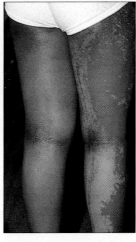

255B

255A–255C Note the linear depigmented areas with hyperpigmentation along side, distributed along Blaschko's lines.

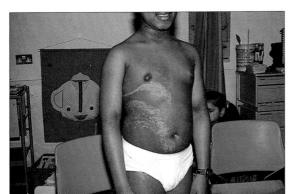

255C

PIEBALDISM
256

Isolated piebaldism can be inherited as an autosomal dominant condition. There are widespread patches of depigmentation which can involve the scalp hair.
Genetic aspects: Autosomal dominant. Mutations have been demonstrated in the c-kit proto-oncogene on 4q. This gene encodes the cellular tyrosine kinase receptor for the mast/stem cell growth factor.

References

Giebel LB, Spritz RA (1991). Mutation of the c-kit (mast/stem cell growth factor receptor) proto-oncogene in human piebaldism. *Proc Nat Acad Sci* **88**:8696–8699.
Spritz RA, Droetto S, Fukushima Y (1992). Deletion of the KIT and PDGFRA genes in a patient with piebaldism. *Am J Med Genet* **44**:492–495.
Winship I, Young K, Martell R *et al.* (1991). Piebaldism: an autonomous autosomal dominant entity. *Clin Genet* **39**:330–337.

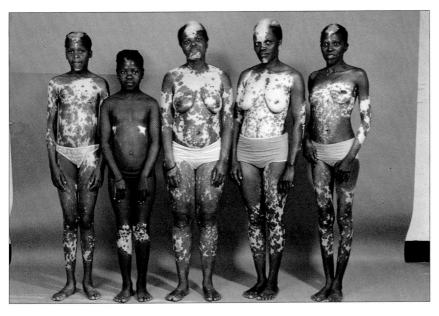

256 Note the patchy skin depigmentation.

WAARDENBURG SYNDROME
257A–257C

There is usually a white forelock, sometimes with more extensive depigmentation of the skin, sensorineural deafness, dystopia canthorum (an increased distance between the inner canthi), heterochromia of the irides, synophrys and a high nasal bridge. Premature greying of the hair, true hyper-telorism, cleft lip and palate, Hirschsprung's disease and congenital heart defects are rarer manifestations. The condition is divided into two main types. In type I there is dystopia canthorum and 25% of patients have deafness; in type II there is no dystopia canthorum and 50% of patients have deafness.

Genetic aspects: Type I has been localised to 2q37. Tassabehji *et al.* (1993) demonstrated mutations in the HuP2 gene (the homologue of mouse Pax-3) in type I cases. The gene for type II Waardenburg syndrome maps to 3p12-p14. Tassabehji *et al.* (1994) demonstrated mutations in the human homologue (MITF) of the mouse mi (microphthalmia) gene. There may be a more severe autosomal recessive type associated with Hirschsprung disease.

References

Badner JA, Chakravarti A (1990). Waardenburg syndrome and Hirschsprung disease: evidence for pleiotropic effects of a single dominant gene. *Am J Med Genet* **35**:100–104.

Tassabehji M, Read AP, Newton VE et al. (1993) Mutations in the PAX3 gene causing Waardenburg syndrome type 1 and type 2. *Nature Genetics* **3**:26–30.

Tassabehji M, Newton VE, Read AP (1994). Waardenburg syndrome type 2 caused by mutations in the human microphthalmia (MITF) gene. *Nature Genetics* **8**:251–255.

da-Silva EO (1991). Waardenburg I syndrome: a clinical and genetic study of two large Brazilian kindreds, and literature review. *Am J Med Genet* **40**:65–74.

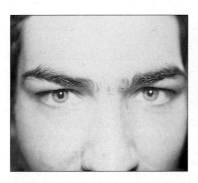 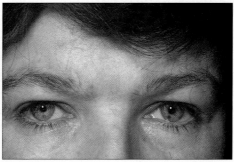 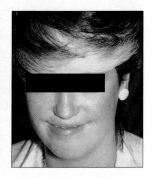

257A and 257B Note the heterochromia of the irises, synophyrs and the dystopia canthorum.

257C Note white forelock.

INCONTINENTIA PIGMENTI   258A–258D

Between birth and 6 weeks of age a linear vesicular eruption appears on the trunk, followed within weeks by a warty (verrucous) eruption which might persist up to the age of 1 year. The classical lesions of whorled hyperpigmentation evolve after this; they may fade in adulthood leaving faintly depigmented atrophic streaks, especially on the legs. It should be noted that some patients have had a recurrence of the vesicles up to 6 years of age. About 40% of cases have eye complications including strabismus, astigmatism, retinal vascular abnormalities, pseudoglioma and retinal detachment. Peg-shaped teeth and hypodontia are common. Some patients have partial alopecia and breast aplasia. The most serious complication is mental retardation, which may occur in no higher than 10% overall of cases, especially in familial cases. 3% of cases are severely retarded (Landy and Donnai). Neonatal seizures are a poor prognostic sign.

Genetic aspects: Many cases are females and inheritance is X-linked dominant. Most affected males are thought to die *in utero*. The mother's skin and teeth should be carefully examined for signs of the disorder and a careful history taken for evidence of neonatal vesicular eruptions.

There may be two loci on the X-chromosome for this disorder. Affected females with X-autosome translocations have been reported where the breakpoint is at Xp11. However, linkage studies locate the gene at Xq28.

References

Carney RG (1976). Incontinentia pigmenti: a world statistical analysis. *Arch Dermatol* **112**:535–542.

Catalano RA (1990). Incontinentia pigmenti. *Am J Ophthalmol* **110**:696–700.

Damstra RJ, Van Duren JA, Van Ginkel CWJ (1991). Incontinentia pigmenti (Bloch–Sulzberger). *Br J Dermatol* **125**:280–281.

Landy SJ, Donnai D (1993). Syndrome of the month. Incontinentia pigmenti (Bloch–Sulzberger syndrome). *J Med Genet* **30**:53–59.

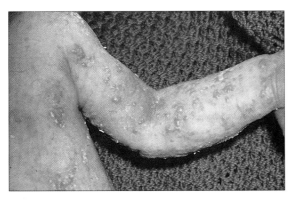

258A Note bullae in the acute phase.

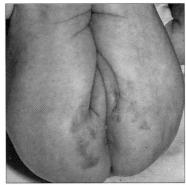

258B The bullae begin to regress after a few weeks.

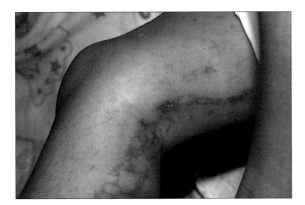

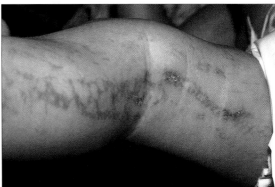

258C and 258D The characteristic linear pigmented lesions develop in infancy.

GOLTZ (FOCAL DERMAL HYPOPLASIA)

259A–259C

The skin lesions are often bilateral but asymmetrical and initially red in colour, patchy and of different shapes and sizes. Papillomas develop around the lips, gums or the side of the nose. Later, fat might herniate through the areas of atrophy. In addition there are often areas of linear or reticular hyper- or hypopigmentation. Scalp hair may be sparse and the nails are frequently dysplastic. Limb defects include syndactyly, polydactyly, or missing fingers or part of a limb. The eyes are also frequently affected, mostly asymmetrically, with chorioretinal or iris colobomata, and microphthalmos or anophthalmos. Microcephaly and mental retardation are frequent.

Genetic aspects: Most cases are female and inheritance is thought to be X-linked dominant with early intrauterine lethality in males.

References

Goltz RW (1990). Focal dermal hypoplasia (Editorial). *Pediatr Dermatol* **7**:313–314.

Goltz RW (1992). Focal dermal hypoplasia syndrome. An update (Editorial comment). *Arch Dermatol* **128**:1108–1111.

Gorski JL (1991). Father-to-daughter transmission of focal dermal hypoplasia associated with nonrandom X-inactivation: support for X-linked inheritance and paternal X chromosome mosaicism. *Am J Med Genet* **40**:332–337.

Marcus DM, Shore JW, Albert DM (1990). Anophthalmia in the focal dermal hypoplasia syndrome. *Arch Ophthalmol* **108**:96–100.

Temple IK, MacDowall P, Baraitser M, Atherton DJ (1990). Syndrome of the month. Focal dermal hypoplasia (Goltz syndrome). *J Med Genet* **27**:180–187.

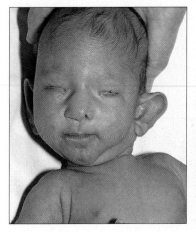

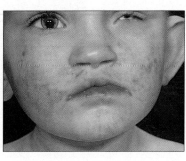

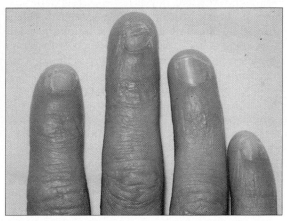

259A and 259B Note the malformed ears, atrophic skin lesions on the face and terminal transverse limb defects. There is microphthalmia and an iris coloboma in **259B**.

259C There is a terminal limb deficiency with fat herniation through areas of skin atrophy.

DYSKERATOSIS CONGENITA

260A–260B

Leucoplakia of mucous membranes, especially the oral mucosa, appears in childhood and similar involvement may be found around the anogenital areas and in the GI tract. The skin manifestations appear around puberty and consist of reticulate hyperpigmentation, usually raindrop in appearance, occurring over the neck, trunk and sometimes the face. Palmoplantar hyperkeratosis, nail dystrophy and sparseness of hair might be other features. On occasions the pigmentation is more generalised. Other features include obliteration of the lacrimal duct, dental problems, dysphagia and premature greying of the hair. The prognosis is poor because of the tendency to develop malignancies, blood dyscrasias (pancytopenia, aplastic anaemia), and carcinoma in the area of the leukoplakia.

Genetic aspects: X-linked recessive. The gene has been assigned to Xq28. Females with the full-blown picture have been described and there is a suggestion that an autosomal recessive type exists.

References
Connor JM, Gatherer D, Gray FC et al. (1986). Assignment of the gene for dyskeratosis congenita to Xq28. *Hum Genet* **72**:348–351.

Connor JM, Teaguf RH (1981). Dyskeratosis congenita: report of a large kindred. *Br J Dermatol* **105**:321–325.

Drachtman RA, Alter BP (1992). Dyskeratosis congenita: clinical and genetic heterogeneity: report of a new case and review of the literature. *Am J Ped Hemat Oncol* **14**:297–304.

Pai GS, Morgan S, Whetsell C (1989). Etiologic heterogeneity in dyskeratosis congenita. *Am J Med Genet* **32**:63–66.

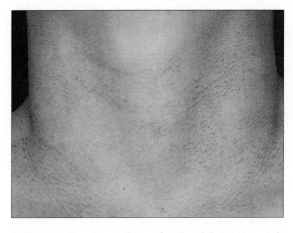

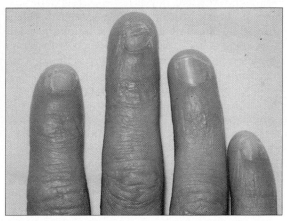

260A Note hyperpigmentation of neck with hypopigmented areas giving a reticular pattern ('rain-drop pigmentation').

260B Note nail dystrophy.

HARLEQUIN BABY

This is the severe form of ichthyosiform erythroderma. In the newborn period affected infants are small and covered with a thick horny skin separated into plaques by ulcerating fissures. Although initially white, the skin becomes grey-yellow. The hands and feet are puffy and the open mouth is 'O'-shaped. Because of the pronounced ectropion, the eyes appear bulbous and staring, and the ears and nose appear to be naked holes. Many cases die in the neonatal period but long-term survival has been reported.

Genetic aspects: Autosomal recessive.

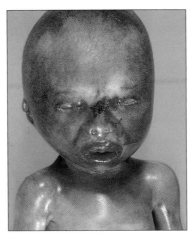

261 Note the thick horny skin and the O-shaped open mouth.

References
Dale BA, Holbrook KA, Fleckman P *et al.* (1990). Heterogeneity in harlequin ichthyosis, an inborn error of epidermal keratinization: variable morphology and structural protein expression and a defect in lamellar granules. *J Invest Dermatol* **94**:6–18.

Lawlor F (1988). Progress of a harlequin fetus to nonbullous ichthyosiform erythroderma. *Pediatrics* **82**:870–873.

Lawlor F, Peiris S (1985). Harlequin fetus successfully treated with etretinate. *Br J Dermatol* **112**:585–590.

Meizner I (1992). Prenatal ultrasonic features in a rare case of congenital ichthyosis (harlequin fetus). *J Clin Ultrasound* **20**:132–134.

Suzumori K, Kanzaki T (1991). Prenatal diagnosis of harlequin ichthyosis by fetal skin biopsy) report of two cases. *Prenatal Diagn* **11**:451–457.

Unamuno P, Pierola JM, Fernandez E *et al.* (1987). Harlequin foetus in four siblings. *Br J Dermatol* **116**:569–572.

ECTODERMAL DYSPLASIA – X-LINKED HYPOHIDROTIC TYPE

This is the commonest of the ectodermal dysplasias. Affected males have sparse scalp hair, eyebrows and eyelashes, and no body hair. They do not sweat and often present in infancy with high fevers. Most teeth are missing and those that do appear are conical in shape. There is often pigmentation and dryness of skin around the eyes and most males have a prominent forehead, a saddle nose, prominent lips and a hoarse voice. Both lacrimation and salivary secretions can be reduced. Intelligence is usually normal, but mild developmental delay can occur.

Genetic aspects: X-linked. The gene has been mapped to Xq12-13 (Zonana *et al.*, 1992). Female carriers can show minor signs of the condition which can be useful for carrier detection. These include sparse hair, missing or abnormally shaped teeth and abnormal sweating patterns, indicating mosaicism for expression of the abnormal gene.

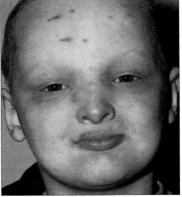

262A and 262B Note the sparse hair and redness around the eyes. The lips are prominent and the scratch marks relate to the dryness of the skin.

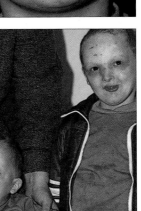

References
Clarke A. (1987) Hypohidrotic ectodermal dysplasia. *J Med Genet* **24**:659–663.

Cunniff C (1990). Hypohidrotic ectodermal dysplasia. *Pediatr Dermatol* **7**:235–236.

Zonana J, Jones M, Browne D *et al.* (1992). High-resolution mapping of the X-linked hypohidrotic ectodermal dysplasia (EDA) locus. *Am J Hum Genet* **51**:1036–1046.

Zonana J, Schinzel A, Upadhyaya M *et al.* (1990). Prenatal diagnosis of X-linked hypohidrotic ectodermal dysplasia by linkage analysis. *Am J Med Genet* **35**:132–135.

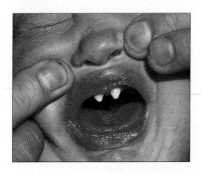

262C Note conically shaped teeth.

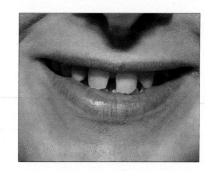

262D Mother of the last child is a carrier by virtue of her hypodontia and abnormally shaped teeth.

RAPP–HODGKIN ECTODERMAL DYSPLASIA   263A–263B

The main features are hypohidrosis, thin wiry hair, absent or sparse eyelashes and eyebrows, absent secondary sexual hair, oligodontia, dystrophic nails and cleft lip and palate. The hair abnormality is pili torti. **Genetic aspects**: Autosomal dominant.

References

Breslau-Siderius EJ, Lavrijsen APM, Otten FWA *et al.* (1991). The Rapp–Hodgkin syndrome. *Am J Med Genet* **38**:107–110.

O'Donnell BP, James WD (1992). Rapp–Hodgkin ectodermal dysplasia. *J Am Acad Dermatol* **27**:323–326.

Rodini EOS, Freitas JAS, Richieri-Costa A (1990). Rapp–Hodgkin syndrome: report of a Brazilian family. *Am J Med Genet* **36**:463–466.

Schroeder HW, Sybert VP (1987). Rapp–Hodgkin ectodermal dysplasia. *J Pediatr* **110**:72–75.

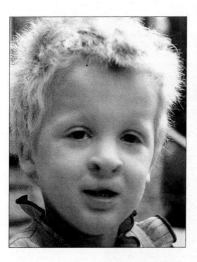
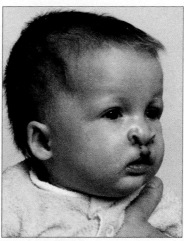

263A and 263B Note the sparse, depigmented hair and the repaired cleft lip and palate.

HAY–WELLS SYNDROME   264A–264D

This condition is also called the ankyloblepharon-ectodermal dysplasia-clefting syndrome, or the AEC syndrome. The ankyloblepharon filiforme adnatum consists of strands bridging the eyelids, made up of a central core of vascular connective tissue surrounded by epithelium. Cleft lip and palate are common. The hair might be totally absent, or sparse and wiry, and the nails absent or dystrophic. The teeth can be pointed and widely spaced, and anhidrosis is usually partial. The condition must be differentiated from Rapp–Hodgkin syndrome, in which clefting also occurs, but not the eyelid fusion.

Genetic aspects: In the original report (Hays and Wells) there were seven patients from four families with clear-cut autosomal dominant transmission.

References

Greene SL, Michels VV, Doyle JA (1987). Variable expression in ankyloblepharon-ectodermal defects-cleft lip and palate syndrome. *Am J Med Genet* **27**:207–212.

Hay RJ, Wells RS (1976). The syndrome of ankyloblepharon, ectodermal defects, and cleft lip and palate. *Br J Dermatol* **94**:277–289.

Shwayder TA, Lane AT, Miller ME (1986). Hay–Wells syndrome. *Pediatr Dermatol* **3**:399–402.

Spiegel J, Colton A (1985). AEC syndrome: ankyloblepharon, ecto-

dermal defects, and cleft lip and palate. Report of two cases. *J Am Acad Dermatol* **12**:810–815.

Weiss AH, Riscile G, Kousseff BG (1992). Ankyloblepharon filiforme adnatum. *Am J Med Genet* **42**:369–373.

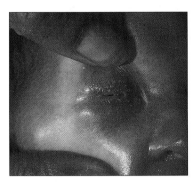

264A–264D
Note the eyelid adhesions and sparse eyelashes. Some nails are absent and some are dystrophic.

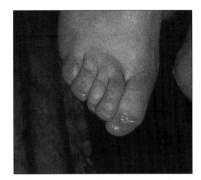

264B

264C

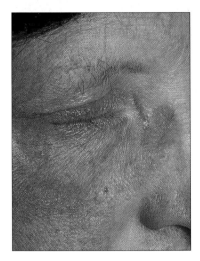

264D

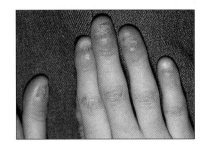

ECTRODACTYLY-ECTODERMAL DYSPLASIA-CLEFTING (EEC)   265A–265F

Limb defects and facial clefting are associated with features of ectodermal dysplasia. The characteristic limb abnormality is a cleft hand or foot, but oligodactyly and syndactyly can also occur. The hair is sparse, fair and dry and the eyebrows and lashes are often absent. Hypohidrosis is variable, although the skin is often dry and hyperkeratosis of palms and feet might occur. The teeth are small and may be partially formed, and hypodontia and anodontia occur. The nails are thin, brittle and ridged, and tear duct abnormalities are common. Urogenital anomalies include megaureter, vesicoureteric reflux, hydronephrosis and hypospadias. Mental development is usually normal.

Genetic aspects: Autosomal dominant. This is a very variable syndrome and care must be taken in examining and counselling parents of an apparently isolated case.

References

Anneren G, Andersson T, Lindgren PG, Kjartansson S (1991). Ectrodactyly-ectodermal dysplasia-clefting syndrome (EEC): the clinical variation and prenatal diagnosis. *Clin Genet* **40**:257–262.

Hasegawa T, Hasegawa Y, Asamura S *et al.* (1991). EEC syndrome (ectrodactyly, ectodermal dysplasia and cleft lip/palate) with a balanced reciprocal translocation between 7q11.21 and 9p12 (or 7p11.2 and 9q12) in three generations. *Clin Genet* **40**:202–206.

McNab AA, Potts MJ, Welham RAN (1989). The EEC syndrome and its ocular manifestations. *Br J Ophthalmol* **73**:261–264.

Nardi AC, Ferreira U, Netto NR Jr *et al.* (1992). Urinary tract involvement in EEC syndrome: a clinical study in 25 Brazilian patients. *Am J Med Genet* **44**:803–806.

Rodini ESO, Richieri-Costa A (1990). EEC syndrome: report on 20 new patients, clinical and genetic considerations. *Am J Med Genet* **37**:42–53.

Tse K, Temple IK, Baraitser M (1990). Dilemmas in counselling: the EEC syndrome. *J Med Genet* **27**:752–755.

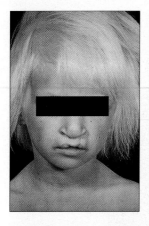
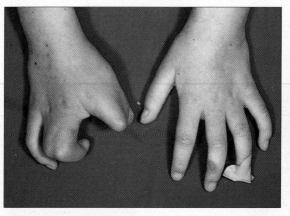
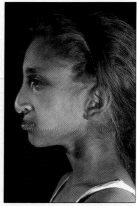

265A–265D Note repaired cleft lip, sparse, dry hair and split hand with partial syndactyly.　　**265C**

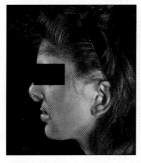
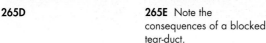
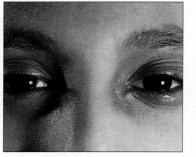
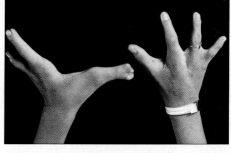

265D

265E Note the consequences of a blocked tear-duct.

265F Note split hands.

EHLERS–DANLOS SYNDROME　　　　　　　　　266A–266G

There are several different clinical and biochemical sub-types:

- EDS I Skin hyperextensible, soft, easily bruised, dystrophic scarring.
- EDS II The same as type I, but milder.
- EDS III Mostly joint hypermobility. Skin stretchy. This is a relatively benign condition.
- EDS IV Severe bruising. Thin skin, prominent veins, vascular rupture and features of premature ageing.
- EDS V X-linked. Cardinal features in a moderate degree.
- EDS VI Eye involvement. Perforation and retinal detachment. Scoliosis.
- EDS VII Dermatosparaxis/arthrochalasis multiplex congenita. The skin is extremely fragile and tears easily.
- EDS VIII Periodontitis type.
- EDS IX (former) Now Occipital horn syndrome.
- EDS X Fibronectin abnormality. Petechiae.

References

Beighton P, Curtis D (1985). X-linked Ehlers–Danlos syndrome type V: the next generation. *Clin Genet* **27**:472–478.

Beighton P, De Paepe A, Danks D et al. (1988). International nosology of heritable disorders of connective tissue, Berlin, 1986. *Am J Med Genet* **29**:581–594.

Beighton P, De Paepe A, Hall JG et al. (1992). Molecular nosology of heritable disorders of connective tissue. *Am J Med Genet* **42**:431–448.

Hogan PA, Krafchik BR (1991). Ehlers–Danlos syndrome. *Pediatr Dermatol* **8**:348–351.

Maroteaux P, Frezal J, Cohen-Solal L (1986). The differential symptomatology of errors of collagen metabolism: a tentative classification. *Am J Med Genet* **24**:219–230.

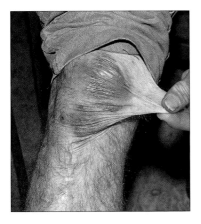 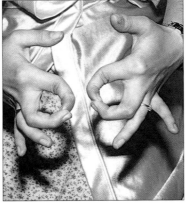 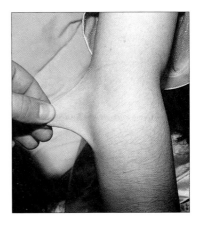

266A–266C Note tissue-paper scars, skin hyperelasticity and joint laxity.　　**266C**

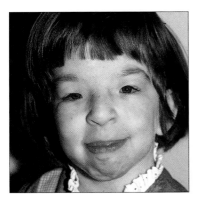

266D–266G This child has Ehlers–Danlos type VII, also called dermatosparaxis, in which the skin is not only lax but fragile and easily torn. Note the premature aged look in **266E** and **266F**.

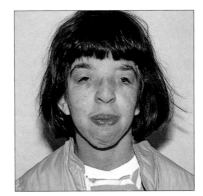

266E

266F

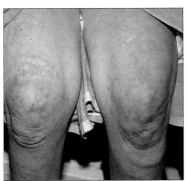 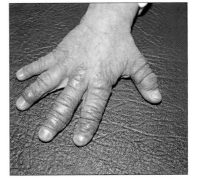

266G

CUTIS LAXA

267A–267B

This entry refers to isolated cutis laxa. The skin is redundant, especially over the dorsum of the hands and feet, and on the face it tends to hang down in folds, causing a prematurely aged appearance. The skin is usually loose but not hyperextensible and is not fragile.

Genetic aspects: Both autosomal dominant and recessive forms of cutis laxa exist (Beighton). Some recessive forms have complications such as bronchomegaly, emphysema and other respiratory problems, dislocated hips and mental retardation (see Gorlin and Cohen for a review).

References
Beighton P (1972). The dominant and recessive forms of cutis laxa. *J Med Genet* **9**:216–221.

Brown FR III, Holbrook KA *et al.* (1982). Cutis laxa. *Johns Hopkins Med J* **150**:148–153.

Damkier A, Brandrup F, Starklint H (1991). Cutis laxa: autosomal dominant inheritance in five generations. *Clin Genet* **39**:321–329.

Fitzsimmons JS, Fitzsimmons EM *et al.* (1985). Variable clinical presentation of cutis laxa. *Clin Genet* **28**:284–295.

Gorlin RJ, Cohen MM Jr (1989). Craniofacial manifestations of Ehlers–Danlos syndromes, cutis laxa syndromes, and cutis laxa-like syndromes. *BDOAS* **25(4)**:39–71.

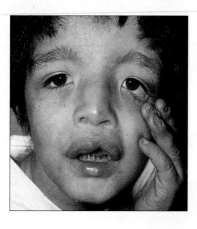

267A Note loose skin, giving an aged appearance.

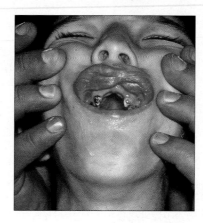

267B The loose skin includes soft tissues inside the mouth.

INFANTILE SYSTEMIC HYALINOSIS

268A–268C

During the first weeks of life affected infants seem to cry with pain when they are moved, and by the age of 2 months flexion contractures develop in the arms and legs. The skin appears thick, especially over the hands, with redness at the creases. The fingers become thickened and there is pigmentation over the knuckles. The gums are hypertrophied and nodules develop on the lips and ears. Pathological examination by EM shows distension of the endoplasmic reticulum and mitochondrial changes. Hyaline deposits are seen in the intestinal wall, the thymus, and to a lesser extent elsewhere. Landing *et al.* described the pathological changes in four infants. Glover *et al.* provide a good review of the literature.

Genetic aspects: Autosomal recessive.

References

Alfi OS, Heuser ET, Landing BH *et al.* (1975). A syndrome of systemic hyalinosis, short-limbed dwarfism and possible thymic dysplasia. *BDOAS* **11(5)**:57–62.

Glover MT, Lake BD, Atherton DJ (1991). Infantile systemic hyalinosis: newly recognized disorder of collagen? *Pediatrics* **87**:228–234.

Glover MT, Lake BD, Atherton DJ (1992). Clinical, histologic, and ultrastructural findings in two cases of infantile systemic hyalinosis. *Pediatr Dermatol* **9**:255–258.

Landing BH, Nadorra R (1986). Infantile systemic hyalinosis: report of four cases of a disease, fatal in infancy, apparently different from juvenile systemic hyalinosis. *Pediatr Pathol* **6**:55–79.

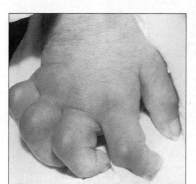

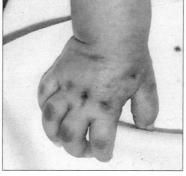

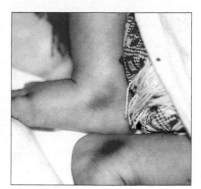

268A Note stiff, swollen, painful fingers.

268B and 268C Dark pigmentation develops over the expanded knuckles and ankle.

SHABBIR – LARYNGO-ONYCHO-CUTANEOUS SYNDROME 269A–269C

The disease starts in infancy with hoarseness of the voice, followed by dystrophic changes of the nails and ulcers of the skin. The skin lesions occur commonly on the face, particularly around the nose and mouth. Although they involve mucocutaneous junctions they do not involve mucous membranes. The limbs, trunk and genitalia are also involved. The nail abnormalities start as a white speck at the end of the nail, followed by thickening, discolouration and loss of the nail. The teeth are notched.

Genetic aspects: Autosomal recessive.

References
Ainsworth JR, Shabbir G, Spencer AF, Cockburn F (1992). Multisystem disorder of Punjabi children exhibiting spontaneous dermal and submucosal granulation tissue formation: LOGIC syndrome. *Clin Dysmorphol* **1**:3–14.
Shabbir G, Hassan M, Kazmi A (1986). Laryngo-onycho-cutaneous syndrome – a study of 22 cases. A new syndrome. *Biomedica* **2**:15–25.

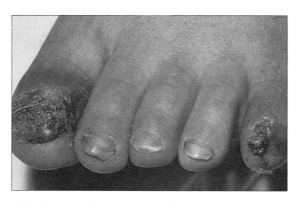

269A Note the ulceration around the nail.

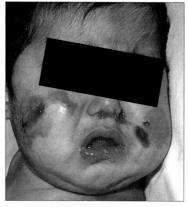

269B Similar ulcerations on the cheeks and lips.

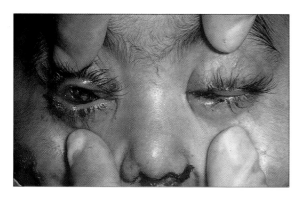

269C Note ulceration of the conjunctiva and lids.

ROTHMUND–THOMSON SYNDROME (POIKILODERMA CONGENITA) 270A–270B

Skin abnormalities appear before 6 months of age with reticular or diffuse erythema on the face, hands and extensor surfaces of the limbs. The trunk is relatively spared. Photosensitivity may manifest with bullae. Older children have dermal atrophy, telangiectasia, patchy increased pigmentation or depigmentation of the skin, hyperkeratosis and scaling. There is also alopecia, photosensitivity, dystrophic nails, abnormal teeth, cataracts, short stature and hypogonadism. The hands may be short and stubby and absent thumbs occur in about 5% of cases.

Genetic aspects: Autosomal recessive.

References
Anonymous (1990). Rothmund–Thomson syndrome. *Pediatr Radiol* **20**:216–217.
Houwing RH, Oosterkamp RF, Berghuis M et al. (1991). Rothmund–Thomson syndrome. *Br J Dermatol* **125**:279–280.
Moss C (1990). Rothmund-Thomson syndrome: a report of two patients and a review of the literature. *Br J Dermatol* **122**:821–829.
Vennos EM, Collins M, James WD (1992). Rothmund-Thomson syndrome: review of the world literature. *J Am Acad Dermatol* **27**:750–762.

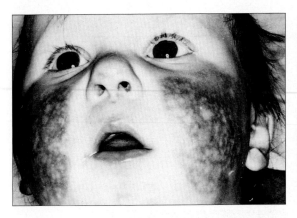

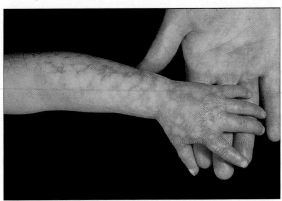

270A Note the telangiectasia and patchy dermal atrophy.

270B Note the marbled appearance of the skin and small thumb.

RESTRICTIVE DERMOPATHY

271A–271B

This condition manifests at birth with aplasia cutis or rigid skin, a characteristic face (hypertelorism, a small nose and mouth, micrognathia, low-set ears), and multiple joint contractures. Death is usually from lack of respiratory effort at birth. Skin histology reveals hyperkeratotic stratum corneum with ortho-keratotic keratinisation, hypoplastic pylosebaceous structures and eccrine sweat glands, absence of dermal rete ridges and a thin dermis (Toriello). Hamel *et al.* reported a false negative prenatal diagnosis by skin biopsy at 20 weeks.

Genetic aspects: Autosomal recessive.

References
Hamel BCJ, Happle R, Steylen PM *et al.* (1992). False-negative pre-natal diagnosis of restrictive dermopathy. *Am J Med Genet* **44**:824–826.
Happle R, Stekhoven JHS, Hamel BCJ *et al.* (1992). Restrictive der-mopathy in two brothers. *Arch Dermatol* **128**:232–235.
Mok Q, Curley R, Tolmie JL *et al.* (1990). Restrictive dermopathy: a report of three cases. *J Med Genet* **27**:315–319.
Toriello HV (1986). Restrictive dermopathy and report of another case. *Am J Med Genet* **24**:625–629.
Verloes A, Mulliez N, Gonzales M *et al.* (1992). Restrictive der-mopathy, a lethal form of arthrogryposis multiplex with skin and bone dysplasias: three new cases and review of the literature. *Am J Med Genet* **43**:539–547.

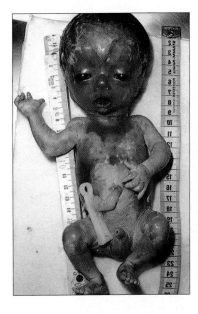

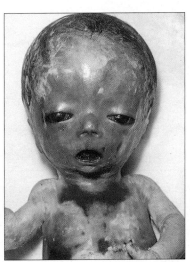

271A and 271B Note contractures of the hips, knees, elbows and ankles, rigid skin, hypertelorism, small pinched nose, and small mouth and jaw.

SJOGREN–LARSSON SYNDROME

272A–272B

Spasticity and mental retardation become evident before the age of 3 years. Ichthyosis is usually present at birth, the scales being usually large and discoloured. Another feature of the condition may be glistening dots in the macula, seen in about 20% of cases. There is a consistent deficiency of alcohol (hexanol) dehydrogenase activity within the epidermis and jejunal mucosa of patients with this syndrome. Prenatal diagnosis has been attempted by examining fetal skin biopsies but there has been one instance where it has been normal at 19 weeks and abnormal at 23.5 weeks.

Genetic aspects: Autosomal recessive.

References

Jagell S, Gustavson K-H, Holmgren G (1981). Sjogren–Larsson syndrome in Sweden: a clinical, genetic and epidemiological study. *Clin Genet* **19**:233–256.

Judge MR, Lake BD, Smith VV *et al.* (1990). Depletion of alcohol (hexanol) dehydrogenase activity in the epidermis and jejunal mucosa in Sjogren–Larsson syndrome. *J Invest Dermatol* **95**:632–634.

Levisohn D, Dintiman B, Rizzo WB (1991). Sjogren–Larsson syndrome: case reports. *Pediatr Dermatol* **8**:217–220.

Tabsh K, Rizzo WB, Holbrook K, Theroux N (1993). Sjogren-Larsson syndrome: technique and timing of prenatal diagnosis. *Obs Gynecol* **82**:700–703.

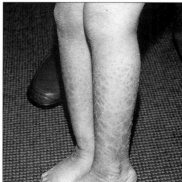

272A and 272B Note ichthyosis on the legs of this child with spasticity.

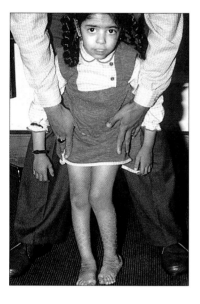

PSEUDOXANTHOMA ELASTICUM (PXE)

273A–273C

A subcutaneous yellow rash occurs in the flexures and around the neck. Ophthalmic features include angioid streaks, chorioretinopathy and blue sclerae. Vascular complications include angina, hypertension and claudication.

Genetic aspects: Pope has suggested that there are two autosomal dominant and two autosomal recessive forms. AR type I manifests with moderate vascular and retinal complications with flexural cutaneous lesions; AR type II has generalised skin involvement but no systemic involvement. AD type I has severe vascular and retinal complications with early blindness and coronary artery disease; AD type II has mild cardiovascular and retinal changes with marfanoid features (hyperextensible joints, blue sclerae, high arched palate).

References

Pope FM (1974). Two types of autosomal recessive pseudoxanthoma elasticum. *Arch Dermatol* **110**:209–212.

Viljoen DL (1988). Syndrome of the month: pseudoxanthoma elasticum (Gronblad–Strandberg syndrome). *J Med Genet* **25**:488–490.

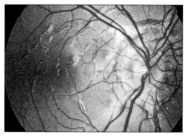

273A Ocular fundus showing angioid streaks and retinal sclerosis.

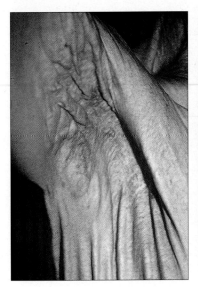
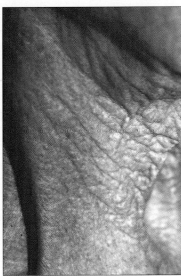

273B and 273C Note redundant skin folds and yellowish, raised skin lesions.

PARRY–ROMBERG SYNDROME (PROGRESSIVE HEMIFACIAL ATROPHY)   274

The condition usually starts in the first or second decade with unilateral facial pigmentation, unilateral atrophy of bone and soft tissue, a midline facial groove and sometimes trigeminal neuralgia and contralateral Jacksonian epilepsy. Occasionally, there is associated localised linear scleroderma of the trunk or limbs. The condition may be a form of linear scleroderma (Lewkonia and Lowry).

Genetic aspects: Mostly sporadic.

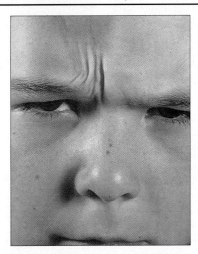

274 Note the hemifacial atrophy.

References
Asher SW, Berg BO (1982). Progressive hemifacial atrophy. Report of three cases, including one observed over 43 years, and computed tomographic findings. *Arch Neurol* **39**:44–46.

Lewkonia RM, Lowry RB (1983). Progressive hemifacial atrophy (Parry–Romberg syndrome) report with review of genetics and nosology. *Am J Med Genet* **14**:385–390.

Miller MT, Sloane H, Goldberg MF *et al.* (1987). Progressive hemifacial atrophy (Parry–Romberg disease). *J Ped Ophthal Strab* **24**:27–36.

PACHYONYCHIA CONGENITA

Many cases manifest with opaque, thickened nails, palmo-plantar hyperkeratosis and hyperhidrosis, oral leukoplakia and follicular hyperkeratosis. In the so-called Jadassohn–Lewandowsky type the above lesions breed true. In the Jackson–Lawler type oral leukoplakia is not present, but neonatal teeth and epidermoid cysts can be a feature.

Genetic aspects: Autosomal dominant. The condition may be genetically heterogeneous. It has been mapped to chromosome 17 and mutations in the keratin 16 and 17 genes have been demonstrated (McLean *et al.*)

References

Besser FS, Moynahan EJ (1971). Pachyonychia congenita with epidermal cysts and teeth at birth: fourth generation. *Br J Dermatol* **84**:95.

Clementi M, Cardin De Stefani E *et al.* (1986). Pachyonychia congenita Jackson–Lawler type: a distinct malformation syndrome. *Br J Dermatol* **114**:367–370.

McLean WHI, Rugg EL, Lunny DP, *et al.*, (1995). Keratin 16 and keratin 17 mutations cause pachyonychia congenita. *Nature Genetics* **9**:273–278.

Rohold AE, Brandrup F 1990). Pachyonychia congenita: therapeutic and immunologic aspects. *Pediatr Dermatol* **7**:307–309.

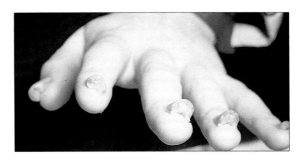

275 Note opaque, thickened nails.

PACHYDERMOPERIOSTOSIS (TOURAINE–SOLENTE–GOLE SYNDROME)   276A–276C

The main features are coarsening of the facial features, clubbing of the digits, and periosteal new bone formation, particularly of the distal ends of the long bones. The condition usually appears around puberty, progresses for about 10 years and then becomes relatively static. Detailed examination of the skin shows marked seborrheic hyperplasia with wide-open sebaceous pores filled with plugs of sebum. The skin becomes thickened on the scalp (sometimes leading to cutis verticis gyrata), on the eyelids (leading to ptosis), and on the hands. Finger clubbing is caused by soft tissue hyperplasia. The main clinical problem is usually hyperhidrosis.

Genetic aspects: Autosomal dominant.

References

Hedayati H, Barmada R, Skosey JL (1980). Acrolysis in pachydermoperiostosis. Primary or idiopathic hypertrophic osteoarthropathy. *Arch Intern Med* **140**:1087–1088.

Lazarus JH, Galloway JK (1973). Pachydermoperiostosis: an unusual cause of finger clubbing. *Am J Roentgenol* **118**:308–313.

Matucci-Cerinic M, Lotti T, Jajic I *et al.* (1991). The clinical spectrum of pachydermoperiostosis (primary hypertrophic osteoarthropathy). *Medicine* **70**:208–214.

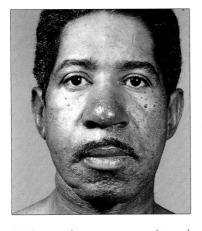

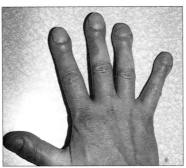

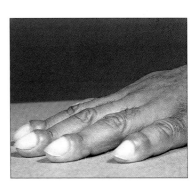

276A Note the coarse greasy skin and acne with hypertrophied sebaceous glands.

276B and 276C Marked clubbing of the fingers.

LIPOID PROTEINOSIS (HYALINOSIS CUTIS ET MUCOSAE)   277

Onset might be in infancy with infiltration of the larynx with amorphous hyaline material. Later the skin and oral cavity are affected. Skin manifestations may take many forms. There is a yellowish papular infiltration, especially around the eyelids and elbows. Seizures and intra-cranial calcification are complications.

Genetic aspects: Autosomal dominant.

References

Burnett JW, Marcy SM (1963). Lipoid proteinosis. *Am J Dis Child* **105**:81–84.

Kleinert R, Cervos-Navarro J et al. (1987). Predominantly cerebral manifestation in Urbach–Wiethe's syndrome (lipoid proteinosis cutis et mucosae): A clinical and pathomorphological study. *Clin Neuropathol* **6**:43–45.

Konstantinov K, Kabakchiev P, Karchev T et al. (1992). Lipoid proteinosis. *J Am Acad Dermatol* **27**:293–297.

Pierard GE, Van Cauwenberge D, Budo J, Lapiere CM (1988). A clinicopathologic study of six cases of lipoid proteinosis. *Am J Dermatopathol* **10**:300–305.

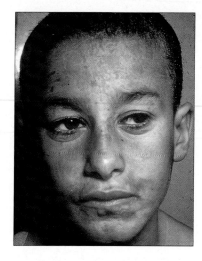

277 Note atrophic scars as the result of healing impetiginous legions, nodules and generally waxy skin.

DISTICHIASIS – LYMPHOEDEMA

Lymphoedema develops around puberty and mostly involves both lower limbs. This is in contrast to Milroy syndrome where the oedema is usually congenital. Distichiasis means a double row of eyelashes. The extra row of lashes occupies the posterior lid margin in the position of the Meibomian gland openings. They scratch the conjunctiva and patients often resort to pulling the lashes out. Other features include webbing of the neck in conjunction with a low hairline, and vertebral defects leading to a kyphosis and back pain. Congenital heart defects can occur and spinal extra-dural cysts are another feature.
Genetic aspects: Autosomal dominant.

References

Byrnes GA, Wilson ME (1991). Congenital distichiasis (Editorial). *Arch Ophthalmol* **109**:1752.

Dale RF (1987). Primary lymphoedema when found with distichiasis is of the type defined as bilateral hyperplasia by lymphography. *J Med Genet* **24**:170–171.

Kolin T, Johns KJ, Wadlington WB et al. (1991). Hereditary lymphedema and distichiasis. *Arch Ophthalmol* **109**:980–981.

Robinow M, Johnson F, Verhagen AD (1970). Distichiasis-lymphedema. A hereditary syndrome of multiple congenital defects. *Am J Dis Child* **119**:343–347.

Schwartz JF, O'Brien MS, Hoffman JC (1980). Hereditary spinal arachnoid cysts, distichiasis, and lymphedema. *Ann Neurol* **7**:340–343.

Shammas HJF, Tabbara KF, Der Kaloustian VM (1979). Distichiasis of the lids and lymphedema of the lower extremities: a report of ten cases. *J Pediatr* **16**:129–132.

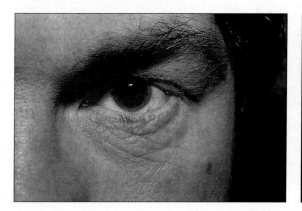

278A Note the double row of eyelashes.

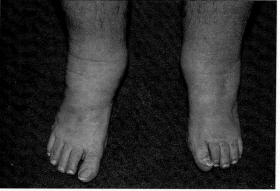

278B The lymphoedema appears at around puberty.

MILROY – HEREDITARY LYMPHOEDEMA

Milroy disease is a congenital form of lymphoedema confined to the lower limbs. The swelling is firm but does pit; it is permanent. In males the oedema may involve the scrotum. The cause is thought to be aplasia or hypoplasia of the lymphatics.

Genetic aspects: Autosomal dominant.

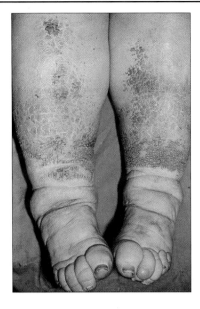

279 Note the lower limb lymphoedema with overlying hyperkeratosis.

References

Dale RF (1985). The inheritance of primary lymphoedema. *J Med Genet* **22**:274–278.

Esterley JR (1965). Congenital hereditary lymphedema. *J Med Genet* **2**:93–98.

Holmes LB, Fields JP, Zabriskie JB (1978). Hereditary late-onset lymphedema. *Pediatrics* **61**:575–579.

Kaariainen H (1984). Hereditary lymphedema: a new combination of symptoms not fitting into present classifications. *Clin Genet* **26**:254–255.

Milroy WF (1928). Chronic hereditary edema: Milroy's disease. *JAMA* **91**:1172–1175.

LIPOMATOSIS, SYMMETRICAL

Onset is around 45 years of age with symmetrical deposition of subcutaneous fat on the upper back, chest and arms, giving the appearance of pseudohypertrophy of the muscles. The face and distal extremities are spared. Overlying telangiectasia and erythema can appear and the skin can be thick, tight and woody. Peripheral neuropathy is an unusual association. There is evidence in some patients of mitochondrial dysfunction. Berkovic *et al.* reported that three patients out of four studied had ragged red fibres on muscle biopsy. This was carried out because of progressive muscle weakness. Silvestri *et al.* reported a 51-year-old male with myoclonus, hearing loss and lipomas who had a mutation at nucleotide 8344 of mtDNA – this is the mutation characteristic for MERRF.

Genetic aspects: The disease is said to be more common in Mediterranean countries, although in familial cases inheritance appears to be autosomal dominant (Kurzweg and Spencer).

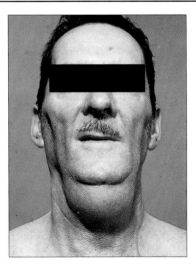

280 Note the symmetrical deposition of subcutaneous fat in the neck.

References

Berkovic SF, Andermann F, Shoubridge EA *et al.* (1991). Mitochondrial dysfunction in multiple symmetrical lipomatosis. *Ann Neurol* **29**:566–569.

Kurzweg FT, Spencer L. Familial multiple lipomatosis. *Am J Surg* 1951)**82**:762–764.

Ross M, Goodman MM (1992). Multiple symmetric lipomatosis (Launois–Bensaude syndrome) (Review). *Int J Dermatol* **31**:80–82.

Silvestri G, Ciafaloni E, Santorelli FM *et al.* (1993), Clinical features associated with the A->G transition at nucleotide 8344 of mtDNA ("MERRF mutation"). *Neurology* **43**:1200–1206.

SYNDROME ASSOCIATIONS

CHARGE ASSOCIATION

CHARGE is an acronym for Coloboma of iris or retina, Heart defects, Atresia of the choanae, Retardation of growth and development, Genital anomalies, and Ear abnormalities. The ears are simple and protruding and may have over-folded helices, and an absent crus of the antihelix. Deafness, which might be sensorineural, conductive, or both, is common. In a significant number of patients there is a unilateral or bilateral facial palsy, which is often partial and needs to be looked for. Genital abnormalities occur mostly in the male where the penis might be small and the testes undescended.

Strictly speaking, to make a diagnosis, four of the major criteria need to be present, but it is not uncommon to encounter patients with only three, and if these are very typical then the diagnosis should still be seriously considered. Renal anomalies and tracheo-oesophageal fistula might occur, suggesting overlap with VATER association.

Genetic aspects: Most cases are sporadic and small (3%) recurrence risks are appropriate, however chromosome analysis should always be carried out, and overlap with Velo-Cardio-Facial syndrome necessitates FISH studies to look for 22q deletions.

References

Blake KD, Russell-Eggitt IM *et al.* (1990). Who's in CHARGE? Multidisciplinary management of patients with CHARGE association. *Arch Dis Child* l**65**:217–223.

Byerly KA, Pauli RM (1993). Cranial nerve abnormalities in CHARGE association. *Am J Med Genet* **45**:751–757.

Harvey AS, Leaper PM, Bankier A (1991). CHARGE association: clinical manifestations and developmental outcome. *Am J Med Genet* **39**:48–55.

Metlay LA, Smythe PS, Miller ME (1987). Familial CHARGE syndrome: clinical report with autopsy findings. *Am J Med Genet* **26**:577–581.

Oley CA, Baraitser M, Grant DB (1988). A reappraisal of the CHARGE association. *J Med Genet* **25**:147–157.

Pagon RA, Graham JM Jr, Zonana J, Yong S-L (1981). Coloboma, congenital heart disease, and choanal atresia with multiple anomalies: CHARGE association. *J Pediatr* **99**:223–227.

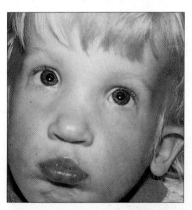

281A–281D Note the cup-shaped, anteverted simple ears.

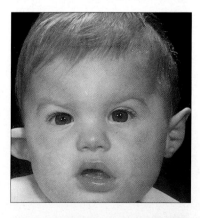

281B

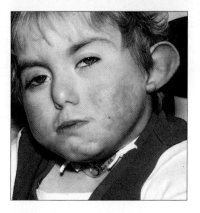

281C

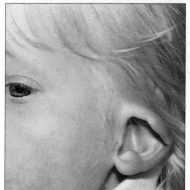

281D

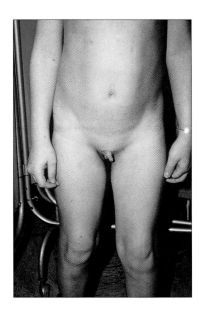

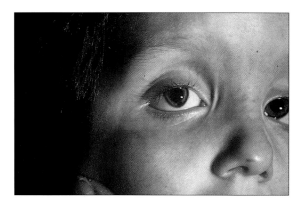

281E Note small genitalia.

281F Note the iris coloboma.

KLIPPEL–FEIL SYNDROME

282A–282C

The main diagnostic features are a short neck, a low posterior hairline and radiological evidence of fusion of the cervical vertebrae. The vertebral anomalies have been classified into three types. In type I there is block fusion of cervical and upper thoracic vertebrae; in type II fusion of one or two cervical vertebrae associated with occipitoatlantal fusion and hemivertebrae; and in type III fusion of cervical and lower thoracic or lumbar vertebrae. Additional features are webbing of the neck, torticollis, and facial asymmetry. An associated finding is deafness, which is unilateral or bilateral, and either conductive or sensorineural. Rarer associations include cleft palate, a cardiovascular lesion (most usually VSD), and renal abnormalities. Note that some patients in this group have features overlapping with the Wildervanck syndrome. A Duane anomaly is characteristic of this latter condition and it should be looked for.

Genetic aspects: Most cases are sporadic, but semidominant inheritance has been described.

References

Gunderson CH, Greenspan RH, Glaser GH *et al.* (1967). The Klippel–Feil syndrome: genetic and clinical reevaluation of cervical fusion. *Medicine* **46**:491–512.

Nagib MG, Maxwell RE, Chou SN (1985). Klippel–Feil syndrome in children: clinical features and management. *Child's Nerv Syst* **1**:255–263.

Nguyen VD, Tyrrel R (1993). Klippel–Feil syndrome: patterns of bony fusion and wasp-waist sign. *Skeletal Radiol* **22**:519–523.

Stewart EJ, O'Reilly BF (1989). Klippel–Feil syndrome and conductive deafness. *J Laryngol Otol* **103**:947–949.

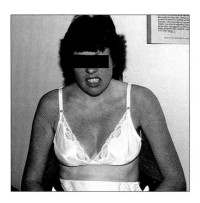

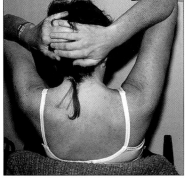

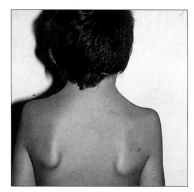

282A–282C Note the short neck with webbing and low hairline.

282C

VATER ASSOCIATION

The well-known acronym, VATER, is used to describe the association of Vertebral defects, Anal atresia or stenosis, Tracheo-Esophageal fistula, Radial defects and Renal anomalies. Some authors have expanded the acronym to VACTERL to include Cardiac defects and non-radial Limb defects.

Genetic aspects: Most cases are sporadic.

References
Corsello G, Maresi E, Corrao AM et al. (1992). VATER/VACTERL association: clinical variability and expanding phenotype including laryngeal stenosis. Am J Med Genet **44**:813–815.
Lubinsky M (1986). Current concepts: VATER and other associations: historical perspectives and modern interpretations. Am J Med Genet **Suppl.2**:9–16.
Weaver DD, Mapstone CL, Yu P-L (1986). The VATER association: analysis of 46 patients. Am J Dis Child **140**:225–229.

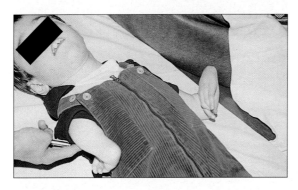

283A Note the bilateral radial aplasia.

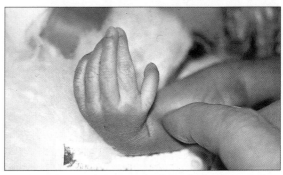

283B Note the proximally placed thumb.

JARCHO–LEVIN (SPONDYLOTHORACIC DYSPLASIA)

The clinical picture is that of an infant with a short trunk and a short immobile neck. Occasionally, there are urogenital abnormalities such as undescended or absent testes, unilateral hydronephrosis and an imperforate anus. Radiographs show crowding of the ribs which gives a fan-like or crab-like appearance to the thorax. The ribs are fused posteriorly and the costo-vertebral articulations are close together. The shortening of the trunk is due to hypoplastic, hemi and fused vertebrae. The majority of cases with this condition do not survive the first year of life. Respiratory problems are the usual cause of death. The differential diagnosis is with other forms of spondylocostal dysostosis where the prognosis is relatively better.

Genetic aspects: Autosomal recessive. Prenatal diagnosis using ultrasound should detect the rib/vertebral body abnormalities.

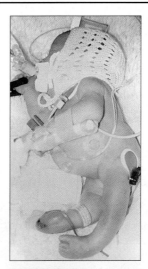

284A Note deformed chest, often resulting in early death due to respiratory failure.

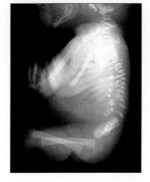

284B Multiple vertebral defects including hemivertebrae and abnormal crowded ribs.

References
Apuzzio JJ, Diamond N, Ganesh V et al. (1987). Difficulties in the prenatal diagnosis of Jarcho–Levin syndrome. Am J Obstet Gynecol **156**:916–918.
Giacoia GP, Say B (1991). Spondylocostal dysplasia and neural tube defects. J Med Genet **28**:51–53.
Karnes PS, Day D, Berry SA, Pierpont MEM (1991). Jarcho–Levin syndrome: four new cases and classification of subtypes. Am J Med Genet **40**:264–270.
Romeo MG, Distefano G, Di Bella D et al. (1991). Familial Jarcho–Levin syndrome. Clin Genet **39**:253–259.

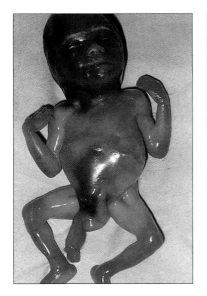

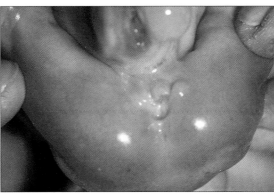

284C and 284D
Similar features in
a 22-week fetus
with anal atresia.

SYNDROMES CAUSED BY TERATOGENESIS

FETAL ALCOHOL SYNDROME

285A–285C

The effects of alcohol on the fetus during pregnancy are variable, and not all children exposed to excessive levels have the full features of the syndrome. Obviously affected infants are of low birth-weight. There is pronounced hypotonia, often a small head, and possibly jitteriness. This is followed by failure to thrive and mild to moderate developmental delay. The facial features consist of mild to moderate microcephaly, short palpebral fissures and a smooth, under-developed philtrum with a thin upper lip. The distal phalanges are small and the fifth fingernail might be hypoplastic. The palmar creases are unusual in that there is often a deep extra line running across the palm from the ulnar side towards the gap between the middle and index fingers. Cardiac lesions occur in about a third of cases and the commonest malformation is a VSD, followed by tetralogy of Fallot and an ASD.

Punctate calcification of the epiphyses, a cleft lip and palate and renal anomalies have all been described. Froster and Baird presented evidence of limb defects in infants exposed to high alcohol levels *in utero*. The limb defects were mainly transverse, but two cases had ulnar defects.

Genetic aspects: Sporadic, but there have been reports of occurrence in siblings when alcohol has been taken in subsequent pregnancies.

References

Autti-Ramo I, Gaily E, Granstrom M-L (1992). Dysmorphic features in offspring of alcoholic mothers. *Arch Dis Child* **67**:712–716.

Autti-Ramo I, Korkman M, Hilakivi-Clarke L *et al.* (1992). Mental development of 2-year-old children exposed to alcohol in utero. *J Pediatr* **120**:740–746.

Day NL, Richardson G, Robles N *et al.* (1990). Effects of prenatal alcohol exposure on growth and morphology of offspring at eight months of age. *Pediatrics* **85**:748–752.

Froster UG, Baird PA (1992). Congenital defects of the limbs and alcohol exposure in pregnancy: data from a population based study. *Am J Med Genet* **44**:782–785.

Spohr H-L, Willms J, Steinhausen H-C (1993). Prenatal alcohol exposure and long-term developmental consequences. *Lancet* **1**:907–910.

Streissguth AP, Aase JM, Clarren SK *et al.* (1991). Fetal alcohol syndrome in adolescents and adults. *JAMA* **265**:1961–1967.

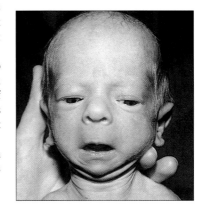

285A–285C Note the profound hypotonia, smooth philtrum, short palpebral fissures and hypoplastic nails.

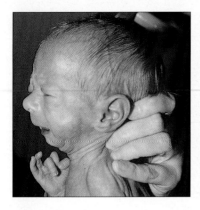

285B

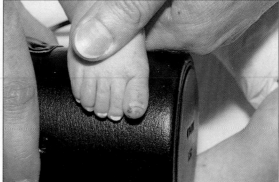

285C

FETAL HYDANTOIN SYNDROME

286A–286C

About one-third of infants exposed to hydantoin *in utero* will have minor craniofacial dysmorphism (mild hypertelorism, a broad depressed nasal bridge, a short nose, broad alveolar ridges, facial hirsutism) and digital anomalies (hypoplasia of the distal phalanges with small, often dysplastic nails). A smaller proportion will have growth and mental retardation. Cleft lip and palate and cardiac defects are the other features. The role of epilepsy itself in the causation of cleft lip and palate has not yet been clarified.

There does not seem on present evidence to be a safe antiepileptic drug during pregnancy. If the patient needs medication, the clinician should aim for monotherapy at the lowest dose possible.

References

D'Souza SW, Robertson IG, Donnai D, Mawer G (1991). Fetal phenytoin exposure, hypoplastic nails, and jitteriness. *Arch Dis Child* **66**:320–324.

Gaily E (1990). Distal phalangeal hypoplasia in children with prenatal phenytoin exposure: results of a controlled anthropometric study. *Am J Med Genet* **35**:574–578.

Hanson JW, Buehler BA (1982). Fetal hydantoin syndrome: current status. *J Pediatr* **101**:816–818.

Meadow R (1991). Anticonvulsants in pregnancy. *Arch Dis Child* **66**:62–65.

Van Dyke DC, Hodge SE, Heide F, Hill LR (1988). Family studies in fetal phenytoin exposure. *J Pediatr* **113**:301–306.

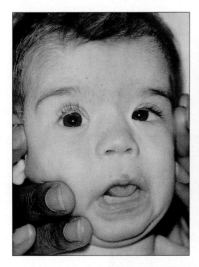
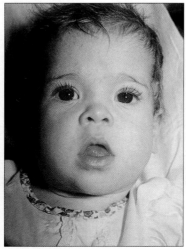
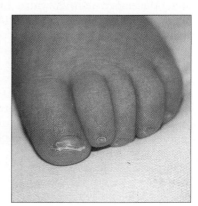

286A–286C Note mid-face hypoplasia, hirsute forehead, prominent epicanthic folds, depressed nasal bridge, broad alveolar ridge and hypoplastic nails.

FETAL VALPROATE SYNDROME

The main worries about maternal valproate therapy have been an increased frequency of neural tube defects, and craniofacial dysmorphism with mild to moderate mental retardation. The proportion of infants affected when the mother is on monotherapy may lie between 2.5 and 10%. However, in one prospective series (Jager-Roman *et al.*) a major malformation occurred in four out of 14 cases. The craniofacial features consist of brachycephaly with a high, trigonocephalic forehead, shallow orbits and prominent eyes. There may be a fold of skin below the lower eyelid. The mouth is small, the philtrum shallow, the upper lip thin and the lower lip prominent. Limb abnormalities can include post-axial polydactyly, pre-axial polydactyly and radial defects (Verloes *et al.*). The other worrying feature has been the high frequency of fetal distress which seems to occur in just under half of the infants.

References

Chitayat D, Farrell K *et al.* (1988). Congenital abnormalities in two siblings exposed to valproic acid in utero. *Am J Med Genet* **31**:369–374.

Jager-Roman E, Deichl A, Jakob S *et al.* (1986). Fetal growth, major malformations, and minor anomalies in infants born to women receiving valproic acid. *J Pediatr* **108**:997–1004.

Martinez-Frias ML (1990). Clinical manifestation of prenatal exposure to valproic acid using case reports and epidemiologic information. *Am J Med Genet* **37**:277–282.

Omtzigt JGC, Los FJ, Hagenaars AM *et al.* (1992). Prenatal diagnosis of spina bifida aperta after first-trimester valproate exposure. *Prenatal Diagn* **12**:893–897.

Verloes A, Frikiche A, Gremillet C *et al.* (1990). Proximal phocomelia and radial ray aplasia in fetal valproic syndrome. *Eur J Pediatr* **149**:266–267.

Winter RM, Donnai D, Burn J *et al.* (1987). Fetal valproate syndrome: is there a recognisable phenotype? *J Med Genet* **24**:692–695.

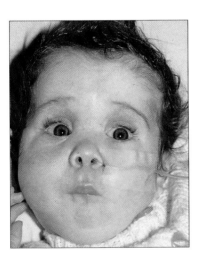 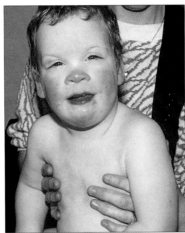

287A and 287B Note the high forehead, prominent eyes, small mouth, long shallow philtrum, thin upper lip and prominent lower lip. There is a characteristic fold of skin below the eyes.

FETAL WARFARIN SYNDROME

The characteristic phenotype is similar to chondrodysplasia punctata. The mid-face is hypoplastic, there is hypertelorism and the nose is small with anteverted nares and a depressed bridge. Radiographs reveal stippling of the unossified epiphyses. Other common abnormalities include congenital heart defects and hypoplastic nails. Cleft palate, cataract, microphthalmos (Wong *et al.*), encephalocele, Dandy–Walker malformation, diaphragmatic hernia and urinary tract abnormalities have all been reported. Exposure in the second or third trimesters can result in severe cerebral abnormalities, probably secondary to haemorrhage. In a review of infants exposed to warfarin during pregnancy Hall *et al.* suggested that one in six may show signs of the embryopathy and of these a significant number were mentally retarded; one in six pregnancies may end in spontaneous abortion or stillbirth. However, Wong *et al.* found that in a series of 29 cases (11 of who were also exposed to heparin) major complications were rare (apart from fetal loss) and the main problems were nasal hypoplasia and low birth-weight.

References

Chong MKB, Harvey D, de Swiet M (1984). Follow-up study of children whose mothers were treated with warfarin during pregnancy. *Br J Obstet Gynaecol* **91**:1070–1073.

Hall JG, Pauli RM, Wilson KM (1980). Maternal and fetal sequelae of anticoagulation during pregnancy. *Am J Med* **68**:122–140.

Pauli RM, Lian JB, Mosher DF, Suttie JW (1987). Association of congenital deficiency of multiple vitamin K-dependent coagulation factors and the phenotype of the warfarin embryopathy: clues to the mechanism of teratogenicity of coumarin derivatives. *Am J Hum Genet* **41**:566–583.

Wong V, Cheng CH, Chan KC (1993). Fetal and neonatal outcome of exposure to anticoagulants during pregnancy. *Am J Med Genet* **45**:17–21.

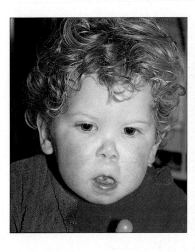
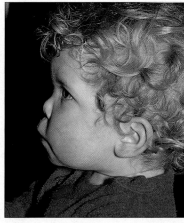

288A and 288B Note small nose, anteverted nares, mid-face hypoplasia, small mouth and flat nasal bridge.

MATERNAL DIABETES SYNDROME

289A–289B

Infants of diabetic mothers have two to three times the average incidence of congenital anomalies. These include neural tube defects, cardiac defects (transposition of the great vessels, coarctation of the aorta, VSD, ASD, cardiomyopathy), renal anomalies (hydronephrosis, renal agenesis, duplication of the renal tracts), intestinal atresias, and forms of caudal regression including sacral agenesis. It has been suggested that pre-axial polydactyly of the feet and proximal insertion of the hallux are important signs. There is also a higher rate of polyhydramnios and neonatal death. Careful diabetic control in the preconceptional period and the first 8 weeks of pregnancy may lower the chances of congenital anomaly.

References

Hernandez JA (1989). Congenital malformations in infants of diabetic mothers. *Curr Opin Obst Gyne* **1**:177–183.

Kousseff BG, Villaveces C, Martinez CR (1991). Unique brain anomalies in an infant of a diabetic mother. *Acta Paediatr Scand* **80**:110–115.

Landon MB, Langer O, Gabbe SG et al. (1992). Fetal surveillance in pregnancies complicated by insulin-dependent diabetes mellitus. *Am J Obstet Gynecol* **167**:617–621.

Molsted-Pedersen L, Pedersen JF (1985). Congenital malformations in diabetic pregnancies. Clinical viewpoints. *Acta Paediatr Scand* **Suppl.320**:79–84.

Swenne I (1988). The fetus of the diabetic mother: growth and malformations. *Arch Dis Child* **63**:1119–1122.

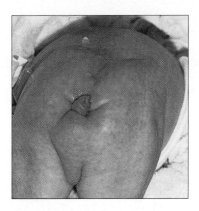

289A Note disorganised sacral region with underlying sacral agenesis and anal atresia.

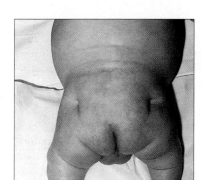

289B There are bilateral skin dimples, indicating sacral agenesis.

MATERNAL PHENYLKETONURIA (PKU) SYNDROME

Offspring of mothers with untreated PKU have a greater than 80% chance of being affected by microcephaly, intrauterine growth retardation, mental retardation and seizures. There is also a 20% chance of malformations such as congenital heart defects, cleft palate and clinodactyly. A characteristic face has been suggested (long simple philtrum, thin upper lip, flattened nasal bridge, epicanthic folds and upturned nose). A collaborative study (Platt *et al.*) showed that optimal outcome occurred when maternal serum phenylalanine levels were maintained below 600 micromoles/L (10mg/dl) from before 6–10 weeks' gestation.

References

Cockburn F, Clark BJ, Byrne A *et al.* (1992). Maternal phenylketonuria: diet, dangers and dilemmas. *Int Pediatr* **7**:67–74.

Levy HL, Lobbregt D, Sansaricq C, Snyderman SE (1992). Comparison of phenylketonuric and nonphenylketonuric siblings from untreated pregnancies in a mother with phenylketonuria. *Am J Med Genet* **44**:439–442.

MRC Working Party on PKU (1993). Phenylketonuria due to phenylalanine hydroxylase deficiency: an unfolding story. *Br Med J* **306**:115–119.

Platt LD, Koch R, Azen C *et al.* (1992). Maternal phenylketonuria collaborative study, obstetric aspects and outcome: the first six years. *Am J Obstet Gynecol* **166**:1150–1162.

Smith I, Glossop J, Beasley M (1990). Fetal damage due to maternal phenylketonuria: effects of dietary treatment and maternal phenylalanine concentrations around the time of conception. *J Inherit Metab Dis* **13**:651–657.

Thompson GN, Francis DEM, Kirby DM *et al.* (1991). Pregnancy in phenylketonuria: dietary treatment aimed at normalising maternal plasma phenylalanine concentration. *Arch Dis Child* **66**:1346–1349.

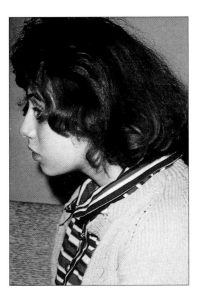
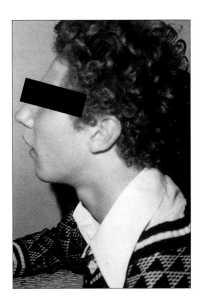

290A and 290B Note microcephaly, which is not phenotypically distinguishable from recessive microcephaly.

INDEX